Thalassemia

Guest Editor

BERNARD G. FORGET, MD

HEMATOLOGY/ONCOLOGY CLINICS OF NORTH AMERICA

www.hemonc.theclinics.com

Consulting Editors
GEORGE P. CANELLOS, MD
NANCY BERLINER, MD

December 2010 • Volume 24 • Number 6

SAUNDERS an imprint of ELSEVIER, Inc.

W.B. SAUNDERS COMPANY
A Division of Elsevier Inc.

1600 John F. Kennedy Blvd. • Suite 1800 • Philadelphia, PA 19103-2899

http://www.theclinics.com

HEMATOLOGY/ONCOLOGY CLINICS OF NORTH AMERICA Volume 24, Number 6
December 2010 ISSN 0889-8588, ISBN 13: 978-1-4377-2531-5

Editor: Kerry Holland
Developmental Editor: Donald Mumford

Hematology/Oncology Clinics (ISSN 0889-8588) is published bimonthly by Elsevier Inc., 360 Park Avenue South, New York, NY 10010-1710. Months of issue are February, April, June, August, October, and December. Business and Editorial Offices: 1600 John F. Kennedy Blvd., Ste. 1800, Philadelphia, PA 19103–2899. Customer Service Office: 3251 Riverport Lane, Maryland Heights, MO 63043. Periodicals postage paid at New York, NY and at additional mailing offices. Subscription prices are $327.00 per year (domestic individuals), $541.00 per year (domestic institutions), $160.00 per year (domestic students/residents), $371.00 per year (Canadian individuals), $662.00 per year (Canadian institutions) $442.00 per year (international individuals), $662.00 per year (international institutions), and $216.00 per year (international and Canadian students/residents). International air speed delivery is included in all *Clinics* subscription prices. All prices are subject to change without notice. **POSTMASTER:** Send address changes to *Hematology/Oncology Clinics of North America*, Elsevier Health Sciences Division, Subscription Customer Service, 3251 Riverport Lane, Maryland Heights, MO 63043. Customer Service (orders, claims, online, change of address): Elsevier Health Sciences Division, Subscription Customer Service, 3251 Riverport Lane, Maryland Heights, MO 63043. Tel: 1-800-654-2452 (U.S. and Canada); 314-447-8871 (outside U.S. and Canada). Fax: 314-447-8029. E-mail: journalscustomerservice-usa@elsevier.com (for print support); journalsonlinesupport-usa@elsevier.com (for online support).

Reprints. For copies of 100 or more, of articles in this publication, please contact the Commercial Reprints Department, Elsevier Inc., 360 Park Avenue South, New York, New York 10010-1710; Tel.: 212-633-3813, Fax: 212-462-1935, E-mail: reprints@elsevier.com.

Hematology/Oncology Clinics of North America is covered in *MEDLINE/PubMed (Index Medicus), EMBASE/ Excerpta Medica, and BIOSIS.*

Contributors

CONSULTING EDITORS

GEORGE P. CANELLOS, MD
William Rosenberg Professor of Medicine, Department of Medical Oncology, Dana-Farber Cancer Institute, Boston, Massachusetts

NANCY BERLINER, MD
Chief, Division of Hematology, Brigham and Women's Hospital; Professor of Medicine, Harvard Medical School, Boston, Massachusetts

GUEST EDITOR

BERNARD G. FORGET, MD
Professor of Medicine and Genetics, Yale University School of Medicine, New Haven, Connecticut

AUTHORS

S.J. ALLEN, MD, MRCP
Professor of Paediatrics and International Health, Institute of Life Sciences, School of Medicine, Swansea University, Singleton Park, Swansea, United Kingdom

GEORGE ATWEH, MD
Professor of Medicine, Division of Hematology and Oncology, Department of Internal Medicine, University of Cincinnati, Cincinnati, Ohio

ARTHUR BANK, MD
Emeritus Professor of Medicine and Genetics and Development, Columbia University, New York, New York

ROSSA W.K. CHIU, MBBS, PhD
Professor, Department of Chemical Pathology; Li Ka Shing Institute of Health Sciences, The Chinese University of Hong Kong, Prince of Wales Hospital, Hong Kong SAR, China

HASSANA FATHALLAH, PhD
Research Assistant Professor, Division of Hematology and Oncology, Department of Internal Medicine, The Vontz Center for Molecular Studies, University of Cincinnati, Cincinnati, Ohio

SARA GARDENGHI, PhD
Postdoctoral Associate, Hematology-Oncology, Department of Pediatrics, Weill Cornell Medical College, New York, New York

JAVID GAZIEV, MD
Clinical Unit, International Center for Transplantation in Thalassemia and Sickle Cell Anemia, Mediterranean Institute of Hematology, Policlinico Tor Vergata, Rome, Italy

RICHARD J. GIBBONS, MD, DPhil
Reader in Clinical Genetics, University of Oxford, John Radcliffe Hospital, Weatherall Institute of Molecular Medicine, Headington, Oxford, United Kingdom

ROBERT W. GRADY, PhD
Associate Professor of Pharmacology, Hematology-Oncology, Department of Pediatrics, Weill Cornell Medical College, New York, New York

DOUGLAS R. HIGGS, MD, DSc
Professor of Molecular Haematology, John Radcliffe Hospital, MRC Molecular Haematology Unit, Weatherall Institute of Molecular Medicine, University of Oxford, Headington, Oxford, United Kingdom

SOHAIL JAHID, BS
Department of Biological Chemistry, University of California, Irvine, Irvine, California

BINDU KANATHEZHATH, MD
Associate Hematologist, Hematology—Oncology, Children's Hospital and Research Center, Oakland, Oakland, California

EUGENE KHANDROS
Cell and Molecular Biology Graduate Group, The Combined Degree Program, University of Pennsylvania School of Medicine, Philadelphia, Pennsylvania

NORALANE M. LINDOR, MD
Department of Medical Genetics, Mayo Clinic, Rochester, Minnesota

STEVEN LIPKIN, MD, PhD
Departments of Medicine and Genetic Medicine, Weill Cornell College of Medicine, Cornell University, New York, New York

Y.M. DENNIS LO, DM, DPhil
Li Ka Shing Professor of Medicine and Professor of Chemical Pathology, Department of Chemical Pathology; Director, Li Ka Shing Institute of Health Sciences, The Chinese University of Hong Kong, Prince of Wales Hospital, Hong Kong SAR, China

GUIDO LUCARELLI, MD
Director, International Center for Transplantation in Thalassemia and Sickle Cell Anemia, Mediterranean Institute of Hematology, Policlinico Tor Vergata, Rome, Italy

DAVID G. NATHAN, MD
Harvard Medical School; Children's Hospital of Boston; Dana-Farber Cancer Institute, Boston, Massachusetts

A. O'DONNELL, PhD
Research Assistant and Honorary Lecturer, Institute of Life Sciences, School of Medicine, Swansea University, Singleton Park, Swansea, United Kingdom

NANCY F. OLIVIERI, MD, FRCP(C)
Professor, Pediatrics Medicine and Public Health Sciences, University of Toronto; Senior Scientist, Toronto General Hospital Research Institute, Toronto, Canada

ZAHRA PAKBAZ, MD
Assistant Clinical Scientist, Children's Hospital Oakland Research Institute, Oakland, California

JOHN B. PORTER, MD
Red Cell Disorders Unit, University College London Hospitals and Whittington Hospital, London, United Kingdom

STEFANO RIVELLA, PhD
Associate Professor of Genetic Medicine, Hematology-Oncology, Department of Pediatrics, Weill Cornell Medical College, New York, New York

VIJAY G. SANKARAN, MD, PhD
Harvard Medical School; Children's Hospital of Boston; Dana-Farber Cancer Institute, Boston; Whitehead Institute for Biomedical Research, Cambridge, Massachusetts

FARRUKH T. SHAH, MD
Red Cell Disorders Unit, University College London Hospitals and Whittington Hospital, London, United Kingdom

NEEL B. SHAH, MB, ChB
Department of Medical Genetics, Mayo Clinic, Rochester, Minnesota

ELLIOTT VICHINSKY, MD
Medical Director, Hematology–Oncology, Children's Hospital and Research Center Oakland, Oakland, California

MARK C. WALTERS, MD
Jordan Family Director, Blood and Marrow Transplant Program, Children's Hospital and Research Center, Oakland, Oakland, California

D.J. WEATHERALL, MD, FRCP, FRS
Regius Professor of Medicine Emeritus, University of Oxford, Weatherall Institute of Molecular Medicine, John Radcliffe Hospital, Headington, Oxford, United Kingdom

MITCHELL J. WEISS, MD, PhD
Associate Professor of Pediatrics, Division of Hematology, Abramson Research Center, Children's Hospital of Philadelphia, Philadelphia, Pennsylvania

T.N. WILLIAMS, MD, MRCP, PhD
Reader in Tropical Medicine, University of Oxford, Oxford, United Kingdom; Kenya Medical Research Institute/Wellcome Trust Programme, Centre for Geographic Medical Research, Kilifi District Hospital, Kilifi, Kenya

Contents

The thalassemias are attributable to the defective production of the α- and β-globin polypeptides of hemoglobin. Significant discoveries have illuminated the pathophysiology and enhanced the prevention and treatment of the thalassemias, and this article reviews many of the advances that have occurred in the past 50 years. However, the application of new approaches to the treatment of these disorders has been slow, particularly in the developing world where the diseases are common, but there is definite progress. This article emphasizes how the increasing knowledge of cellular and molecular biology are facilitating the development of more effective therapies for these patients.

The inherited disorders of hemoglobin, including the thalassemias, are by far the commonest monogenic diseases. Although several factors are responsible for their very high frequency, the major mechanism seems to be natural selection mediated by heterozygote protection against severe forms of malaria. Recent work has highlighted the complexity of the interplay among the different hemoglobin variants themselves and among different levels of malaria resistance, and is helping to explain the extraordinary heterogeneity in the distribution of the hemoglobin disorders even within short geographical distances. Some progress has also been made toward understanding the cellular and immune mechanisms that may underlie heterozygote protection against malaria in these conditions. In addition to providing valuable information about human evolutionary biology, work in this field has an increasingly important influence on the development of programs for the better management of the hemoglobin disorders, particularly in the poorer countries of the tropical world.

Down-regulation of α-globin synthesis causes α-thalassemia with underproduction of fetal (HbF, $\alpha_2\gamma_2$) and adult (HbA, $\alpha_2\beta_2$) hemoglobin. This article focuses on the human α-globin cluster, which has been characterized in great depth over the past 30 years. In particular the authors describe how the α genes are normally switched on during erythropoiesis and switched off as hematopoietic stem cells commit to nonerythroid lineages. In addition, the principles by which α-globin expression may be perturbed by natural mutations that cause α-thalassemia are reviewed.

Hemoglobin E thalassemia accounts for about one-half of all cases of severe beta thalassemia. There is marked variability in its clinical severity ranging from an asymptomatic to a transfusion-dependent phenotype. The phenotypic variability and inadequate longitudinal data present challenges in determining the optimal management of patients. This article summarizes findings on the natural history of Hemoglobin E thalassemia and some factors responsible for its clinical heterogeneity. Major genetic factors include the type of beta thalassemia mutation, the co-inheritance of alpha thalassemia, and polymorphisms associated with increased synthesis of fetal hemoglobin. Other factors, including response to anemia, and the influence of infection with malaria and other environmental influences, may be important. The remarkable variation and instability of clinical phenotypes in Hemoglobin E thalassemia require individual management plans for each patient, which should be reassessed over time.

Erythrocytes must regulate hemoglobin synthesis to limit the toxicities of unstable free globin chain subunits. This regulation is particularly relevant in β-thalassemia, in which β-globin deficiency causes accumulation of free α-globin, which forms intracellular precipitates that destroy erythroid precursors. Experimental evidence accumulated over more than 40 years indicates that erythroid cells can neutralize moderate amounts of free α-globin through generalized protein quality control mechanisms, including molecular chaperones, the ubiquitin-proteasome system, and autophagy. In many ways, β-thalassemia resembles protein aggregation disorders of the nervous system, liver, and other tissues, which occur when levels of unstable proteins overwhelm cellular compensatory mechanisms. Information gained from studies of nonerythroid protein aggregation disorders may be exploited to further understand and perhaps treat β-thalassemia.

β-Thalassemia is a genetic disorder caused by mutations in the β-globin gene and characterized by chronic anemia caused by ineffective erythropoiesis, and accompanied by a variety of serious secondary complications such as extramedullary hematopoiesis, splenomegaly, and iron overload. In the past few years, numerous studies have shown that such secondary disease conditions have a genetic basis caused by the abnormal expression of genes with a role in controlling erythropoiesis and iron metabolism. In this article, the most recent discoveries related to the mechanism(s) responsible for anemia/ineffective erythropoiesis and iron overload are discussed in detail. Particular attention is paid to the pathway(s) controlling the expression of hepcidin, which is the main regulator of iron metabolism, and the Epo/EpoR/Jak2/Stat5 signaling pathway, which regulates erythropoiesis. Better understanding of how these pathways function and are altered in β-thalassemia has revealed several possibilities for development of new therapeutic approaches to treat of the complications of this disease.

Transfusional iron loading inevitably results in hepatic iron accumulation, with variable extrahepatic distribution that is typically less pronounced in sickle cell disease than in thalassemia disorders. Iron chelation therapy has the goal of preventing iron-mediated tissue damage through controlling tissue iron levels, without incurring chelator-mediated toxicity. Historically, target levels for tissue iron control have been limited by the increased frequency of deferoxamine-mediated toxicity and low levels of iron loading. With newer chelation regimes, these limitations are less evident. The reporting of responses to chelation therapies has typically focused on average changes in serum ferritin in patient populations. This approach has three limitations. First, changes in serum ferritin may not reflect trends in iron balance equally in all patients or for all chelation regimens. Second, this provides no information about the proportion of patients likely respond. Third, this gives insufficient information about iron trends in tissues such as the heart. Monitoring of iron overload has advanced with the increasing use of MRI techniques to estimate iron balance (changes in liver iron concentration) and extrahepatic iron distribution (myocardial T2*). The term nonresponder has been increasingly used to describe individuals who fail to show a downward trend in one or more of these variables. Lack of a response of an individual may result from inadequate dosing, high transfusion requirement, poor treatment adherence, or unfavorable pharmacology of the chelation regime. This article scrutinizes evidence for response rates to deferoxamine, deferiprone (and combinations), and deferasirox.

Reactivation of fetal hemoglobin (HbF) expression is an important therapeutic option in adult patients with hemoglobin disorders. The understanding of the developmental regulation of γ-globin gene expression was followed by the identification of a number of chemical compounds that can reactivate HbF synthesis in vitro and in vivo in patients with hemoglobin disorders. These HbF inducers can be grouped in several classes based on their mechanisms of action. This article focuses on pharmacologic agents that were tested in humans and discusses current knowledge about the mechanisms by which they induce HbF.

Hematopoietic stem cell transplantation (HSCT) offers potentially curative therapy for patients with thalassemia major and sickle cell disease (SCD). Current myeloablative treatment protocols allow the cure of 78% to 90%

of patients with thalassemia and 72% to 96% with SCD, depending on disease status at the time of transplantation. The major limitation to successful transplantation is the lack of a suitable HLA-matched family donor. Unrelated donor HSCT is now extensively used to treat thalassemia, with results similar to those obtained following transplantation using HLA-matched sibling donors. Patients who lack a matched related or unrelated donor can now benefit from successful transplantation using haploidentical donors.

Hematopoietic cell transplantation is curative therapy for thalassemia major. Although the clinical application of hematopoietic cell transplantation has relied on marrow collected from related and unrelated donors as the primary source of donor hematopoietic cells, umbilical cord blood (UCB) is an alternative source of hematopoietic cells and represents a suitable allogeneic donor pool in the event that a marrow donor is not available. Progress in developing UCB transplantation for thalassemia is reviewed and the most likely areas of future clinical investigation are discussed.

Fetal DNA is present in the plasma of pregnant women and can be used for noninvasive prenatal diagnosis. Early work had focused on the detection of paternally inherited fetal mutations in maternal plasma. Recent advances in single-molecule counting approaches have allowed the mutation dosage of the fetus to be analyzed in maternal plasma. These developments have been demonstrated as feasible for noninvasive prenatal diagnosis of several hemoglobinopathies, including β-thalassemia and hemoglobin E disease.

Allogeneic stem cell transplantation currently is the only curative option for severe β-thalassemia and sickle cell disease. Human globin gene therapy with autotransplantation of transduced human hematopoietic stem cells is an exciting alternative approach to a potential cure. One patient with thalassemia has recently been reported to have clinical benefit after lentiviral human β-globin gene therapy. He has not required blood transfusions for almost 2 years. Most of the patient's gene correction and new human β-globin gene expression is caused by the expansion of a single clone in which the corrective transgene is inserted into an *Hmga2* gene.

Animal models of cancer have been instrumental in understanding the progression and therapy of hereditary cancer syndromes. The ability to alter the genome of an individual mouse cell in both constitutive and inducible approaches has led to many novel insights into their human counterparts. In this review, knockout mouse models of inherited human cancer syndromes are presented and insights from the study of these models are highlighted.

Although inherited predisposition to colorectal cancer (CRC) has been suspected for more than 100 years, definitive proof of Mendelian syndromes had to await maturation of molecular genetic technologies. Since the 1980s, the genetics of several clinically distinct entities has been revealed. Five disorders that share a hereditary predisposition to CRC are reviewed in this article.

THE CLINICS ARE NOW AVAILABLE ONLINE!

Access your subscription at:
www.theclinics.com

Preface

Thalassemia

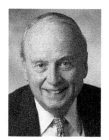

Bernard G. Forget, MD
Guest Editor

Over the years, study of the thalassemia syndromes has served as a paradigm for gaining insights into the cellular and molecular biology, as well as the pathophysiology, of inherited genetic disorders. The thalassemias constitute a heterogeneous group of naturally occurring, inherited mutations characterized by abnormal globin gene expression, resulting in total absence or quantitative reduction of α- or β-globin chain synthesis in human erythroid cells. α-Thalassemia is associated with absent or decreased production of α chains, whereas in the β thalassemias, there is absent or decreased production of β chains. The articles that follow describe in detail the knowledge and the latest progress that have accrued on our understanding of the pathophysiology, the molecular genetics, the clinical manifestations, the management and prevention of the various thalassemia syndromes, with an emphasis on β thalassemia. The overview by Sankaran and Nathan provides an excellent summary of these advances.

A very important pathophysiological process is responsible for the major clinical manifestations in β thalassemia major. The continued synthesis in normal amounts of normal α-globin chains results in the accumulation, within the erythroid cells, of excessive amounts of these chains. Not finding complementary globin chains with which to bind, these unpaired α chains form insoluble aggregates or inclusion bodies that precipitate within the cell, causing membrane damage and premature destruction of the red cells. The process of inclusion body formation occurs not only in mature erythrocytes, but in particular in the erythroid precursor cells of the bone marrow. As a result, there is extensive intramedullary destruction of erythroid precursor cells, a process that is called ineffective erythropoiesis. This process is not only responsible for the severe anemia leading to massive erythropoietic stress, marrow expansion, and extramedullary hematopoiesis, but it is also an important contributing factor to the abnormal iron metabolism and iron overload observed in the disorder, as discussed in the article by Gardenghi and colleagues.

Hematol Oncol Clin N Am 24 (2010) xiii–xv
doi:10.1016/j.hoc.2010.08.014
0889-8588/10/$ – see front matter © 2010 Elsevier Inc. All rights reserved.

hemonc.theclinics.com

The severity of the clinical manifestations in β thalassemia generally correlates well with the size of the free α chain pool and the degree of α- to non-α-globin chain imbalance. Therefore, the fortuitous coinheritance of α thalassemia together with homozygous β thalassemia reduces the degree of α- to non-α-globin chain imbalance and leads to a milder clinical course. Similarly, coinheritance of β thalassemia with conditions that are associated with increased levels of synthesis of γ chains of HbF ($\alpha_2\gamma_2$) leads to less imbalance between α- and non-α-globin chain synthesis, resulting in decreased formation of α chain inclusion bodies, increased effective production of red cells, and their prolonged survival in the circulation. Thus, a considerable amount of research has been devoted to attempts to increase fetal hemoglobin synthesis as a therapeutic measure in patients with β thalassemia major. This topic is discussed in detail in the article by Atweh and Fathallah. Other studies have focussed on the process of α chain catabolism as a possible therapeutic target, as discussed in the article by Khandros and Weiss.

The clinical course in most cases of homozygous β thalassemia is severe. Although anemia is not evident at birth, severe hypochromic, microcytic, hemolytic anemia develops during the first year of life and a regular transfusion program must be undertaken to maintain an adequate circulating hemoglobin level. The clinical manifestations of homozygous β thalassemia in childhood have changed considerably over the last 3–4 decades, owing to changes in the philosophy and practice of transfusion therapy. With modern transfusion therapy, most children will develop normally, with few or no skeletal abnormalities, and will have a reasonably good quality of life. However, transfusional iron overload is a virtually inevitable consequence of this life-saving therapy. Therefore, transfusion therapy needs to be coupled with a vigorous program of iron chelation, typically using parenterally administered deferoxamine and/or, more recently, orally effective iron-chelating agents. Although it is theoretically possible to maintain iron balance with such a management program, compliance is often difficult to achieve. Significant iron overload eventually develops in most patients and is the major cause of morbidity and mortality in young adults. The topics of iron overload and iron chelation therapy are discussed in detail in the article by Porter and Shah.

The one therapy that is curative is bone marrow or hematopoietic stem cell transplantation (HSCT), which is being increasingly practiced when feasible. However, only a minority of patients who could benefit from HSCT have an HLA-compatible sibling as stem cell donor. Therefore, the use of alternative donors has become the focus of increasing investigation, including the use of partially mismatched related or unrelated adult or umbilical cord blood sources of stem cells. The current status of HSCT for β thalassemia, including the use of umbilical cord blood, is discussed in detail in the article by Gaziev and Lucarelli as well as that by Kanathezhath and Walters.

For many years, it was hoped that advances in the fields of molecular biology and gene transfer, including elucidation of the molecular basis of β thalassemia and the successful transfer of globin genes in animal model systems, would provide the basis for carrying out gene therapy for the disorder by substituting a functional globin gene to replace the defective one. A number of technical difficulties have greatly delayed actual attempts to carry out globin gene therapy in man. However, very recently such a procedure has been successfully accomplished, as discussed in the article by Dr Arthur Bank.

There have been a number of important developments in recent years that have greatly increased our understanding and management of thalassemia, as detailed in the various articles published in this issue of *Hematology/Oncology Clinics of North America*. Hopefully, this momentum will continue and lead to even greater achievements in coming years.

Bernard G. Forget, MD
Yale University School of Medicine
333 Cedar Street, PO Box 208021
New Haven, CT 06520-8021, USA

E-mail address:
bernard.forget@yale.edu

Thalassemia: An Overview of 50 Years of Clinical Research

Vijay G. Sankaran, MD, PhD[a,b,c,d], David G. Nathan, MD[a,b,c],*

KEYWORDS

• Thalassemia • Hemoglobin • Erythrocyte • Transfusion

The thalassemias are a group of disorders that are attributable to the defective production of hemoglobin (Hb). The mature Hb molecule is a tetramer composed of 2 α-globin and 2 β-globin polypeptides, which assemble, along with a heme prosthetic group, to form the complete molecule. In the α-thalassemias, sufficiently defective production of α-globin chains results in decreased red cell (erythrocyte) Hb content and free β-globin polypeptides, which can assemble to form a moderately unstable Hb known as HbH. This unstable Hb causes a mild to moderate hemolytic and hypochromic anemia.[1] In the β-thalassemias, impaired production of β-globin chains result in unpaired α-globin chains, which are unstable in erythroid precursors, where they precipitate and cause membrane injury and unfolded protein responses and thereby lead to toxicity and death of these cells. This in turn causes ineffective erythropoiesis and the numerous clinical features of the disease.[2,3]

In the last 5 decades, a significant set of discoveries has illuminated the pathophysiology and enhanced the prevention and treatment of the thalassemias. This article briefly reviews many of the important advances in thalassemia that have occurred in this period. The study of the thalassemia syndromes has greatly enhanced the development and application of molecular biology to biomedical research. Patients with the thalassemia syndromes have contributed enormously to understanding of the molecular basis of health and disease. However, the application of these new approaches to the treatment of these disorders has been slow, particularly in the developing world where the diseases are common, but there is definite progress. The articles in this issue emphasize how ever increasing knowledge of cellular and molecular biology is facilitating the development of more effective therapies for these patients.

[a] Harvard Medical School, Boston, MA 02115, USA
[b] Children's Hospital of Boston, Boston, MA 02115, USA
[c] Dana-Farber Cancer Institute, Boston, MA 02115, USA
[d] Whitehead Institute for Biomedical Research, Cambridge, MA 02142, USA
* Corresponding author. Harvard Medical School, Boston, MA 02115.
E-mail address: david_nathan@dfci.harvard.edu

Hematol Oncol Clin N Am 24 (2010) 1005–1020
doi:10.1016/j.hoc.2010.08.009
0889-8588/10/$ – see front matter © 2010 Elsevier Inc. All rights reserved.

THE MOLECULAR PATHOPHYSIOLOGY OF THALASSEMIA

Although the first clinical descriptions of the thalassemia syndromes were published by Cooley, Rietti, Greppi, and Micheli in 1925,[4] it took many more years before the pathophysiology of these diseases began to be elucidated. The first clues came from research in the 1950s that used protein chemistry to assess various Hb variants. Based on the extensive studies by numerous groups in this era, Ingram and Stretton[5] suggested that there were 2 groups of thalassemias, α and β, which were caused by defects in the synthesis of α- and β-globin polypeptides, respectively. Several years later, Fessas[6] suggested that the cause of the β-thalassemia syndromes could be attributable to unbalanced globin chain synthesis, with the disease manifestations resulting from the presence of intraerythroblastic inclusions of unpaired α-globin molecules. His prescient idea was confirmed by spectrographic observations with Thorell that the inclusions were indeed comprised largely of α-globin chains.[7] Several other workers, including Clegg, Weatherall, Marks, Weissman, and Nathan, came to similar conclusions about the pathophysiology of this disease and provided a great deal of experimental support for this hypothesis.[8–11]

However, with only the tools of protein chemistry available, the exact molecular basis of these diseases remained an enigma and a great deal of speculation took place in the era following these observations.[12–14] After much experimental work, an era of RNA analysis ushered in important new approaches to this problem and several seminal experimental observations followed. In the early 1970s, Benz, Forget, Kan, Nathan, Lodish, Marks, Bank, and Nienhuis showed that β-globin mRNA translation was reduced in patients with β-thalassemia, suggesting that this defect was caused by impaired or defective production of a functional mRNA.[15–18] With the discovery and isolation of reverse transcriptase, newer approaches to this problem became available because cDNA could be synthesized, and this rapidly led to the elucidation by Housman, Benz, Forget, Bank, and numerous others that the thalassemias appeared to be generally attributable to decreased globin mRNA levels.[19,20] Kan, Weatherall, and their colleagues, used α-globin cDNA probes to identify the first genetic mutations in thalassemia by showing that the α-globin genes were deleted in certain forms of α-thalassemia.[21,22]

Soon afterward, a highly productive period began with the identification of various thalassemia mutations and deletions. Numerous clinical scientists, including Kan, Forget, Weatherall, Orkin, Higgs, Kazazian, were empowered by the tools and insight provided by basic scientists such as David Baltimore, Phil Sharp, Tom Maniatis, Phil Leder, Harvey Lodish, and Daniel Nathans. The work began with the use of Southern blotting to elucidate deletions resulting in thalassemia. Although this was highly successful in the α-thalassemias,[23,24] it was of limited use in β-thalassemia, and only in specific instances.[25] This problem was solved with the use of gene cloning and DNA sequencing to identify point mutations that result in the thalassemias. In most instances, recurrent common mutations were found in many patients, making routine sequencing laborious and limited in its ability to identify new mutations. However, the finding that different β-globin gene mutations exist on haplotype blocks, at least at the β-globin locus, at first by Kan in sickle cell anemia and then by Antonarakis, Kazazian, and Orkin in β-thalassemia, helped to surmount this limitation.[26–28] This resulted in the discovery of hundreds of mutations that cause the thalassemia syndromes. Not only was a large set of mutations identified that result in the thalassemias, but this also led to the elucidation of many mechanisms that can impair mRNA production or function in the cell. Insights were gained into processes as diverse as transcription, mRNA modification, splicing, and translation.[1,4] These findings presaged the period that would follow with the identification of mutations in various genes that cause a diverse group of mendelian disorders. Even in the past few years, new lessons on the molecular lesions that can cause human disease continue to be learned from the thalassemias, as exemplified by a Melanesian form of α-thalassemia that is attributable to the creation of a new promoter, which competes during transcription with the endogenous α-globin promoters.[29]

Even before the insights from molecular biology began to be used to elucidate the pathophysiology of the thalassemia syndromes, an effort was initiated to use measurements of globin chain imbalance for prenatal diagnosis. The methods pioneered by several scientists, including Clegg, Weatherall, Huehns, Stamatoyannopoulos, and Kazazian, led directly to the first successful prenatal diagnosis by Kan and colleagues.[30,31] Advances in these techniques were made by Chang and colleagues,[32] leading to more feasible diagnostic methods. Cao, Loukopoulos, and others in the Mediterranean region helped to apply these methods in their respective populations, resulting in a large reduction in the incidence of new patients with thalassemia in those populations.[33,34] With the discovery of the molecular basis for many of the common thalassemia mutations, DNA-based prenatal genetic diagnostic methods were soon applied and supplanted the older methods.[35–37] This allowed earlier detection in the first trimester and, as a result, these methods were more widely adopted in a variety of countries. However, there is still controversy surrounding these approaches, limiting their use to populations in which prenatal genetic diagnosis or premarital genetic counseling is accepted.[38]

TRANSFUSION THERAPY AND IRON CHELATION

Although the elucidation of the molecular pathophysiology of the thalassemia syndromes proceeded rapidly, therapeutic advances were slower. Many patients with β-thalassemia, and occasional patients with severe forms of α-thalassemia, require regular transfusions to survive. In the case of β-thalassemia, this therapy had an important effect in reducing the massive ineffective erythropoiesis and attendant bone destruction and organ infiltration that characterized untreated β-thalassemia. Initial work, started by Wolman[39] and later Piomelli and colleagues[40] in the 1960s, suggested the importance of maintaining the Hb level of patients at least at 6 to 8 g per deciliter.[39,40] Subsequent studies suggested that considerably higher levels of Hb may be desirable,[41] but newer evidence suggests that a target of 9 to 10 g per deciliter seems to be most effective.[42] In the 1970s, several additional advances in transfusion techniques occurred. Filtration of blood to remove leukocytes began to be used and allowed for a reduction in severe febrile reactions and decreased alloimmunization to human leukocyte antigens.[43] In addition, the concept of starting transfusions early in life and sustaining these transfusions without interruption appeared to be helpful in achieving immune tolerance.[42]

However, a major problem became evident in patients who were regularly transfused during the 1960s and 1970s. Although many of the patients survived past childhood as a result of these transfusions, the patients were often severely affected as a result of iron overload. Most commonly, these patients were dying as a result of heart failure. The extent of hepatic iron appeared to correlate most closely with the occurrence of heart failure, whereas cardiac iron levels did not seem to relate to the presence of heart failure. Such observations have been supported by studies of patients with thalassemia and also studies on hemochromatosis.[42,44] This phenomenon seems to be attributable to free non–transferrin-bound iron being most toxic to cardiomyocytes.[45] Therefore, the presence of low levels of cardiac iron does not prevent heart failure from free circulating iron.

There has been a great deal of work in the past few years to find newer and better methods to measure noninvasively the burden of iron in the heart, liver, and other tissues. Some work has suggested that newer magnetic resonance imaging (MRI)–based methods of cardiac iron measurement may be useful.[46] However, as discussed earlier, cardiac iron does not necessarily provide a good surrogate for the iron burden that is likely to result in heart failure. Therefore, in spite of these developments, care needs to be taken to ensure that clinical practices are based on adequate evidence of efficacy. Other methods show promise, such as the superconducting quantum interface device that has the potential to provide an integrated measurement of liver iron.[47] However, this technology is both cumbersome and expensive, and there are questions of reproducibility between centers. Hepatic MRI provides an integrated measurement of liver iron burden.[48] However, this method is also expensive, and the signal is dependent on the chemical state of iron. Hepatic MRI is becoming the gold standard for measurement of total body iron and has supplanted liver biopsy because the latter is adversely affected by uneven iron distribution. Computed tomography has not been clinically developed for this purpose because of justifiable concerns for radiation dosage.[49]

In the 1970s, a major advance occurred in treating the iron overload present in these chronically transfused patients. Propper and colleagues[50,51] developed a clinically effective method for continuous subcutaneous infusion of deferoxamine, an effective but nonabsorbable iron chelator with a short plasma half-life, through the use of a portable pump. Pippard and colleagues[52] then modified this regimen for increased compliance. In the following decades, 3 major independent clinical trials showed markedly improved cardiac disease–free survival in patients who followed modified versions of the protocols for the use of deferoxamine.[53–55] However, in spite of these promising results with deferoxamine, many therapeutic obstacles remained for dealing with iron chelation. In the period immediately following the development of these protocols, it became evident that, for many patients, deferoxamine would only have limited efficacy, because these patients had already been iron overloaded for too long. Therefore, it took a couple of decades to see the results of this treatment in the patients who began these regimens from an early age. It was also evident that the use of an iron chelator that required continuous subcutaneous infusion was limited by compliance in many patients.

As a result of these limitations, a search for orally available iron chelators was initiated. The first such compound to become available was deferiprone, an absorbable and more cell-penetrable agent with a short plasma half-life.[56] Although the history of this iron chelator, and the fallout from clinical trials to evaluate its efficacy, is a controversial and complicated area in the history of iron chelation, it is evident that there has never been a demonstration of superiority for this chelation method compared with the use of deferoxamine.[57] Deferiprone has been shown to be unable to prevent accumulation or reduce the iron burden in most patients in whom it was tested.[58] This drug has not been approved by the US Food and Drug Administration (FDA) for any use in the United States. Nonetheless, a potentially important observation was made by Giardina and Grady[59] regarding this iron chelator. They suggested that deferiprone may be useful as a shuttle to assist in the removal of cardiac iron by transferring this iron to deferoxamine. Although this has been suggested as a potentially useful approach and clinical trials are being set up to properly test the efficacy of this regimen, it is not clear that this will solve the compliance issues facing the use of deferoxamine alone.

In the intervening years, Novartis developed deferasirox, an alternative orally available and rationally designed iron chelator with a long plasma half-life. This chelator showed clear efficacy in initial small clinical trials.[60] Since that time, several larger trials have shown its efficacy and comparability with deferoxamine.[61–63] This drug is now FDA approved for use in patients with β-thalassemia, as well as patients requiring blood transfusions for other diseases including sickle cell disease, myelodysplastic syndrome, and other chronic anemias. The drug is useful, but variations in bioavailability create important dosing considerations, and the drug is expensive.[64] The topics of iron overload and chelation therapy are discussed in greater detail in the article by Porter and Shah elsewhere in this issue.

Although the development and clinical use of deferasirox has been promising, more work is needed. Iron overload is still a problem, even when the best and strictest iron chelation regimens are used. It is likely that highly effective methods will be developed from a more sophisticated understanding of the physiologic regulation of iron. This topic is reviewed in depth in the article by Gardenghi and colleagues elsewhere in this issue. In the past few years, understanding of this regulatory process has expanded enormously and the therapeutically intervening with this regulation now seems possible. In 2000, the peptide hormone hepcidin was discovered by Ganz and colleagues.[65] Hepcidin seems to be a master regulator of iron homeostasis by directly inhibiting the activity of the major iron transporter, ferroportin. Ferroportin is necessary for iron release from intestinal cells and macrophages into the blood[66] Miller and colleagues[67] recently suggested that ineffective erythropoiesis in thalassemia causes an increase in the level of a protein known as GDF15, which inhibits the activity of hepcidin. If this observation is confirmed, it may, in part, explain why patients with thalassemia intermedia become iron overloaded so readily. This work, along with several other studies, suggests that hepcidin may be a key therapeutic target that could reduce iron overload in patients with thalassemia.[68] There have also been recent efforts to use other strategies to reduce the toxicity of free iron, such as through the use of transferrin, in mouse models of thalassemia.[69] Although this seems to be beneficial in these mouse models, it is unclear whether this will be a viable therapeutic strategy, given the need for regular expensive infusion treatments in patients. Nonetheless, it is clear that recent work in this field will assist in increasing understanding of normal and pathologic iron metabolism, and this will lead to more effective strategies to control iron overload in chronically transfused patients.

REGULATION OF FETAL HB AND ITS MODULATION IN THERAPY

Higher levels of fetal Hb (HbF) are able to ameliorate the severity of β-thalassemia by improving the balance of α- and non–α-globin chains and thereby preventing inclusion body formation. This finding was particularly evident from careful clinical observations in rare patients with highly increased levels of HbF who had a significantly milder clinical course and from the observation of infants with β-thalassemia who only begin showing symptoms after the expression of HbF declines in the months following birth.[1,70] Such findings have also been subsequently confirmed in larger epidemiologic studies of numerous thalassemia populations.[71–73] As a result of this, several investigators have attempted to establish how the regulation of the fetal to adult Hb switch in humans occurs and how this can be therapeutically modulated.[74,75]

The human globin genes were among the first to be cloned and the structure of the entire β-globin cluster was soon elucidated and sequenced.[76] Around that time, it became evident that the silenced HbF genes in the β-globin cluster underwent DNA methylation in adult erythroid cells, whereas this was not the case in erythroid cells from embryonic and fetal life. As a result, in the early 1980s, DeSimone and colleagues[77] tested whether a DNA hypomethylating agent, 5-azacytidine, might allow reactivation of the HbF genes in adult erythroid cells of monkeys. These experiments were successful and showed the usefulness of this approach to increase HbF levels. Ley and colleagues[78-80] and Nienhuis then went on to test this approach in patients with β-thalassemia and sickle cell disease. These small trials were successful and experts in the field, such as Edward Benz, editorially remarked at that time that "molecular biology has come to the bedside."[81] However, there was concern about the long-term sequelae of a potentially mutagenic compound like 5-azacytidine. Nathan[82] and Stamatoyannopoulos[75] suggested that the effect of 5-azacytidine on HbF induction might relate to its ability to act as an S-phase cell cycle inhibitor, rather than through an epigenetic effect on the fetal globin gene promoters. With their colleagues, both Nathan and Stamatoyannopoulos went on to prove that numerous S-phase inhibitors, including hydroxyurea, were all highly effective as inducers of HbF in monkeys.[83-85] Platt and colleagues[86] then tested hydroxyurea, which had the safest side effect profile, in patients with sickle cell disease and showed a clear HbF response. The response does not have to be large because HbF is a powerful antisickling agent. The exploratory observations of Platt and colleagues[87] were then examined in large clinical trials initially conducted by Charache and Dover and their associates.[88,89] The results have led to FDA approval of hydroxyurea for use in patients with sickle cell disease. However, hydroxyurea has not provided the same effectiveness in patients with β-thalassemia, who require much more HbF to achieve globin chain balance.[90,91] It may be more effective in some select populations with β-thalassemia, particularly those with an XmnI polymorphism at position −158 in the γ-globin gene promoter. Additionally, other S-phase inhibitors or safer derivatives of 5-azacytidine may also show promise for this purpose.

Around the time that these studies were being performed, in the mid-1980s, Perrine and colleagues[92] reported another important observation. Along with Bard,[93] they showed that infants of diabetic mothers have a delayed fetal to adult Hb switch. Because it was known that hydroxybutyrate is increased in mothers with diabetes, Perrine and colleagues[94] went on to test the idea that butyrate, or other similar short-chain fatty acids, may be effective as inducers of HbF first in sheep and then in patients. Although initial trials showed promise,[95,96] these therapies were not particularly effective.[97] However, a subset of patients did show responses in these trials and in independent studies performed by Dover, Atweh, and their colleagues.[97-99] Although hydroxybutyrate is increased in diabetic mothers, numerous other metabolites are also increased in this ketotic state and therefore further investigation of this phenomenon is worthwhile. It has been suggested that these short-chain fatty acids are likely to induce HbF through the inhibition of histone deacetylases (HDACs).[100] Various HDAC inhibitors can be potent inducers of HbF in vitro and so these compounds may show clinical efficacy in vivo.[101,102] Pharmacologic induction of HbF production is discussed in greater detail in the article by Atweh and Fatallah elsewhere in this issue.

Molecular regulators of the fetal to adult Hb switch have been sought with the idea that targeted approaches could be developed if such molecules were identified. Although numerous regulators of erythropoiesis and globin gene expression had been identified, none appeared to directly explain the fetal to adult switch that occurs in ontogeny.[103] Recently, new insight into this process has occurred as a result of human genetic association studies.[104] By examining genetic polymorphisms in the human genome that were associated with HbF levels in adults, 3 major loci associated with HbF levels were found.[105-107] These loci included the β-globin locus on chromosome 11, a region between the genes *HBS1L* and *MYB* on chromosome 6, and the *BCL11A* gene on chromosome 2. The gene *BCL11A* had previously been studied for its role as a zinc-finger transcription factor necessary for B lymphocyte production. However, a role in erythroid progenitors had not previously been appreciated. The role of this transcription factor in regulating HbF levels was therefore examined, given the compelling genetic association observed.[108] This gene was found to be expressed in an inversely correlated manner with the expression of the HbF genes seen in the course of human ontogeny, as well as in humans with different HbF-associated *BCL11A* genetic variants. This finding led to the hypothesis that this gene may function as a repressor of the HbF genes in humans. Using a proteomic approach, BCL11A was found to interact with the erythroid transcription factors, GATA-1 and FOG-1, as well as a repressor complex known as NuRD. The NuRD complex contains 2 HDACs, suggesting that these may be the targets of short-chain fatty acids and other HDAC inhibitors that induce HbF. The role of BCL11A in directly regulating the HbF genes was shown by knocking this gene down using siRNA and shRNA methods in primary human erythroid cells. These results showed that this knockdown results in robust increases in the level of HbF without causing a major perturbation of erythroid differentiation. Consistent with a direct role in regulating the HbF genes, it was shown that BCL11A directly interacts with the β-globin cluster in human erythroid cells. Together these findings identified BCL11A as a major regulator of the fetal to adult Hb switch in humans. Subsequently, it was shown that BCL11A also plays a critical role in the evolutionarily divergent globin gene switches that occur in mammals, suggesting a critical conserved role of this factor in this phenomenon.[109] Collectively, these studies established BCL11A or its interacting partners as potentially important therapeutic targets to induce HbF levels. Moreover, BCL11A is unique in that human genetic association studies suggested that it plays a major role in vivo in the regulation of HbF levels in humans. Indeed, studies have shown that polymorphisms in *BCL11A* play an important role in ameliorating the severity of both sickle cell disease and β-thalassemia.[72,73,105,107] It is likely that further study of this factor and others that will find similar results and may assist in developing targeted therapeutic approaches to increase HbF in patients with β-thalassemia. Other genetic variants that have not been as well studied seem to ameliorate β-thalassemia to as great an extent (or perhaps even more so) than the polymorphisms in *BCL11A*, suggesting that further studies of these other factors could lead to fruitful new insight into how HbF could be therapeutically modulated.[72,73]

The presence of concomitant α-globin gene mutations with β-thalassemia can result in a much milder clinical syndrome. This finding is attributable to a reduction in the extent of globin chain imbalance.[110] Although not as much effort has been focused on the modulation of α-globin levels in β-thalassemia,[111] this may represent another valuable therapeutic strategy, in addition to the efforts to stimulate HbF production. Studies of cohorts of patients with β-thalassemia confirm the ameliorating effects of α-globin gene deletions on the clinical course in these populations.[71,72,111]

STEM CELL TRANSPLANTATION & GENE THERAPY

Although a variety of therapeutic approaches have been used in the thalassemia syndromes, only bone marrow or stem cell transplantation offers the hope of a complete cure. This is a theoretic possibility, but many difficulties face patients who consider this treatment route. Although claims are often made about the broad potential to treat patients with thalassemia throughout the world, it is likely that many of the claims ignore the practicality of these therapies in settings such as the developing world.[112] Patients face the potentially dangerous occurrence of graft failure, graft versus host disease, or other complications of this therapy. Although some centers seem to have extremely high success rates,[113,114] this has not been more broadly reproducible and it is unclear to what extent this may reflect variations in technical approach or patient selection.

Despite the limitations to this approach, there is nonetheless promise in this work. Recent studies from Tisdale and colleagues[115] have described improved, milder conditioning regimens for patients with sickle cell disease that allow disease amelioration through the presence of mixed chimeric transplants. Few studies have reported such reduced-intensity conditioning regimens in patients with disorders of Hb, but it is likely that more reports of this sort will be seen in the future.[116] It remains to be seen how effective these approaches will be as larger clinical trials are performed. One concern with this approach is that there is a substantial chance of graft failure, although, with improvements in conditioning regimens, this may be surmountable. There are also certain clinical observations that have occurred in the context of such graft failure. In at least 2 reported cases, there seems to be sustained amelioration of disease following graft failure that is attributable to increased HbF production following host hematopoietic stem cell (HSC) reconstitution.[117,118] The basis of these observations is unclear, but it suggests that, if this mechanism could be understood, it may be possible to use this insight to develop better treatments for patients with thalassemia. Stem cell transplantation is discussed in greater detail in the articles by Gaziev and Lucarelli and by Kanathezhath and Walters elsewhere in this issue.

From the mid-1980s, when the transduction of HSCs by retroviruses in mice was first described by Williams, Mulligan, and their colleagues, it seemed as though gene therapy was imminent.[119] However, more than 2 decades has passed since that time and only limited progress has been made. There has been a variety of setbacks, including the untoward events that occurred in Philadelphia[120] and the leukemia that emerged in patients with X-linked severe combined immunodeficiency in France.[121] Nonetheless, there is promise that such approaches may become a clinical reality in the near future.[122] Improvements in vector design, viral transduction protocols, use of various target cell populations, and monitoring of patients suggests that these approaches are becoming safer and more effective. The complete amelioration of mouse models of β-thalassemia by gene therapy has been reported in the past few years.[123–126] Small-scale human trials of patients who are severely affected have been initiated or are soon to begin.[127,128] Although a trial by the group at St Jude Children's Research Hospital is planned for the near future, a trial has been underway in France by Leboulch and colleagues[122] (see the article by Bank elsewhere in this issue). This clinical trial has so far involved the treatment of 2 patients with β-thalassemia. The first patient became cytopenic following the conditioning and transplant regimen and had to be rescued with backup CD34 cells. The second patient in this trial became transfusion independent almost a year after the transplant with a Hb level of 9 g per deciliter. However, it is unclear whether this was attributable to the success of gene therapy alone, because only one-third of the total Hb was derived from the gene therapy vector. The HbF level in this patient has been highly and consistently increased after recovery, suggesting that, akin to the patients discussed earlier with HbF increases after allogeneic stem cell graft failure, a mechanism may be at play to cause such phenomena. However, this patient was also reported to have clonal dominance, with the clonal cells having viral integration in the HMGA2 oncogenic gene locus.[122] Major hurdles still exist for such gene therapy approaches.

Although a pessimistic view may be taken of the future of gene therapy, there are promising basic science developments that suggest that the problems being faced may be surmountable. Targeted integration approaches that are being developed by Porteus and others suggest that there may be ways to avoid random and potentially oncogenic viral integration events.[129–131] In addition, there is great hope that advances in the use of cell therapy may allow many of these hurdles to be overcome. Thanks to the pioneering work of Yamanaka and the subsequent advances by Thompson, Jaenisch, Daley, and others, there is hope that the use of human induced pluripotent cells or other stem cells may eventually yield advances in our clinical approach to these problems.[132] However, although these approaches are promising based on work in model systems,[133] there are many limitations that need to be overcome before this work can begin to enter the clinic.[134]

CONCLUDING REMARKS

Nearly 50 years have passed since Phaedon Fessas made his seminal observations on the molecular pathophysiology of the thalassemia syndromes. A great deal has been learned since that time. The molecular basis for these diseases is now understood, survival in these patients has improved thanks to highly effective iron chelation regimens, the problem of HbF induction is now approached in a targeted manner, and the reality of improved stem cell or gene therapy may be imminent. All of these advances will continue to rely on close relationships between basic scientists and their clinical colleagues, who are as well versed in the molecular sciences as they are in medicine.[135,136] Patients depend on such vital interactions for important therapeutic advances.

There are important limitations and areas in which a great deal of work still remains to be done. Most patients with these diseases live in the developing world.[137] It has been convenient to ignore this fact while important advances in the molecular sciences were made, but this is no longer possible. Partnerships must be established between more developed countries and the developing world. How these diseases can best be approached in the developing world is still unclear, but more work in this area is likely to show what strategies will work. More careful clinical studies of these diseases must be considered in regions where they are prevalent. The importance of this is shown by the recent studies showing the previously unappreciated extent of phenotypic diversity in HbE-β-thalassemia[71] (see the article by Olivieri and colleagues elsewhere in this issue). Such work is likely to show how little is truly understood about the natural history of these diseases. It is important to focus our effort not only on making scientific advances in this field but also on ensuring that these findings can be brought to bear to benefit patients worldwide.

In this issue, the many scientific and medical advances that hold great promise for the many patients with thalassemia syndromes are described. Medicine has benefited greatly from the thousands of patients with these diseases. They deserve our best efforts to use the recent advances in the biomedical sciences to bring them, and their families, real relief.

REFERENCES

1. Weatherall DJ, Clegg JB. The thalassaemia syndromes. 4th edition. Oxford; Malden (MA): Blackwell Science; 2001.
2. Olivieri NF. The beta-thalassemias. N Engl J Med 1999;341:99–109.
3. Rund D, Rachmilewitz E. Beta-thalassemia. N Engl J Med 2005;353:1135–46.
4. Weatherall DJ. Thalassaemia: the long road from bedside to genome. Nat Rev Genet 2004;5:625–31.

5. Ingram VM, Stretton AO. Genetic basis of the thalassaemia diseases. Nature 1959;184:1903–9.

6. Fessas P. Inclusions of hemoglobin erythroblasts and erythrocytes of thalassemia. Blood 1963;21:21–32.

7. Fessas P, Loukopoulos D, Thorell B. Absorption spectra of inclusion bodies in beta-thalassemia. Blood 1965;25:105–9.

8. Weatherall DJ, Clegg JB, Naughton MA. Globin synthesis in thalassaemia: an in vitro study. Nature 1965;208:1061–5.

9. Nathan DG, Gunn RB. Thalassemia: the consequences of unbalanced hemoglobin synthesis. Am J Med 1966;41:815–30.

10. Heywood JD, Karon M, Weissman S. Amino acids: incorporation into alpha- and beta-chains of hemoglobin by normal and thalassemic reticulocytes. Science 1964;146:530–1.

11. Marks PA, Burka ER. Hemoglobins A and F: formation in thalassemia and other hemolytic anemias. Science 1964;144:552–3.

12. Gabuzda TG, Nathan DG, Gardner FH, et al. Hemoglobin F and beta thalassemia. Science 1967;157:1079.

13. Clegg JB, Weatherall DJ. Haemoglobin synthesis in alpha-thalassaemia (haemoglobin H disease). Nature 1967;215:1241–3.

14. Clegg JB, Weatherall DJ, Na-Nakorn S, et al. Haemoglobin synthesis in beta-thalassaemia. Nature 1968;220:664–8.

15. Nienhuis AW, Anderson WF. Isolation and translation of hemoglobin messenger RNA from thalassemia, sickle cell anemia, and normal human reticulocytes. J Clin Invest 1971;50:2458–60.

16. Benz EJ Jr, Forget BG. Defect in messenger RNA for human hemoglobin synthesis in beta thalassemia. J Clin Invest 1971;50:2755–60.

17. Nathan DG, Lodish HF, Kan YW, et al. Beta thalassemia and translation of globin messenger RNA. Proc Natl Acad Sci U S A 1971;68:2514–8.

18. Bank A, Marks PA. Hemoglobin synthesis in thalassemia. Semin Hematol 1971; 4:97–115.

19. Housman D, Forget BG, Skoultchi A, et al. Quantitative deficiency of chain-specific globin messenger ribonucleic acids in the thalassemia syndromes. Proc Natl Acad Sci U S A 1973;70:1809–13.

20. Kacian DL, Gambino R, Dow LW, et al. Decreased globin messenger RNA in thalassemia detected by molecular hybridization. Proc Natl Acad Sci U S A 1973;70:1886–90.

21. Ottolenghi S, Lanyon WG, Paul J, et al. The severe form of alpha thalassaemia is caused by a haemoglobin gene deletion. Nature 1974;251:389–92.

22. Taylor JM, Dozy A, Kan YW, et al. Genetic lesion in homozygous alpha thalassaemia (hydrops fetalis). Nature 1974;251:392–3.

23. Orkin SH, Old J, Lazarus H, et al. The molecular basis of alpha-thalassemias: frequent occurrence of dysfunctional alpha loci among non-Asians with Hb H disease. Cell 1979;17:33–42.

24. Embury SH, Lebo RV, Dozy AM, et al. Organization of the alpha-globin genes in the Chinese alpha-thalassemia syndromes. J Clin Invest 1979;63:1307–10.

25. Orkin SH, Old JM, Weatherall DJ, et al. Partial deletion of beta-globin gene DNA in certain patients with beta 0-thalassemia. Proc Natl Acad Sci U S A 1979;76:2400–4.

26. Kan YW, Dozy AM. Polymorphism of DNA sequence adjacent to human beta-globin structural gene: relationship to sickle mutation. Proc Natl Acad Sci U S A 1978;75:5631–5.

27. Antonarakis SE, Boehm CD, Giardina PJ, et al. Nonrandom association of poly-morphic restriction sites in the beta-globin gene cluster. Proc Natl Acad Sci U S A 1982;79:137–41.

28. Orkin SH, Kazazian HH Jr, Antonarakis SE, et al. Linkage of beta-thalassaemia mutations and beta-globin gene polymorphisms with DNA polymorphisms in human beta-globin gene cluster. Nature 1982;296:627–31.

29. De Gobbi M, Viprakasit V, Hughes JR, et al. A regulatory SNP causes a human genetic disease by creating a new transcriptional promoter. Science 2006;312: 1215–7.

30. Kan YW, Golbus MS, Trecartin R. Prenatal diagnosis of homozygous beta-thal-assaemia. Lancet 1975;2:790–1.

31. Kan YW, Golbus MS, Klein P, et al. Successful application of prenatal diagnosis in a pregnancy at risk for homozygous beta-thalassemia. N Engl J Med 1975; 292:1096–9.

32. Chang H, Hobbins JC, Cividalli G, et al. In utero diagnosis of: hemoglobinopa-thies. Hemoglobin synthesis in fetal red cells. N Engl J Med 1974;290:1067–8.

33. Aleporou-Marinou V, Sakarelou-Papapetrou N, Antsaklis A, et al. Prenatal diag-nosis of thalassemia major in Greece: evaluation of the first large series of attempts. Ann N Y Acad Sci 1980;344:181–8.

34. Cao A, Rosatelli C, Pirastu M, et al. Thalassemias in Sardinia: molecular pathology, phenotype-genotype correlation, and prevention. Am J Pediatr Hem-atol Oncol 1991;13:179–88.

35. Orkin SH, Alter BP, Altay C, et al. Application of endonuclease mapping to the analysis and prenatal diagnosis of thalassemias caused by globin-gene dele-tion. N Engl J Med 1978;299:166–72.

36. Boehm CD, Antonarakis SE, Phillips JA 3rd, et al. Prenatal diagnosis using DNA polymorphisms. Report on 95 pregnancies at risk for sickle-cell disease or beta-thalassemia. N Engl J Med 1983;308:1054–8.

37. Old JM, Ward RH, Petrou M, et al. First-trimester fetal diagnosis for haemoglo-binopathies: three cases. Lancet 1982;2:1413–6.

38. Colah R, Surve R, Wadia M, et al. Carrier screening for beta-thalassemia during pregnancy in India: a 7-year evaluation. Genet Test 2008;12:181–5.

39. Wolman IJ. Transfusion therapy in Cooley's anemia: growth and health as related to long-range hemoglobin levels. A progress report. Ann N Y Acad Sci 1964; 119:736–47.

40. Piomelli S, Danoff SJ, Becker MH, et al. Prevention of bone malformations and cardiomegaly in Cooley's anemia by early hypertransfusion regimen. Ann N Y Acad Sci 1969;165:427–36.

41. Propper RD, Button LN, Nathan DG. New approaches to the transfusion management of thalassemia. Blood 1980;55:55–60.

42. Nathan DG. Thalassemia: the continued challenge. Ann N Y Acad Sci 2005; 1054:1–10.

43. Rebulla P. Blood transfusion in beta thalassaemia major. Transfus Med 1995;5: 247–58.

44. Sonakul D, Thakerngpol K, Pacharee P. Cardiac pathology in 76 thalassemic patients. Birth Defects Orig Artic Ser 1988;23:177–91.

45. Link G, Pinson A, Hershko C. Heart cells in culture: a model of myocardial iron overload and chelation. J Lab Clin Med 1985;106:147–53.

46. Kirk P, Roughton M, Porter JB, et al. Cardiac T2* magnetic resonance for predic-tion of cardiac complications in thalassemia major. Circulation 2009;120:1961–8.

47. Brittenham GM, Farrell DE, Harris JW, et al. Magnetic-susceptibility measurement of human iron stores. N Engl J Med 1982;307:1671–5.

48. St Pierre TG, Clark PR, Chua-anusorn W, et al. Noninvasive measurement and imaging of liver iron concentrations using proton magnetic resonance. Blood 2005;105:855–61.

49. Goldberg HI, Cann CE, Moss AA, et al. Noninvasive quantitation of liver iron in dogs with hemochromatosis using dual-energy CT scanning. Invest Radiol 1982;17:375–80.

50. Propper RD, Cooper B, Rufo RR, et al. Continuous subcutaneous administration of deferoxamine in patients with iron overload. N Engl J Med 1977;297:418–23.

51. Propper RD, Shurin SB, Nathan DG. Reassessment of the use of desferrioxamine B in iron overload. N Engl J Med 1976;294:1421–3.

52. Pippard MJ, Callender ST, Weatherall DJ. Chelation regimens with desferrioxamine. Lancet 1977;1:1101.

53. Olivieri NF, Nathan DG, MacMillan JH, et al. Survival in medically treated patients with homozygous beta-thalassemia. N Engl J Med 1994;331:574–8.

54. Brittenham GM, Griffith PM, Nienhuis AW, et al. Efficacy of deferoxamine in preventing complications of iron overload in patients with thalassemia major. N Engl J Med 1994;331:567–73.

55. Borgna-Pignatti C, Rugolotto S, De Stefano P, et al. Survival and complications in patients with thalassemia major treated with transfusion and deferoxamine. Haematologica 2004;89:1187–93.

56. Cunningham MJ, Nathan DG. New developments in iron chelators. Curr Opin Hematol 2005;12:129–34.

57. Cohen AR, Galanello R, Piga A, et al. Safety and effectiveness of long-term therapy with the oral iron chelator deferiprone. Blood 2003;102:1583–7.

58. Hoffbrand AV, AL-Refaie F, Davis B, et al. Long-term trial of deferiprone in 51 transfusion-dependent iron overloaded patients. Blood 1998;91:295–300.

59. Giardina PJ, Grady RW. Chelation therapy in beta-thalassemia: an optimistic update. Semin Hematol 2001;38:360–6.

60. Nisbet-Brown E, Olivieri NF, Giardina PJ, et al. Effectiveness and safety of ICL670 in iron-loaded patients with thalassaemia: a randomised, double-blind, placebo-controlled, dose-escalation trial. Lancet 2003;361:1597–602.

61. Cappellini MD, Pattoneri P. Oral iron chelators. Annu Rev Med 2009;60:25–38.

62. Porter J, Galanello R, Saglio G, et al. Relative response of patients with myelodysplastic syndromes and other transfusion-dependent anaemias to deferasirox (ICL670): a 1-yr prospective study. Eur J Haematol 2008;80:168–76.

63. Vichinsky E, Onyekwere O, Porter J, et al. A randomised comparison of deferasirox versus deferoxamine for the treatment of transfusional iron overload in sickle cell disease. Br J Haematol 2007;136:501–8.

64. Chirnomas D, Smith A, Braunstein J, et al. Oral chelators deferasirox and deferiprone for transfusional iron overload in thalassemia major: new data, new questions. Blood 2006;107:3436–41.

65. Ganz T. Hepcidin, a key regulator of iron metabolism and mediator of anemia of inflammation. Blood 2003;102:783–8.

66. Nemeth E, Ganz T. The role of hepcidin in iron metabolism. Acta Haematol 2009; 122:78–86.

67. Tanno T, Bhanu NV, Oneal PA, et al. High levels of GDF15 in thalassemia suppress expression of the iron regulatory protein hepcidin. Nat Med 2007; 13:1096–101.

68. Gardenghi S, Marongiu MF, Ramos P, et al. Ineffective erythropoiesis in beta-thalassemia is characterized by increased iron absorption mediated by down-regulation of hepcidin and up-regulation of ferroportin. Blood 2007;109:5027–35.
69. Li H, Rybicki AC, Suzuka SM, et al. Transferrin therapy ameliorates disease in beta-thalassemic mice. Nat Med 2010;16:177–82.
70. Weatherall DJ. Phenotype-genotype relationships in monogenic disease: lessons from the thalassaemias. Nat Rev Genet 2001;2:245–55.
71. Premawardhena A, Fisher CA, Olivieri NF, et al. Haemoglobin E beta thalassaemia in Sri Lanka. Lancet 2005;366:1467–70.
72. Galanello R, Sanna S, Perseu L, et al. Amelioration of Sardinian beta0 thalassemia by genetic modifiers. Blood 2009;114:3935–7.
73. Nuinoon M, Makarasara W, Mushiroda T, et al. A genome-wide association identified the common genetic variants influence disease severity in beta(0)-thalassemia/hemoglobin E. Hum Genet 2010;127:303–14.
74. Bank A. Regulation of human fetal hemoglobin: new players, new complexities. Blood 2006;107:435–43.
75. Stamatoyannopoulos G. Control of globin gene expression during development and erythroid differentiation. Exp Hematol 2005;33:259–71.
76. Fritsch EF, Lawn RM, Maniatis T. Molecular cloning and characterization of the human beta-like globin gene cluster. Cell 1980;19:959–72.
77. DeSimone J, Heller P, Hall L, et al. 5-Azacytidine stimulates fetal hemoglobin synthesis in anemic baboons. Proc Natl Acad Sci U S A 1982;79:4428–31.
78. Ley TJ, Anagnou NP, Young NS, et al. 5-Azacytidine for beta thalassaemia? Lancet 1983;1:467.
79. Ley TJ, DeSimone J, Anagnou NP, et al. 5-Azacytidine selectively increases gamma-globin synthesis in a patient with beta+ thalassemia. N Engl J Med 1982;307:1469–75.
80. Ley TJ, DeSimone J, Noguchi CT, et al. 5-Azacytidine increases gamma-globin synthesis and reduces the proportion of dense cells in patients with sickle cell anemia. Blood 1983;62:370–80.
81. Benz EJ Jr. Clinical management of gene expression. N Engl J Med 1982;307:1515–6.
82. Nathan DG. Regulation of fetal hemoglobin synthesis by cell cycle specific drugs. Prog Clin Biol Res 1985;191:475–500.
83. Letvin NL, Linch DC, Beardsley GP, et al. Influence of cell cycle phase-specific agents on simian fetal hemoglobin synthesis. J Clin Invest 1985;75:1999–2005.
84. Letvin NL, Linch DC, Beardsley GP, et al. Augmentation of fetal-hemoglobin production in anemic monkeys by hydroxyurea. N Engl J Med 1984;310:869–73.
85. Papayannopoulou T, Torrealba de Ron A, Veith R, et al. Arabinosylcytosine induces fetal hemoglobin in baboons by perturbing erythroid cell differentiation kinetics. Science 1984;224:617–9.
86. Platt OS, Orkin SH, Dover G, et al. Hydroxyurea enhances fetal hemoglobin production in sickle cell anemia. J Clin Invest 1984;74:652–6.
87. Platt OS. Hydroxyurea for the treatment of sickle cell anemia. N Engl J Med 2008;358:1362–9.
88. Charache S, Terrin ML, Moore RD, et al. Effect of hydroxyurea on the frequency of painful crises in sickle cell anemia. Investigators of the Multicenter Study of Hydroxyurea in Sickle Cell Anemia. N Engl J Med 1995;332:1317–22.
89. Steinberg MH, Barton F, Castro O, et al. Effect of hydroxyurea on mortality and morbidity in adult sickle cell anemia: risks and benefits up to 9 years of treatment. JAMA 2003;289:1645–51.

90. Yavarian M, Karimi M, Bakker E, et al. Response to hydroxyurea treatment in Iranian transfusion-dependent beta-thalassemia patients. Haematologica 2004;89:1172–8.

91. Alebouyeh M, Moussavi F, Haddad-Deylami H, et al. Hydroxyurea in the treatment of major beta-thalassemia and importance of genetic screening. Ann Hematol 2004;83:430–3.

92. Perrine SP, Greene MF, Faller DV. Delay in the fetal globin switch in infants of diabetic mothers. N Engl J Med 1985;312:334–8.

93. Bard H, Prosmanne J. Relative rates of fetal hemoglobin and adult hemoglobin synthesis in cord blood of infants of insulin-dependent diabetic mothers. Pediatrics 1985;75:1143–7.

94. Perrine SP, Rudolph A, Faller DV, et al. Butyrate infusions in the ovine fetus delay the biologic clock for globin gene switching. Proc Natl Acad Sci U S A 1988;85: 8540–2.

95. Perrine SP, Ginder GD, Faller DV, et al. A short-term trial of butyrate to stimulate fetal-globin-gene expression in the beta-globin disorders. N Engl J Med 1993; 328:81–6.

96. Perrine SP, Olivieri NF, Faller DV, et al. Butyrate derivatives. New agents for stimulating fetal globin production in the beta-globin disorders. Am J Pediatr Hematol Oncol 1994;16:67–71.

97. Sher GD, Ginder GD, Little J, et al. Extended therapy with intravenous arginine butyrate in patients with beta-hemoglobinopathies. N Engl J Med 1995;332:1606–10.

98. Dover GJ, Brusilow S, Charache S. Induction of fetal hemoglobin production in subjects with sickle cell anemia by oral sodium phenylbutyrate. Blood 1994;84: 339–43.

99. Dover GJ, Brusilow S, Samid D. Increased fetal hemoglobin in patients receiving sodium 4-phenylbutyrate. N Engl J Med 1992;327:569–70.

100. Fathallah H, Weinberg RS, Galperin Y, et al. Role of epigenetic modifications in normal globin gene regulation and butyrate-mediated induction of fetal hemoglobin. Blood 2007;110:3391–7.

101. Cao H, Stamatoyannopoulos G, Jung M. Induction of human gamma globin gene expression by histone deacetylase inhibitors. Blood 2004;103:701–9.

102. Quek L, Thein SL. Molecular therapies in beta-thalassaemia. Br J Haematol 2007;136:353–65.

103. Cantor AB, Orkin SH. Transcriptional regulation of erythropoiesis: an affair involving multiple partners. Oncogene 2002;21:3368–76.

104. McCarthy MI, Abecasis GR, Cardon LR, et al. Genome-wide association studies for complex traits: consensus, uncertainty and challenges. Nat Rev Genet 2008; 9:356–69.

105. Uda M, Galanello R, Sanna S, et al. Genome-wide association study shows BCL11A associated with persistent fetal hemoglobin and amelioration of the phenotype of beta-thalassemia. Proc Natl Acad Sci U S A 2008;105:1620–5.

106. Menzel S, Garner C, Gut I, et al. A QTL influencing F cell production maps to a gene encoding a zinc-finger protein on chromosome 2p15. Nat Genet 2007;39:1197–9.

107. Lettre G, Sankaran VG, Bezerra MA, et al. DNA polymorphisms at the BCL11A, HBS1L-MYB, and beta-globin loci associate with fetal hemoglobin levels and pain crises in sickle cell disease. Proc Natl Acad Sci U S A 2008;105:11869–74.

108. Sankaran VG, Menne TF, Xu J, et al. Human fetal hemoglobin expression is regulated by the developmental stage-specific repressor BCL11A. Science 2008;322:1839–42.

109. Sankaran VG, Xu J, Ragoczy T, et al. Developmental and species-divergent globin switching are driven by BCL11A. Nature 2009;460:1093–7.
110. Kan YW, Nathan DG. Mild thalassemia: the result of interactions of alpha and beta thalassemia genes. J Clin Invest 1970;49:635–42.
111. Higgs DR. Gene regulation in hematopoiesis: new lessons from thalassemia. Hematology Am Soc Hematol Educ Program 2004;1–13.
112. Bordignon C. Stem-cell therapies for blood diseases. Nature 2006;441:1100–2.
113. Gaziev J, Sodani P, Polchi P, et al. Bone marrow transplantation in adults with thalassemia: treatment and long-term follow-up. Ann N Y Acad Sci 2005;1054: 196–205.
114. Chandy M. Stem cell transplantation in India. Bone Marrow Transplant 2008;42- (Suppl 1):S81–4.
115. Hsieh MM, Kang EM, Fitzhugh CD, et al. Allogeneic hematopoietic stem-cell transplantation for sickle cell disease. N Engl J Med 2009;361:2309–17.
116. Locatelli F. Reduced-intensity regimens in allogeneic hematopoietic stem cell transplantation for hemoglobinopathies. Hematology Am Soc Hematol Educ Program 2006;398–401.
117. Paciaroni K, Gallucci C, De Angelis G, et al. Sustained and full fetal hemoglobin production after failure of bone marrow transplant in a patient homozygous for beta 0-thalassemia: a clinical remission despite genetic disease and transplant rejection. Am J Hematol 2009;84:372–3.
118. Ferster A, Corazza F, Vertongen F, et al. Transplanted sickle-cell disease patients with autologous bone marrow recovery after graft failure develop increased levels of fetal haemoglobin which corrects disease severity. Br J Haematol 1995;90:804–8.
119. Williams DA, Lemischka IR, Nathan DG, et al. Introduction of new genetic material into pluripotent haematopoietic stem cells of the mouse. Nature 1984;310: 476–80.
120. Woo SL. Policy statement of the American Society of Gene Therapy on reporting of patient adverse events in gene therapy trials. Mol Ther 2000;1:7–8.
121. Fischer A, Abina SH, Thrasher A, et al. LMO2 and gene therapy for severe combined immunodeficiency. N Engl J Med 2004;350:2526–7 [author reply: 2526–7].
122. Cavazzana-Calvo M, Payen E, Negre O, et al. Transfusion independence and HMGA2 activation after gene therapy of human β-thalassaemia. Nature 2010; 467(7313):318–22.
123. Imren S, Payen E, Westerman KA, et al. Permanent and panerythroid correction of murine beta thalassemia by multiple lentiviral integration in hematopoietic stem cells. Proc Natl Acad Sci U S A 2002;99:14380–5.
124. Rivella S, May C, Chadburn A, et al. A novel murine model of Cooley anemia and its rescue by lentiviral-mediated human beta-globin gene transfer. Blood 2003; 101:2932–9.
125. May C, Rivella S, Callegari J, et al. Therapeutic haemoglobin synthesis in beta-thalassaemic mice expressing lentivirus-encoded human beta-globin. Nature 2000;406:82–6.
126. May C, Rivella S, Chadburn A, et al. Successful treatment of murine beta-thalassemia intermedia by transfer of the human beta-globin gene. Blood 2002; 99:1902–8.
127. Lisowski L, Sadelain M. Current status of globin gene therapy for the treatment of beta-thalassaemia. Br J Haematol 2008;141:335–45.

128. Bank A, Dorazio R, Leboulch P. A phase I/II clinical trial of beta-globin gene therapy for beta-thalassemia. Ann N Y Acad Sci 2005;1054:308–16.
129. Porteus MH, Baltimore D. Chimeric nucleases stimulate gene targeting in human cells. Science 2003;300:763.
130. Porteus MH, Carroll D. Gene targeting using zinc finger nucleases. Nat Biotechnol 2005;23:967–73.
131. Urnov FD, Miller JC, Lee YL, et al. Highly efficient endogenous human gene correction using designed zinc-finger nucleases. Nature 2005;435:646–51.
132. Belmonte JC, Ellis J, Hochedlinger K, et al. Induced pluripotent stem cells and reprogramming: seeing the science through the hype. Nat Rev Genet 2009;10:878–83.
133. Hanna J, Wernig M, Markoulaki S, et al. Treatment of sickle cell anemia mouse model with iPS cells generated from autologous skin. Science 2007;318:1920–3.
134. Daley GQ. Stem cells: roadmap to the clinic. J Clin Invest 2010;120:8–10.
135. Nathan DG. The several Cs of translational clinical research. J Clin Invest 2005;115:795–7.
136. Goldstein JL, Brown MS. The clinical investigator: bewitched, bothered, and bewildered–but still beloved. J Clin Invest 1997;99:2803–12.
137. Weatherall D, Akinyanju O, Fucharoen S, et al. Inherited disorders of hemoglobin. Disease control priorities in developing countries. 2nd edition. New York: Oxford University Press; 2006. p. 663–80.

The Population Genetics and Dynamics of the Thalassemias

D.J. Weatherall, MD, FRCP, FRS[a],*, T.N. Williams, MD, MRCP, PhD[b], S.J. Allen, MD, MRCP[c], A. O'Donnell, PhD[c]

KEYWORDS

- Thalassemia • Malaria • Population genetics
- Natural selection

The inherited disorders of hemoglobin are by far the commonest monogenic diseases. Recent estimates show that up to 350,000 babies are born each year with a serious disorder of this type, approximately 20% of which are a form of thalassemia. Approximately 90% of these births occur in low- or middle-income countries.[1] Although the high rate of consanguineous marriage in some of these countries undoubtedly plays a role in the high frequency of births of these Mendelian recessive disorders,[2] little doubt now exists that natural selection through heterozygote advantage against malaria is the major factor underlying their extremely high frequency and distribution.

Information collected over the past 20 years show that the high frequencies of at least some forms of thalassemia reflect heterozygote, or in some cases homozygote, protection against *Plasmodium falciparum* malaria, the most severe form of the disease, and some progress has been made toward understanding the cellular mechanisms involved.[3–5] Recently, however, evidence has been obtained for complex epistatic interactions among the different inherited hemoglobin disorders with respect to malaria protection, at least partly explaining some profound differences in their distribution among different populations.[6] Furthermore, it appears that some forms of thalassemia may be characterized by an increased susceptibility to infection by *P vivax* in early childhood. Although this form of malaria was neglected for many years

The work of the authors quoted in this review was supported by the Wellcome Trust, United Kingdom, and the March of Dimes.

[a] Weatherall Institute of Molecular Medicine, University of Oxford, John Radcliffe Hospital, Headington, Oxford, OX3 9DS, UK

[b] Kenya Medical Research Institute/Wellcome Trust Programme, Centre for Geographic Medical Research, Kilifi District Hospital, Kilifi, Kenya

[c] Institute of Life Sciences, School of Medicine, Swansea University, Singleton Park, Swansea, SA2 8PP, UK

* Corresponding author.

E-mail address: liz.rose@imm.ox.ac.uk

and thought to be of much less clinical importance, recent work has suggested that it causes a high level of mortality and major morbidity in many parts of Asia and South America.[7,8] Therefore, in addition to considerable importance with respect to explaining the current high frequency and distribution of the different forms of thalassemia, a better understanding of their interactions with different forms of malaria may have important implications for their management in the future.

This article reviews recent developments in this field and attempts to anticipate their place in future thalassemia research.

THE EVOLUTION OF THE MALARIA HYPOTHESIS

Early population studies of the gene frequency for thalassemia in the Mediterranean region and United States soon raised the fundamental question as to why the condition is so high in Mediterranean populations, and not found in those of North European origin. In 1947 Neel and Valentine[9] suggested that this might reflect variation in mutation rates between different ethnic groups. In 1949, Haldane[10] proposed an alternative hypothesis., suggesting that, because the red cells of thalassemia carriers are smaller than normal, they might also be more resistant to attacks by the sporozoa that cause malaria, a disease that was prevalent in southern Europe until World War II. This proposal intimated that a state of balanced polymorphism exists, in which in malarious areas thalassemia carriers will tend to have more children and hence the gene frequency will increase until it is balanced by its loss in homozygotes, who die before reproductive age.

Paradoxically, shortly after Haldane's proposal, Allison[11] obtained independent evidence that, in the case of sickle cell disease, heterozygotes are protected against severe malaria, thus accounting for the high frequency of this condition in Africa. However, progress in determining whether Haldane's hypothesis might be correct in the case of thalassemia was much slower. Studies in Sardinia showed that the frequency of the thalassemia gene was considerably higher in the low-lying coastal regions than in villages in the hills at an altitude at which malaria transmission does not occur.[12,13] Similar evidence suggesting a relationship between the distribution of malaria and thalassemia was obtained from Italy,[14] but when these correlations were sought in other parts of the world they were not found.[15] All of these studies were bedevilled by problems of founder effects and gene drift, together with lack of knowledge about the origins of the thalassemia genes: had they arisen in Europe and carried east by population movement, or had they arisen in the east and moved west through a similar mechanism[16]? Only after it was possible to study the molecular basis for the thalassemias did it become feasible to answer some of these fundamental questions.

THALASSEMIA AND *P FALCIPARUM*
α *Thalassemia*

The first studies in the molecular era of the interplay between thalassemia and *P falciparum* malaria investigated this interaction in the Southwest Pacific. Previous demographic data had shown that malaria reaches its highest frequency in Papua New Guinea and then declines in a south-easterly direction. The frequency of α^+ thalassemia was found to also have a clinal distribution across this region, being highest in the coastal regions of Papua New Guinea, with a carrier rate of approximately 70%, and shifting to less than 5% in New Caledonia.[17] Of course, this slowly declining frequency of α thalassemia mirroring a fall in the frequency of malaria transmission could be explained by the gene having been introduced from the Asian mainland

and carried south by the early populations that spread across this region, hence being diluted as they moved further south. However, analysis of the molecular forms of α thalassemia and their particular *HBA* haplotypes provided clear evidence that the form of α thalassemia in this region was different from that of the Asian mainland and that it had almost certainly arisen locally and been amplified by a locally acting mechanism, presumably malaria.[17] The same form of α thalassemia was found in some, but not all, of the Pacific islands in which malaria had never been recorded. However, it was always the same mutation that had been found in the Vanuatu Islands and hence seemed to have been distributed around the Pacific as its islands were populated.[18,19]

The causal relationship of the high gene frequencies of α thalassemia to protection against *P falciparum* malaria was confirmed by case-control studies in Papua New Guinea, which provided clear evidence that both heterozygotes and homozygotes for α^+ thalassemia are protected against the more serious complications of *P falciparum* malaria infection.[20] Later, similar studies performed in Africa confirmed that α thalassemia offers considerable protection against the complications of *P falciparum* infection[21] and that protection against malaria-associated anemia is also mediated in mild *P falciparum* infections accompanied by inflammation.[22] In addition, an unexpected finding was that α thalassemia seems to protect children against infections other than malaria, both in Papua New Guinea[20] and Kenya.[23]

Several mechanisms have been described that at least partly explain the protective effect of α thalassemia against malarial infection. Studies of a large cohort of children in Vanuatu, an island with an extremely high rate of transmission of both *P falciparum* and *P vivax* malaria, suggested that babies with uncomplicated malaria and enlargement of the spleen had a higher frequency of α^+ thalassemia than age-matched normal babies. It was suggested that the early susceptibility to *P vivax*, which may reflect the more rapidly turning over population of red cells in α^+ thalassemic infants, may be acting as a natural vaccine by inducing cross-species protection against later *P falciparum* infection.[24] Of course, this protective mechanism would only be relevant to populations in which both varieties of parasite exist.

At the cellular level, no evidence shows a reduced rate of invasion or growth of *P falciparum* in the red cells of individuals with α^+ or α^0 thalassemia. It has been found, however, that these cells consistently bind more malaria-immune globulin than normal cells.[25,26] Furthermore, α thalassemic red cells infected with parasites are more susceptible to phagocytosis in vitro, and are less able than normal red cells to form rosettes, an in vitro phenomena whereby uninfected red cells bind to infected cells. Experts have observed that complement receptor 1 (CR1) expression, which is essential for rosette formation, is reduced on α thalassemia red cells, offering a plausible explanation for reduced rosetting and, because the amount of rosetting strongly correlates with the severity of malaria infection, for a protective mechanism.[27] Furthermore, infected α thalassemic red cells are less able to adhere to human umbilical endothelial cells and are less susceptible to phagocytosis.[28,29] Because rosetting and cytoadherence are mechanisms that may be involved in the sequestration of infected red blood cells, these findings together suggest that abnormalities of the α thalassemic red cell membrane may be of fundamental importance in protecting against the severe complications of malaria.

It has also been suggested that the relatively high red cell counts in heterozygotes, or particularly homozygotes, for α^+ thalassemia may provide a further mechanism for protection, notably against the profound anemia that characterizes severe *P falciparum* infection in young infants.[30]

The mechanism involved in protection against nonmalarial infections is unclear. It could be mediated through prevention of malaria-associated immune suppression or acquisition of nonspecific immunity against malaria that also protects against other diseases.

β Thalassemia

Apart from an early case-control study in northern Liberia, which suggested that the β thalassemia trait is protective against severe malaria,[31] no further studies of this type have been performed. However, extremely suggestive evidence shows that the β thalassemias have reached their high frequency through selection against malaria. The comparative altitude studies mentioned earlier have been confirmed, showing a higher frequency of β thalassemia in the low-lying coastal regions of Papua New Guinea compared with frequencies in the mountainous regions.[32]

In evolutionary terms, it seems likely that P falciparum is a fairly recent human pathogen. A finding favoring β thalassemia being a relatively recently acquired polymorphism is the fact that every population in which this disease is common has a different set of mutations. Furthermore, studies of HBB haplotypes and their relationship to thalassemia mutations has provided further information in this respect. Unlike the HBA haplotypes, a "hot-spot" exists for recombination in the HBB cluster, resulting in distinct 5' and 3' haplotypes. Admixture between these haplotypes seems to have occurred among human populations, but this is not observed in the case of β thalassemia. The thalassemia mutations, which occur in the 3' haplotype, are almost always associated with the same 5' haplotype, indicating that they arose much more recently in evolutionary terms and that there has not been time for admixture of the haplotypes that carry these genes.[15] This theory suggests a very recent selective pressure, approximately 5000 years, which agrees with current estimations of the time that human populations have been exposed to the pathogenic forms of Plasmodium.

In vitro culture studies have shown that the rates of invasion and growth of P falciparum in β thalassemic red cells do not differ significantly from those in normal cells. However, early studies showed that parasite growth is significantly retarded in red cells that contain more than 5pg/HbF per cell,[33] an observation that was confirmed later using a transgenic mouse model carrying human γ genes.[34] Because good evidence shows that the rate of decline of HbF production after birth is delayed in β thalassemia heterozygotes,[15] this could provide a mechanism of protection during the first year of life.

Hemoglobin E

Because HbE is synthesized at a slightly reduced rate, homozygotes have the hematologic phenotype of the β thalassemia trait, whereas heterozygotes have very slightly reduced red cell indices. Because this variant reaches extremely high frequencies throughout parts of India and southeast Asia, reaching up to a 70% carrier frequency in parts of northern Thailand,[15] it is highly likely that it has been influenced by strong selection, at least at some time during human evolution.

No formal case control studies have analyzed the putative protective effect of the HbE trait against malaria. However, extended linkage disequilibrium in the region of the HBB gene carrying the HbE variant provides strong evidence that this mutation has come under intense and relatively recent selective pressure. The HbE trait was found to be significantly associated with a reduced severity of disease in adults admitted with severe P falciparum malaria.[35] In vitro culture evidence also shows that red cells from HbE heterozygotes, although not homozygotes, are more resistant to invasion by P falciparum.[36]

Therefore, although the evidence is still incomplete, relative heterozygote resistance against severe malaria seems to be at least one of the important mechanisms responsible for the extraordinarily high gene frequencies of this variant in many Asian countries.

EPISTATIC INTERACTIONS AMONG THE THALASSEMIAS, HEMOGLOBIN VARIANTS, AND MALARIA

One of the curious features of the different forms of thalassemia is how their gene frequency may vary very considerably even over short geographical distances. Although this may partly reflect the equally uneven distribution of present or past malaria transmission, recent studies suggest that the situation may be much more complicated.

In East Africa, although heterozygotes for α^+ thalassemia or the sickle cell trait have been found to be significantly more resistant to the severe complications of malaria, this protective effect is canceled out completely in those who have received both genes; that is, they are heterozygous for both the α^+ thalassemia and sickle-cell determinants.[37] The reason for this remarkable effect is not yet absolutely clear, although it may partly reflect the lower mean cell HbS level that is well documented in the sickle cell trait when it is accompanied by an α thalassemia trait.[15] Very recently, the use of models derived from this epistatic interaction and a second interaction of this type (ie, the ameliorating effect of the inheritance of α thalassemia on the phenotype of β thalassemia) have made it possible to provide a convincing mechanism explaining why the sickle-cell gene is so common in Africa but not in the Mediterranean population, where α and β thalassemia predominate.[38] Little doubt seems to exist that further analysis of the complex epistatic interactions of this type will provide invaluable information about the current world distribution of the thalassemias and related disorders.

THE THALASSEMIAS AND P VIVAX INFECTION

Until recently, malaria caused by P vivax infection was thought to be a relatively mild condition and of less clinical importance than infection caused by P falciparum. However, this view has changed, and it has become apparent that this disease may be much more severe than was formerly realized, and is causing an increasingly serious public health problem in many parts of Asia and South America.[7,8] Furthermore, unlike P falciparum, P vivax is able to survive in the liver for long periods, leading to repeated attacks of malaria and chronic ill health.

Epidemiologic studies, first in populations of African origin[39] and much later in those of Papua New Guinea,[40] showed a high frequency of the Duffy-negative blood group phenotype in populations in which malaria is common. The finding that red cells lacking the Duffy antigen are resistant to invasion by P knowlesi, although not P falciparum, suggested that the Duffy blood group antigen might be the receptor for the related parasite, P vivax.[41] Although this is undoubtedly the case, very recent studies in Madagascar[42] have confirmed an earlier suspicion[43,44] that human red cells may possess another receptor for P vivax. Studies have established that the Duffy antigen/chemokine receptor (DARC) is not expressed on red cells when a mutation is present in the promoter that changes a GATA-1 binding site.[45] In cells carrying this mutation, DARC expression on the surface is abolished, and thereby inhibiting DARC-mediated entry of P vivax. Reflecting the greater expression of DARC on younger red cells, evidence shows that P vivax has a particular predilection for reticulocytes and young red cells.[46] This finding is in distinction to P falciparum, which invades red cells of all ages. However, contrary to the long-held belief that cell age has no effect on invasion by *P falciparum*, differential centrifugation and in vitro culture studies have shown that even this parasite has a predilection for younger red cells.[47]

The relationship between the DARC polymorphism and protection against invasion of red cells by *P vivax* has had extraordinary consequences. Presumably because of its protective effect, the polymorphism reached fixation in some populations, so that very large regions of Africa are now inhabited by Duffy-negative individuals, as is the case for the many thousands who emigrated to other parts of the world from these regions. The recent findings in Madagascar,[42] which clearly showed that Duffy-negative individuals can be infected by *P vivax*, provide clear confirmation that a second receptor for the parasite exists, although its identity has not yet been determined. Together with the remarkable ability of malarial parasites to achieve drug resistance, these recent observations are yet another example of its remarkable genetic adaptability.

The first indication that thalassemic red cells might be more susceptible to invasion by *P vivax* came from studies of babies in Vanuatu, who seemed to be more susceptible to vivax malaria very early in their lives.[24] These observations were confirmed a few years later in studies on the north coast of Papua New Guinea.[20] Studies also found that, at least as judged by soluble transferrin receptor levels, children who are heterozygous or, particularly, homozygous for α^+ thalassemia have an increased rate of red cell turnover, and therefore a slightly younger mean red cell population, thus providing a plausible explanation for their increased propensity to invasion by *P vivax*.[48]

A recent study found that, at least as judged by antibody levels to *P vivax*, children with HbE β thalassemia in Sri Lanka are more prone to *P vivax* infection than age-matched controls, and that they tend to have a more severe phenotype and larger spleens than those with the same condition who do not have serologic evidence of such high exposure to *P vivax*.[49] Again, the fact that these patients have a rapid red cell turnover and elevated reticulocyte counts provides a possible mechanism for increased susceptibility to this parasite.

Of course, other possible explanations exist for these findings, which must be explored further. For example, nothing is yet known about the immune response to *P vivax* in the HbE trait or other forms of thalassemia associated with HbE. One possibility is that, as has been suggested in the case of the sickle-cell trait,[50] part of the protective mechanism against malaria may be reflected in a more active immune response, although in the case of the thalassemias this remains to be fully explored. Recent studies in Papua New Guinea[51] and the authors' unpublished data from the same region suggest that this is not the case in α^+ thalassemia. However, if this were the case for the HbE trait, this might be reflected in compound heterozygotes for HbE and β thalassemia, although it is difficult to reconcile this possibility with the observation that those with more severe disease tend to have higher antibody levels than those with a milder phenotype.

Another possibility is that the more severe forms of thalassemia, such as HbE β thalassemia, are associated with increased propensity to some forms of malaria for reasons that are distinct from the hemoglobin constitution in these conditions. For example, these patients are subject to recurrent bouts of fever, and this may be associated with a body odor that is more attractive to the mosquito.[52] However, because of the possibility of potentiating the severity of the disease, these interactions among *P vivax* and severe forms of malaria in Asia must be studied further.

POPULATION GENETICS AND EVOLUTIONARY IMPLICATIONS

In evolutionary terms, the expansion of the genes for thalassemia and other hemoglobin disorders seems to have been a fairly recent event. It is believed that, although the ancestral forms of the species of malarial parasites that infect humans arose many millions of years ago,[53] P falciparum only arose from its closest ancestor approximately 10 million years ago. After some 10 million years of development in Africa, modern humans emigrated out of the region 40 to 10,000 years ago, possibly carrying some of the polymorphisms that evolved from selection against P falciparum.[54] Death from malaria may have increased very rapidly between 5000 to 10,000 years ago because of the development of agriculture and village settlements that would have greatly facilitated transmission of malaria by mosquitoes.[55] This time scale is compatible with data suggesting that the expansion of malaria-resistant polymorphisms only began to occur somewhere around 5000 years ago.

If these interpretations are correct, they help explain the current world distribution of thalassemia and other hemoglobin variants. For example, these conditions are virtually nonexistent in the indigenous Amero-Indian populations of the Americas. Presumably the selective polymorphisms leading to their high frequency in current Asian populations were not present before the early migrations of these populations into the New World. When malaria reached this region is still uncertain, although it is suggested that it may have been as recently as the early Spanish Conquest. If this is the case, there may have been insufficient time for selection to generate high frequencies of thalassemia or other resistant polymorphisms in these populations.

These findings also offer a convincing basis for the remarkable heterogeneity in the distribution and frequency of the genes for thalassemia and related disorders, even within short geographic distances. Maps of the current or past distribution of P falciparum malaria frequently coincide with regions of high gene frequency for one or another inherited hemoglobin disorder.[56] These observations, taken together with the complex epistatic interactions among malaria and different hemoglobin variants, undoubtedly provide the basis for the uneven distribution of the malaria-resistant polymorphisms and, incidentally, make it extremely difficult to determine their gene frequencies in populations without rather tedious micromapping studies, which are the analysis of samples from many different regions within high-frequency countries.

CLINICAL IMPLICATIONS AND DIRECTIONS FOR FUTURE WORK

Although the frequency of malaria caused by P falciparum is declining in many countries because of the development of malaria control programs, it is likely to remain a considerable global health problem for the foreseeable future because of the continuous evolution of drug-resistant parasites, continued poverty, and the likelihood of global warming. And even if it were eradicated, it would take many generations for the frequency of malaria-resistant polymorphisms to decline significantly. Furthermore, as countries proceed through the demographic and epidemiologic transitions, whereby neonatal and childhood mortality rates decline, many children with thalassemia and related disorders who would hitherto have died early in life are now surviving to present for diagnosis and management. Furthermore, because the bulk of these diseases occur in low-income countries in which the populations are increasing, the high frequency of the hemoglobin disorders is likely to persist or even increase further.

Because of the heterogeneous distribution of these conditions, and the necessity to provide governments and international health agencies with more accurate data about the health burden that they will produce in the future, further micromapping studies of their frequency and distribution are urgently required, particularly in the high-frequency populations.[57]

The increasing evidence that at least some forms of thalassemia may be associated with an increased susceptibility to P vivax malaria is of considerable importance, particularly as this condition is now thought to be a much more serious global health problem than previously thought. In addition to a need for an understanding of the potential immunizing effect of this form of malaria against P falciparum early in life, more evidence must be obtained about the interaction of this parasite with the more severe forms of thalassemia in Asia, particularly HbE β thalassemia. For example, if, as suggest by preliminary studies in Sri Lanka,[49] P vivax infection has a deleterious effect on the course of this condition, prophylaxis against this form of malaria may be necessary in many Asian countries in which both it and HbE β thalassemia are prevalent. Because of the potential expense and difficulty in providing prophylaxis and radical treatment for P vivax malaria, these issues require urgent attention.

Finally, there is clearly still a relatively limited understanding of the cellular and potential immune mechanisms through which different forms of thalassemia and related hemoglobin disorders offer protection against malaria. A better understanding of the mechanisms might offer new approaches to the prevention or treatment of malaria. For example, the finding that DARC is the major receptor for the malarial parasite on red cells led to the discovery of the malarial protein that binds to this receptor, a promising target for future vaccine development. The recent finding that populations of Duffy-negative individuals exist who are susceptible to P vivax therefore requires an urgent search for the identity of this second receptor.

More than half a century has elapsed since Haldane's remarkable insights led to what became known as the *malaria hypothesis* to explain the extremely high frequencies of thalassemia and related genetic disorders of the red cell. Considering what has been learned about the remarkable genetic adaptability of the malarial parasite, the complex epistatic interplay between malaria-resistant genes, and the multiple cellular and immune mechanisms that may underlie malaria resistance, it is not surprising that it has taken so long to get this far in the development of this complex field. But some reasonably clear-cut directions and priorities for future work are now known, which, in addition to shedding some valuable light on the mechanisms of human evolution, have important implications for the better control of malaria and the common inherited disorders of the red cell in the poorer populations of the world.

ACKNOWLEDGMENTS

The work of the authors quoted in this review was supported by the Wellcome Trust, UK, and the March of Dimes. We thank Jeanne Packer and Liz Rose for their help in preparing this manuscript.

REFERENCES

1. Modell B, Darlison M. Global epidemiology of haemoglobin disorders and derived service indicators. Bull World Health Organ 2008;86:480.
2. Bittles AH, Mason WM, Greene J, et al. Reproductive behavior and health in consanguineous marriages. Science 1991;252:789.
3. Kwiatkowski DP. How malaria has affected the human genome and what human genetics can teach us about malaria. Am J Hum Genet 2005;77:171.
4. Williams TN. Red blood cell defects and malaria. Mol Biochem Parasitol 2006; 149:121.

5. Weatherall DJ. Genetic variation and susceptibility to infection: the red cell and malaria. Br J Haematol 2008;141:276.
6. Weatherall DJ. The inherited diseases of hemoglobin are an emerging global health burden. Blood 2010;115:4331.
7. Mendis K, Sina BJ, Marchesini P, et al. The neglected burden of Plasmodium vivax malaria. Am J Trop Med Hyg 2001;64:97.
8. Rogerson SJ, Carter R. Severe vivax malaria: newly recognised or rediscovered. PLoS Med 2008;5:e136.
9. Neel JV, Valentine WN. Further studies on the genetics of thalassaemia. Genetics 1947;32:38.
10. Haldane JBS. The rate of mutation of human genes. In: Proceedings of the Eighth International Congress of Genetics. Hereditas 1949;35:267.
11. Allison AC. Protection afforded by sickle-cell trait against subtertian malarial infection. Br Med J 1954;1(4857):290.
12. Carcassi V, Ceppellini R, Pitzus F. [Frequenza della talassemia in quattro popolazioni sarde e suoi rapporti con la distribuzione dei gruppi sanguini e della malaria]. Boll Ist Sieroter Milan 1957;36:206 [in Italian].
13. Siniscalco M, Bernini L, Latte B, et al. Favism and thalassaemia in Sardinia and their relationship to malaria. Nature 1961;190:1179.
14. Vezzoso B. [Influenza della malaria sulla mortalita infantile per anemia con speciale riguardo al morbo di Cooley]. Riv Malariol 1946;XXV:61 [in Italian].
15. Weatherall DJ, Clegg JB. The Thalassaemia syndromes. 4th edition. Oxford (UK): Blackwell Science; 2001.
16. Todd D. Genes, beans and Marco Polo. University of Hong Kong Gazette; 1978. 26:1.
17. Flint J, Hill AVS, Bowden DK, et al. High frequencies of α thalassaemia are the result of natural selection by malaria. Nature 1986;321:744.
18. Hill AVS, Gentile B, Bonnardot JM, et al. Polynesian origins and affinities: globin gene variants in Eastern Polynesia. Am J Hum Genet 1987;40:453.
19. O'Shaughnessy DF, Hill AVS, Bowden DK, et al. Globin genes in Micronesia: origins and affinities of Pacific Island peoples. Am J Hum Genet 1990;46:144.
20. Allen SJ, O'Donnell A, Alexander NDE, et al. α^+-thalassaemia protects children against disease due to malaria and other infections. Proc Natl Acad Sci U S A 1997;94:14736.
21. Williams TN, Wambua S, Uyoga S, et al. Both heterozygous and homozygous alpha+ thalassemias protect against severe and fatal Plasmodium falciparum malaria on the coast of Kenya. Blood 2005;106:368.
22. Veenemans J, Andang'o PE, Mbugi EV, et al. Alpha+ -thalassaemia protects against anemia associated with asymptomatic malaria: evidence from community-based surveys in Tanzania and Kenya. J Infect Dis 2008;198:401.
23. Wambua S, Mwangi TW, Kortok M, et al. The effect of alpha+-thalassaemia on the incidence of malaria and other diseases in children living on the coast of Kenya. PLoS Med 2006;3:e158.
24. Williams TN, Maitland K, Bennett S, et al. High incidence of malaria in α-thalassaemic children. Nature 1996;383:522.
25. Luzzi GA, Merry AH, Newbold CI, et al. Surface antigen expression on *Plasmodium falciparum*-infected erythrocytes is modified in α- and β-thalassemia. J Exp Med 1991;173:785.
26. Williams TN, Weatherall DJ, Newbold CI. The membrane characteristics of Plasmodium falciparum-infected and -uninfected heterozygous alpha(0)thalassaemic erythrocytes. Br J Haematol 2002;118:663.

27. Cockburn IA, Mackinnon MJ, O'Donnell A, et al. A human complement receptor 1 polymorphism that reduces *Plasmodium falciparum* rosetting confers protection against severe malaria. Proc Natl Acad Sci U S A 2004;101:272.

28. Udomsangpetch R, Sueblinvong T, Pattanapanyasat K, et al. Alteration in cytoadherence and rosetting of *Plasmodium falciparum*-infected thalassemic red blood cells. Blood 1993;82:3752.

29. Yuthavong Y, Butthep P, Bunyaratvej A, et al. Impaired parasite growth and increased susceptibility to phagocytosis of *Plasmodium falciparum* infected alpha-thalassemia and hemoglobin Constant Spring red blood cells. Am J Clin Pathol 1988;89:521.

30. Fowkes FJ, Allen SJ, Allen A, et al. Increased microerythrocyte count in homozygous alpha(+)-thalassaemia contributes to protection against severe malarial anaemia. PLoS Med 2008;5:e56.

31. Willcox MC, Bjorkman A, Brohult J, et al. A case-control study in northern Liberia of *Plasmodium falciparum* malaria in haemoglobin S and β-thalassaemia traits. Ann Trop Med Parasitol 1983;77:239.

32. Hill AVS, Bowden DK, O'Shaughnessy DF, et al. β-thalassemia in Melanesia: association with malaria and characterization of a common variant (IVSI nt 5 G-C). Blood 1988;72:9.

33. Pasvol G, Weatherall DJ, Wilson RJ. Effects of foetal haemoglobin on susceptibility of red cells to *Plasmodium falciparum*. Nature 1977;270:171.

34. Shear HL, Grinberg L, Gilman J, et al. Transgenic mice expressing human fetal globin are protected from malaria by a novel mechanism. Blood 1998;92:2520.

35. Hutagalung R, Wilairatana P, Looareesuwan S, et al. Influence of hemoglobin E trait on the severity of Falciparum malaria. J Infect Dis 1999;179:283.

36. Chotivanich K, Udomsangpetch R, Pattanapanyasat K, et al. Hemoglobin E: a balanced polymorphism protective against high parasitemias and thus severe *P falciparum* malaria. Blood 2002;100:1172.

37. Williams TN, Mwangi TW, Wambua S, et al. Negative epistasis between the malaria-protective effects of alpha+-thalassemia and the sickle cell trait. Nat Genet 2005;37:1253.

38. Penman BS, Pybus OG, Weatherall DJ, et al. Epistatic interactions between genetic disorders of hemoglobin can explain why the sickle-cell gene is uncommon in the Mediterranean. Proc Natl Acad Sci U S A 2009;106:21242.

39. Miller LH, Mason SJ, Clyde DF, et al. The resistance factor to *Plasmodium vivax* in Blacks. N Engl J Med 1976;295:302.

40. Zimmerman PA, Woolley I, Masinde GL, et al. Emergence of FY*A(null) in a Plasmodium vivax-endemic region of Papua New Guinea. Proc Natl Acad Sci U S A 1999;96:13973.

41. Miller LH, Haynes JD, McAuliffe FM, et al. Evidence for differences in erythrocyte surface receptors for the malarial parasites, *Plasmodium falciparum* and *Plasmodium knowlesi*. J Exp Med 1977;146:277.

42. Menard D, Barnadas C, Bouchier C, et al. Plasmodium vivax clinical malaria is commonly observed in Duffy-negative Malagasy people. Proc Natl Acad Sci U S A 2010;107:5967.

43. Cavasini CE, Mattos LC, Couto AA, et al. *Plasmodium vivax* infection among Duffy antigen-negative individuals from the Brazilian Amazon region: an exception? Trans R Soc Trop Med Hyg 2007;101:1042.

44. Ryan JR, Stoute JA, Amon J, et al. Evidence for transmission of Plasmodium vivax among a Duffy antigen negative population in Western Kenya. Am J Trop Med Hyg 2006;75:575.

45. Tournamille C, Colin Y, Cartron JP, et al. Disruption of a GATA motif in the *Duffy* gene promoter abolishes erythroid gene expression in Duffy-negative individuals. Nat Genet 1995;10:224.
46. Woolley IJ, Hotmire KA, Sramkoski RM, et al. Differential expression of the Duffy antigen receptor for chemokines according to RBC age and FY genotype. Transfusion 2000;40:949.
47. Pasvol G, Weatherall DJ, Wilson RJ. The increased susceptibility of young red cells to invasion by the malarial parasite *Plasmodium falciparum*. Br J Haematol 1980;45:285.
48. Rees DC, Williams TN, Maitland K, et al. Alpha thalassemia is associated with increased soluble transferrin receptor levels. Br J Haematol 1998;103:365.
49. O'Donnell A, Premawardhena A, Arambepola M, et al. Interaction of malaria with a common form of severe thalassemia in an Asian population. Proc Natl Acad Sci U S A 2009;106:18716.
50. Williams TN, Mwangi TW, Roberts DJ, et al. An immune basis for malaria protection by the sickle cell trait. PLoS Med 2005;2:e128.
51. Fowkes FJ, Michon P, Pilling L, et al. Host erythrocyte polymorphisms and exposure to *Plasmodium falciparum* in Papua New Guinea. Malar J 2008;7:1.
52. Lindsay S, Ansell J, Selman C, et al. Effect of pregnancy on exposure to malaria mosquitoes. Lancet 1972;355:1972.
53. Rich SM, Ayala FJ. Evolutionary origins of human malaria parasites. In: Dronamraju KR, Arese P, editors. Malaria: genetic and evolutionary aspects. New York: Springer; 2006. p. 190.
54. Cavalli-Sforza LL, Feldman MW. The application of molecular genetic approaches to the study of human evolution. Nat Genet 2003;33(Suppl):266.
55. Carter R, Mendis KN. Evolutionary and historical aspects of the burden of malaria. Clin Microbiol Rev 2002;15:564.
56. de Silva S, Fisher CA, Premawardhena A, et al. Thalassaemia in Sri Lanka: implications for the future health burden of Asian populations. Sri Lanka Thalassaemia Study Group. Lancet 2000;355:786.
57. Weatherall DJ. The importance of micromapping the gene frequencies for the common inherited disorders of haemoglobin. Br J Haematol 2010;149:635.

The Molecular Basis of α-Thalassemia: A Model for Understanding Human Molecular Genetics

Douglas R. Higgs, MD, DSc*, Richard J. Gibbons, MD, DPhil

KEYWORDS

- α-Thalassemia • α-Globin gene cluster • Hemoglobin
- Genetic mutations

Over the past 50 years, our understanding of the normal production of hemoglobin and how errors in this process give rise to α- and β-thalassemia has been at the center of many developments that have established the principles underlying normal globin gene regulation and how this may be perturbed by natural mutations. This field has advanced as a 2-way process; improved understanding of normal globin gene expression has guided the search for mutations, and the identification of genetic variation associated with specific red cell phenotypes has often provided unexpected insights into the normal mechanisms underlying globin gene regulation. Although the globin genes are often considered as a "special case" with respect to our understanding of gene regulation, on the contrary, there is very little that we have learnt from this system that has not been of general relevance to human molecular genetics.

This review concentrates on the human α-globin cluster, which has been characterized in great depth over the past 30 years. In particular the authors describe how the α genes are normally switched on during erythropoiesis and switched off as hematopoietic stem cells commit to nonerythroid lineages. In addition, the principles by which α-globin expression may be perturbed by natural mutations that cause α-thalassemia are reviewed.

Down-regulation of α-globin synthesis causes α-thalassemia with underproduction of fetal (HbF, $\alpha_2\gamma_2$) and adult (HbA, $\alpha_2\beta_2$) hemoglobin.[1] The considerable diversity of mutations that have been identified is explained by the fact that carriers for

John Radcliffe Hospital, MRC Molecular Haematology Unit, Weatherall Institute of Molecular Medicine, University of Oxford, Headington, Oxford OX3 9DS, UK
* Corresponding author.
E-mail address: doug.higgs@imm.ox.ac.uk

Hematol Oncol Clin N Am 24 (2010) 1033–1054
doi:10.1016/j.hoc.2010.08.005
0889-8588/10/$ – see front matter
hemonc.theclinics.com

α-thalassemia are (to some extent) protected from falciparum malaria in a manner that we still do not fully understand (reviewed in Ref.[2]). Consequently, in tropical and subtropical regions of the world (where malaria is endemic) α-thalassemia reaches very high frequencies, making it one of the most common of all human genetic disease traits.[2] Amongst people originating from these areas, compound heterozygotes and homozygotes for some mutations may have severe hematologic phenotypes. When α-globin synthesis is reduced to around 25% or less, patients may suffer from a moderately severe hemolytic anemia associated with readily detectable excess β-globin chains in the form of β_4 tetramers (referred to as HbH); hence the condition is called HbH disease.[3] When α-globin synthesis is even further reduced (or even abolished), this gives rise to a severe intrauterine anemia associated with excess γ-globin chains in the form of γ_4 tetramers (referred to as Hb Bart's); hence this condition is referred to as the Hb Bart's hydrops fetalis syndrome (BHFS).[4]

The high frequency of α-thalassemia trait, HbH disease, and Hb Bart's hydrops fetalis means that tens of thousands of patient samples have been analyzed and that probably most of the natural mutations affecting these genes are now known. However, when all known mutations have been excluded, new often rare but informative genetic variants are still being found. Nevertheless, in most instances accurate genetic counseling and (when appropriate) prenatal testing can be made available in countries where the health care infrastructure is able to support this.

In clinical practice α-thalassemia is much less of a problem than β-thalassemia.[5] When genetic counseling is available, most families choose to avoid continuing pregnancies in which the fetus has the BHFS, although rare infants with this condition survive and have been treated with lifelong blood transfusion or bone marrow transplantation.[4] Most patients with HbH disease can lead a relatively normal life, blood transfusion and iron chelation being rarely required. In fact a major clinical interest in α-thalassemia comes from its interaction with β-thalassemia. In some circumstances, the coinheritance of α-thalassemia appears to have a significant impact on the clinical phenotype of compound heterozygotes and homozygotes for β-thalassemia (reviewed in Refs.[6,7]), presumably by reducing the production of free α-globin chains (the main cause of red cell damage in β-thalassemia). Understanding in detail how expression of the α-globin genes is normally regulated may therefore identify pathways by which α-globin synthesis could be down-regulated and thereby ameliorate the phenotype of β-thalassemia.

NORMAL STRUCTURE AND REGULATION OF THE HUMAN α-GLOBIN GENE CLUSTER

Expression of the α-like and β-like globin chains is regulated by clusters of genes on chromosomes 16 and 11, respectively.[8,9] The α-like gene cluster is located close to the telomere of chromosome 16 (16p13.3) including an embryonic gene (ζ) and 2 fetal/adult genes arranged along the chromosome in the order telomere-ζ-α2-α1-centromere, surrounded by widely expressed genes (**Fig. 1**). The normal cluster is denoted $\alpha\alpha$. Approximately 25 to 65 kb upstream of the α-globin genes there are 4 highly conserved noncoding sequences, or multispecies conserved sequences (MCS), called MCS-R1 to -R4, which are thought to be involved in the regulation of the α-like globin genes (see **Fig. 1**). It is of interest that 3 of these elements (MCS-R1–3) lie within the introns of the adjacent widely expressed gene c16orf35. Of these elements, only MCS-R2 (also known as HS-40) has been shown to be essential for α-globin expression.[8]

As multipotent hemopoietic progenitors commit to the erythroid lineage and begin to differentiate to form mature red blood cells, key erythroid transcription factors (eg, GATA-2, GATA-1, SCL, SpXKLF, NF-E2) and various cofactors (eg, FOG, pCAF, p300) progressively bind to the upstream MCS-R elements and the promoters of the α-like globin genes (**Fig. 2**). Binding of these factors is associated with widespread modifications of the associated chromatin reflecting activation (eg, histone acetylation). Finally, RNA polymerase II (PolII) is recruited to both the upstream regions and the globin promoters as transcription starts in early erythroid progenitors.[10,11] At the same time, the upstream elements and promoters of the globin genes interact with each another via the formation of chromatin loops. It has recently been shown that HS-40 is critically required for looping to occur and for the stable recruitment of PolII to the α-globin promoters.[11,12]

It has become clear that this series of up-regulatory events taking place in erythroid cells is only a part of the complete story of α-globin regulation. Although the α-globin genes are expressed in a strictly tissue-specific manner, they are contained in a large chromosomal region which is broadly transcriptionally active and bears the hallmarks of constitutively active chromatin.[13,14] Therefore, it was predicted that within such a region, mechanisms should exist to maintain the α-globin genes in a silent state in nonerythroid cells. An extensive survey of chromatin modifications in erythroid and nonerythroid cells showed that the α-globin cluster is marked by a specific signature (H3K27me3) in nonerythroid cells but less so in erythroid cells.[15] The H3K27me3 mark is imposed by a histone methyltransferase (EZH2), which forms part of a repressive Polycomb complex called PRC2.[16] Consistent with this, components of this complex (EZH2 and SUZ12) have also been found at the α-globin cluster in nonerythroid cells. The PRC2 complex recruits histone deacetylases (HDACs) and another repressive Polycomb complex (called PRC1; Lynch and colleagues, unpublished data, 2009). Experimental data suggest that together, these complexes (PRC1, PRC2, and HDACs) maintain the silence of the α genes in multipotent cells and differentiated nonerythroid cells[15] but that they are cleared from the α-globin promoter before the activation steps described (see **Fig. 2**).

Activation of the α-globin genes can thus be thought of as a multistep process in which transcription of α-globin is at first somewhat leaky, albeit expressed at very low levels, in hematopoietic stem cells when the α genes are partially repressed by the Polycomb system. As cells differentiate down the nonerythroid pathway, the genes become increasingly silenced by Polycomb so that in mature nonerythroid cells no transcription can be detected. By contrast, as cells differentiate along the erythroid pathway, Polycomb silencing is removed as the activating events are played out on the cluster (see **Fig. 2**). All results to date have been obtained by analyzing populations of cells so that we only see the average effects. Seeing the true order of events in single cells is a challenge for the future.

NORMAL VARIATION WITHIN THE HUMAN α-GLOBIN CLUSTER

Over the past few years whole genome analysis has revealed the scale of variation across the human genome in apparently normal individuals.[17,18] Such variation results from single nucleotide polymorphisms (SNPs), variations in the numbers of tandem repeats (VNTRs), variations in microsatellites, copy number variants (CNVs, caused by homologous or illegitimate recombination), segmental duplications and deletions, and chromosomal translocations.[17,18] Although heralded as a surprise, in fact the extent of variation and mechanisms underlying such polymorphic changes were anticipated from detailed characterization of the regions containing the globin loci in large numbers (thousands) of nonthalassemic individuals. In addition to SNPs forming ancestral haplotypes,[19] it had been shown that extensive polymorphic variation

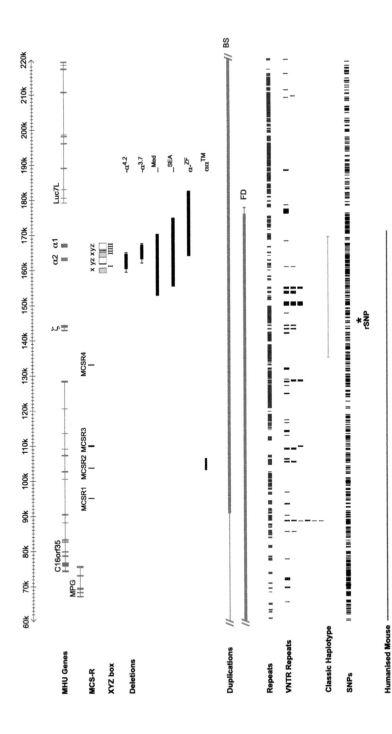

caused by genomic rearrangements were found in hematologically normal individuals. These variants are summarized in detail in Ref.[20] but the most notable small-scale variations in the α cluster occur in the many G-rich VNTRs in this region[14] together with the large-scale variation commonly observed in the subtelomeric region of chromosome 16.[21] Studies of the different arrangements of these polymorphisms and VNTRs in various population samples have made it possible to define a series of α-globin-gene haplotypes that have been of considerable value both in the analysis of evolutionary aspects of the gene clusters and in defining the origins of many of the α-thalassemia mutations.[2,19] In addition to their value as genetic markers, these variants have been useful in distinguishing functionally important areas of the α-globin cluster from regions that appear to be of little functional significance.[22]

α-THALASSEMIA CAUSED BY SEQUENCE VARIATIONS IN THE STRUCTURAL GENES

Although most sequence variants in the α-globin cluster (including variation with HS-40) are caused by neutral SNPs, the authors currently know of 69 point mutations or oligonucleotide variants that alter gene expression, referred to as nondeletional forms of α-thalassemia (denoted $\alpha^T\alpha$ or $\alpha\alpha^T$ depending on whether the α_2 or α_1 gene is affected). As for many other human genetic diseases, these mutations may affect the canonical sequences that control gene expression, including the CCAAT and TATA box sequences associated with the promoter, the initiation codon (ATG), splicing signals (GT/AG), the termination codon (TAA), and the poly(A) adenylation signal (AATAAA). In addition to these mutations, α-thalassemia may also be caused by in-frame deletions, frameshift mutations, and nonsense mutations (often leading to nonsense-mediated decay of the RNA) and/or to the production of abnormal protein. Some variants alter the structure of the hemoglobin molecule making the dimer ($\alpha\beta$) or tetramer ($\alpha_2\beta_2$) unstable. Such molecules may precipitate in the red cell, forming insoluble inclusions that damage the red cell membrane. Over the past few years it has become apparent that some α-globin structural variants are so unstable that they undergo very rapid postsynthetic degradation and thereby cause the phenotype of α-thalassemia. A full list of sequence variations in the structural genes that cause α-thalassemia is available.[20]

TRANSLOCATIONS AND DUPLICATIONS OF THE α-GLOBIN CLUSTER

Rarely, chromosomal translocations involving 16p13.3 place the α-globin locus at the tip of another chromosome, as seen, for example, in some relatives of patients with the

---

Fig. 1. The human α-globin cluster (5′ζ-α2-α1-3′) surrounded by widely expressed genes (*MPG*, *C16orf35*, and *Luc7L*) on chromosome 16 (16p13.3). Below this the multispecies conserved elements (MCS-Rs) are shown. The X, Y, and Z boxes are the regions of duplication that play a part in the generation of the common α-thalassemias, as discussed in the text. The most common deletions removing one (-$\alpha^{3.7}$ and -$\alpha^{4.2}$) or both (--^{Med} and --^{SEA}) α genes and causing thalassemia are shown as horizontal bars, as are the unusual deletions α-^{ZF} and ($\alpha\alpha$)^{TM}. The duplications of the cluster, BS and FD, are also indicated. For a full catalog of all deletions that cause α-thalassemia see Ref.[20] At the bottom of the figure the positions of common repeats, variable number random repeats (VNTRs) and SNPs are shown. The region containing all SNPs and VNTRs corresponding to the classic haplotype used in population studies (as discussed in the text) is illustrated as a thin horizontal line. The regulatory SNP (rSNP) that creates new functional GATA1 binding site seen in the Melanesian nondeletional α-thalassemia is shown with an asterisk. The extent of the α-globin locus present in the humanized mouse is shown as a thin line.

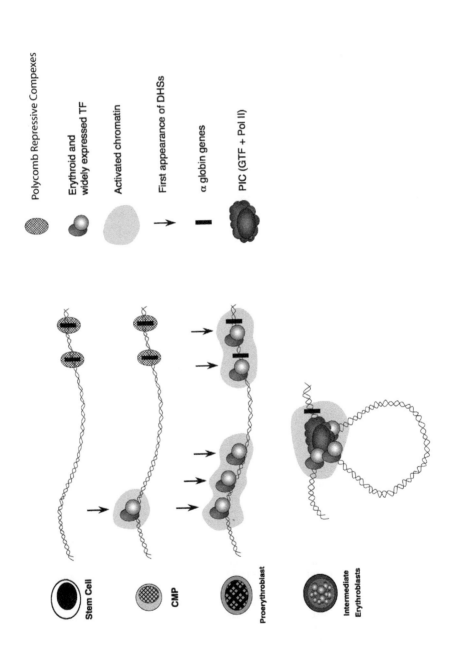

Polycomb Repressive Compexes

Erythroid and
widely expressed TF

Activated chromatin

First appearance of DHSs

α globin genes

PIC (GTF + Pol II)

Stem Cell

CMP

Proerythroblast

Intermediate
Erythroblasts

ATR-16 syndrome (see later discussion). To date the authors know of 16 individuals with such balanced translocations and none of them has α-thalassemia. Because the closest centromeric breakpoint of these chromosomal translocations lies only 1.2 Mb from the α-globin genes, these findings demonstrate that the cis-acting sequences required for full α-globin regulation are contained within this region and that expression is not perturbed by rearrangements on this scale. In 2 individuals with unbalanced translocations, and 3 copies of 16p13.3, the α/β globin chain synthesis ratios were 1.5 and 1.6 (Refs.[23,24] and Fichera M, unpublished data, 1998), again indicating that the additional, mis-localized copy of the α complex is expressed even though its genomic position has been altered.

Two large duplications of the terminal region of chromosome 16 have also been described in patients with β-thalassemia intermedia. Because these patients are simply heterozygotes for the β-thalassemia mutations, the implication is that their relatively severe phenotype results from the production of excess α-globin chains from the α genes in the duplicated regions. In one pedigree, 3 α clusters (αα:αα:αα) are present on one copy of chromosome 16 (Ref.[25] and unpublished data). Provisional data suggest that at least 2 and possibly all 3 clusters in the duplicated region are fully active. A carrier for this abnormal chromosome (αα:αα:αα/αα), with a total of 8 α genes, has an α/β-globin chain synthesis ratio of 2.7.[25] A recent study has more fully characterized what appears to be a very similar rearrangement in another Italian family with β-thalassemia intermedia[26] revealing a duplication of approximately 260 kb (see BS in **Fig. 1**). These investigators also characterized another duplication of approximately 175 kb of chromosome 16 lying between the end of the α cluster and the telomere (see FD in **Fig. 1**). Again the phenotype of a compound heterozygote for this rearrangement (αα:αα/αα) and β-thalassemia trait suggested that the additional α clusters in the duplicated segment are fully active, indicating that all sequences required for fully regulated α-globin expression lie in this duplicated segment of chromosome 16.

These findings, delimiting the region required to direct fully regulated expression of the human α-globin cluster, are consistent with experimental data from a mouse model in which the mouse α-globin cluster was replaced with approximately 135 kb of the human α-globin cluster.[27] This region contains all sequences within a region of conserved synteny between the human and mouse, including the globin genes and their regulatory elements. The pattern and levels of expression of the human transgenes in this segment of DNA suggest that this region of approximately 135 kb contains all of the sequences required to express the α-globin genes correctly from an appropriate chromosomal environment, although, as discussed previously,[27] the level of expression in a mouse environment is less than in the human.

Fig. 2. In stem cells and early progenitors the cluster is silenced by the Polycomb repressive complex. In multipotent cells (CMP), the cluster is primed in the upstream region (MCSR-2) by multiprotein complexes containing SCL and NF-E2 nucleated by GATA-2. In committed erythroid progenitors (U-MEL, proerythroblast stage), additional remote regulatory sequences are bound by multiprotein complexes containing various combinations of SCL, NF-E2, and GATA1 replacing GATA2. At this stage, the α-globin promoter is also occupied by a combination of factors including NF-Y and is poised for expression. In differentiating erythroid cells the preinitiation complex (PIC), including PolII, is recruited to the enhancers in a cooperative manner but independently of the promoter. Krüppel-like transcription factors are also recruited, independently of the upstream elements and to the promoter. At this final stage, the α-globin promoter is now occupied by a multiprotein complex that represents a docking site for the recruitment of the PIC, which is entirely dependent on the presence of the upstream elements that interact with the promoter, forming a loop.

α-THALASSEMIA CAUSED BY DELETIONS REMOVING ONE OF THE DUPLICATED STRUCTURAL GENES

Heteroduplex and DNA sequence analysis has shown that the duplicated α-globin genes (αα) are embedded within 2 highly homologous, 4-kb duplication units whose sequence identity appears to have been maintained throughout evolution by gene conversion and unequal crossover events.[28–31] These regions are divided into homologous subsegments (X, Y, and Z) by nonhomologous elements (I, II, and III, see **Fig. 1; Fig. 3**). Reciprocal homologous recombination between Z segments, which are 3.7 kb apart, produces chromosomes with only one α gene (-$\alpha^{3.7}$, rightward deletion, see **Figs. 1** and **3**)[32] that cause α-thalassemia and others with 3 α genes (ααα$^{anti3.7}$).[33] Recombination between homologous X boxes, which are 4.2 kb apart, also gives rise to an α-thalassemia determinant (-$\alpha^{4.2}$, leftward deletion, see **Figs. 1** and **3**)[32] and an ααα$^{anti4.2}$ chromosome.[34] Further recombination events between the resulting chromosomes (α, αα, ααα) may give rise to quadruplicated α genes (αααα),[35] or quintuplicated (ααααα)[36] or other unusual patchwork rearrangements.

Although these long-standing observations have pointed to the mechanism by which -α and ααα chromosomes arise, it has only recently been shown (using single DNA molecule polymerase chain reaction) how they may occur in vivo.[37] From this work, the overall picture is one of reciprocal recombination (and unequal exchange) occurring in mitosis (premeiotic) in the germ line. The estimated frequencies of -α and ααα arrangements in sperm are in the order of 1–5 × 10^{-5}. Deletions and duplications may also occur in somatic tissues by related mechanisms, although deletions detected in blood occur by intrachromosomal rather than interchromosomal recombination.

In addition to the common -α chromosomes, several rare deletions that remove either the α_1 or α_2 gene (leaving one gene intact, -α) have been described. In general these remove either the α_1 or α_2 gene by nonhomologous recombination. All of these deletions leave one α gene intact, and it is therefore possible to assess the influence of these deletions on expression of the remaining gene. When all of the data from these deletions that cause α-thalassemia are considered alongside the observations from nonthalassemic variants (see above), it appears that large segments of the α-globin cluster are not essential for α-globin expression.[22] Figures showing the full list of currently known deletions removing a single α gene are presented by Rugless and colleagues.[22]

α-THALASSEMIA CAUSED BY DELETIONS REMOVING BOTH OF THE DUPLICATED STRUCTURAL GENES

The authors currently know of approximately 50 deletions from the α-globin cluster that either completely or partially delete both α-globin genes, and therefore that no α-chain synthesis is directed by these chromosomes in vivo. Examples of 2 common deletions --^{MED} and --^{SEA} are shown in **Fig. 1**. Homozygotes for such chromosomes (--/--) have the Hb BHFS. Compound heterozygotes for these deletions and deletions removing a single α gene (see above) have HbH disease (--/-α).

With completion of the DNA sequence of 16p13.3[13] and beyond,[38] it has been possible to define the full extent of many of the deletions that remove both α genes (--). These deletions can be grouped into those (like --^{MED} and --^{SEA}, see **Fig. 1**) that lie entirely within the α-globin cluster and deletions that extend up to approximately 800 kb beyond the α cluster to include the flanking genes. Although these deletions remove other genes, affected heterozygotes appear phenotypically normal, apart from their α-thalassemia: in some patients α-thalassemia trait (--/αα) and in others

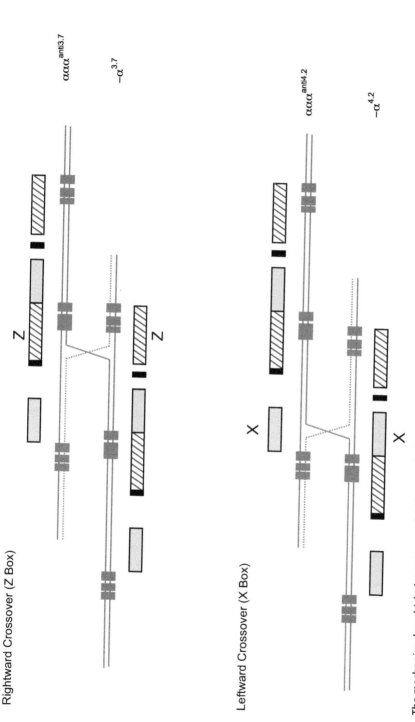

Fig. 3. The mechanism by which the common deletions underlying α-thalassemia occur. Crossovers between misaligned Z boxes give rise to the -α$^{3.7}$ and αααanti3.7 chromosomes. Crossovers between misaligned X boxes give rise to -α$^{4.2}$ and αααanti4.2 chromosomes.

HbH disease (--/-α). In patients with more extensive deletions with monosomy for a large segment of 16p13.3, α-thalassemia is associated with developmental abnormalities and mental retardation (so-called ATR-16 syndrome, see later discussion). It is interesting to note that all of the α-thalassemia deletions that occur at polymorphic frequencies in human populations are limited to the α cluster and do not extend into the surrounding genes, suggesting that deletion of these genes (even in heterozygotes) may result in a selective disadvantage.

Detailed analysis of several of these determinants of α-thalassemia indicates that they often result from illegitimate or nonhomologous recombination events (eg, Refs.[22,39]). Such events may involve short regions of partial sequence homology at the breakpoints of the molecules that are rejoined, but they do not involve the extensive sequence-matching required for homologous recombination as described in the previous section.

Sequence analysis has shown that members of the dispersed family of Alu repeats are frequently found at or near the breakpoints of these deletions. Alu-family repeats occur frequently in the genome (3 $\times$ 10^5 copies) and seem to be particularly common in and around the α-globin cluster, where they make up approximately 25% of the entire sequence. These repeats may simply provide partially homologous sequences that promote DNA-strand exchanges during replication, or possibly a subset of Alu sequences may be more actively involved in the process. Detailed sequence analysis of the junctions of the α-globin deletions has revealed several interesting features including palindromes, direct repeats, and regions of weak homology. Some deletions involve more complex rearrangements that introduce new pieces of DNA bridging the 2 breakpoints of the deletion. In 2 deletions this inserted DNA originates from upstream of the α cluster, and appears to have been incorporated into the junction in a manner suggesting that the upstream segment lies close to the breakpoint regions during replication.[22,39] Orphan sequences from unknown regions of the genome are frequently found bridging the sequence breakpoints of other α-thalassemia deletions. At least 2 of the deletions result from chromosomal breaks in the 16p telomeric region that have been "healed" by the direct addition of telomeric repeats (TTAGGG)$_n$.[40] This mechanism is described later in further detail. All currently known deletions that remove both α genes are summarized in Ref.[20]

A RARE MUTATION CAUSING α-THALASSEMIA VIA AN ANTISENSE RNA

During a study to identify thalassemia in families from the Czech Republic, Indrak and colleagues[41] reported a novel deletion (>18 kb) involving the α_1 and θ gene (denoted α-^{ZF}; see Fig. 1; Fig. 4). Heterozygotes for this deletion have a mild hypochromic microcytic anemia with a reduced α/β globin chain biosynthesis ratio and Hb H inclusions. These findings suggested that although the α_2 gene appeared to be intact, it had been inactivated by the deletion.

Barbour and colleagues[42] and Tufarelli and colleagues[43] further characterized this mutation and showed that the deletion juxtaposes a downstream gene (Luc7L) next to the structurally normal α_2 globin gene. Although this α_2 gene retains all of its local (eg, promoter) and remote (eg, MCS-R2/HS-40) cis-acting elements, its expression is silenced and its associated CpG island (see Fig. 4) becomes completely methylated during early development, and the chromatin associated with the promoter remains inactive and inaccessible, even in erythroid cells. From the analysis of experimental models recapitulating this deletion and from further characterization of the affected individual,[43] it was shown that transcription of antisense mRNA from Luc7L, through the α_2 globin gene, was responsible for methylation of the associated CpG island and silencing of α-globin expression.

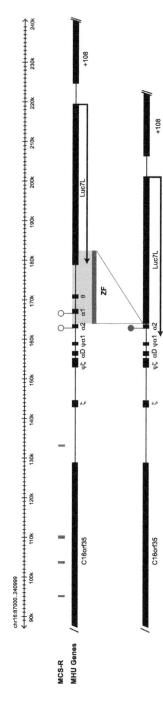

Fig. 4. The key features of the α^{ZF} mutation. In the normal cluster the promoters of the α-globin genes lie in unmethylated CpG-rich islands. Partial deletion of Luc7L juxtaposes this truncated gene next to the remaining α_2-globin gene and RNA transcripts from Luc7L extend through the α_2-globin gene. This process is thought to attract de novo DNA methylases early in development, methylating the α_2 CpG island and silencing it.

Since this original report the authors have identified 2 other individuals (also from Poland) with the same mutation. The mutation is not only important for understanding the molecular basis for this rare form of thalassemia, but also illustrates a new mechanism underlying human genetic disease. Since this description there has been a report of a similar mechanism silencing the mismatch repair gene *MSH2* in patients with susceptibility to colorectal cancer (Lynch syndrome).[44]

DELETIONS REMOVING THE UPSTREAM REGULATORY ELEMENTS OF THE α-GLOBIN GENE CLUSTER

As discussed earlier, expression of the α genes is critically dependent on a multispecies conserved, noncoding regulatory sequence (MCS-R) that lies 40 kb upstream of the ζ2 globin gene. This region (called MCS-R2) is associated with an erythroid-specific DNase I hypersensitive site, referred to as HS-40. Detailed analysis of MCS-R2 has shown that it contains multiple binding sites for the erythroid-restricted *trans*-acting factors GATA-1 and NF-E2, and binding sites for the ubiquitously expressed SpXKLF family of transcription factors.[45] The role(s) of other upstream MCS elements (MCS-R1, -R3, and -R4) that contain similar combinations of binding sites are not yet clear.

The first indication that remote regulatory sequences controlling α-globin expression might exist came from observations on a patient with α-thalassemia.[46] Analysis of the abnormal chromosome (αα)^{RA} from this patient demonstrated a 62-kb deletion from upstream of the α complex that includes HS-40. Although both α genes on this chromosome are intact and entirely normal, they appear to be nonfunctional. Since this original observation, many more patients with α-thalassemia caused by deletions of HS-40 and a variable amount of the flanking DNA have been described, summarized in Ref.[8] Recently the smallest of these, which removes approximately 3.3 kb of DNA including MCS-R2 but no other MCS-R element, was described[47] (see **Fig. 1**) in a patient whose phenotype is consistent with both *cis*-linked α genes being down-regulated, again suggesting that MCS-R2 is the major (if not the only) upstream α-globin enhancer element.

Interspecific hybrids each containing an abnormal copy of chromosome 16 from such patients have been made by fusing Epstein-Barr virus transformed cell lines with mouse erythroleukemia (MEL) cells. In contrast to normal copies of chromosome 16, the abnormal chromosomes produce severely reduced (often <1% of normal) levels of human α-globin mRNA, indicating that these deletions severely down-regulate expression of the α genes and are responsible for the associated α-thalassemia. A specific knockout of MCS-R2 (HS-40) alone[48] from such a chromosome together with many experiments in transgenic mice strongly suggests that MCS-R2 is the major active element deleted by these arrangements. More recently, this observation was further strengthened by showing that removal of just MCS-R2 from a mouse model that recapitulates human α-globin expression severely reduces α-globin expression.[27]

The mechanisms by which these natural mutations have arisen are quite diverse. In one the deletion resulted from a recombination event between partially homologous Alu repeats that are normally 62 kb apart.[46] In another the deletion arose via a subtelomeric rearrangement.[49] The chromosomal breakpoint was found in an Alu element located approximately 105 kb from the 16p subtelomeric region. The broken chromosome was stabilized with a new telomere acquired by recombination between this Alu element and a subtelomeric Alu repeat associated with the newly acquired chromosome end. In at least 5 cases the chromosomes appear to have been broken and then stabilized by the direct addition of telomeric repeats to nontelomeric DNA.[40]

Sequence analysis suggests that these chromosomes are "healed" via the action of telomerase, an enzyme that is normally involved in maintaining the integrity of telomeres. In the remaining cases the mechanism has not yet been established. However, it is interesting that some (eg, $(\alpha\alpha)^{IJ}$, $(\alpha\alpha)^{Sco}$),[50,51] but not all, of these mutations appear to have arisen *de novo*, because neither parent has the abnormal chromosome.

α-THALASSEMIA RESULTING FROM COMPETITION FOR THE UPSTREAM REGULATORY ELEMENTS

α-Thalassemia is common throughout Melanesia and is frequently caused by the known $-\alpha^{3.7}$ and $-\alpha^{4.2}$ mutations. However, it is also documented that in some Melanesian patients (from Papua New Guinea and Vanuatu) with α-thalassemia (α-thalassemia trait and HbH disease) the α-globin genes are intact, suggesting a nondeletional form of α-thalassemia ($\alpha^T\alpha/\alpha\alpha$ or $\alpha^T\alpha/\alpha^T\alpha$) (**Fig. 5**). In these patients detailed mapping and DNA sequence analysis of the α genes and all of the upstream MCS elements was normal, and yet further studies showed that this form of α-thalassemia is linked to the α-globin cluster at 16p13.3. To identify the mutation responsible for this unusual form of α-thalassemia, De Gobbi and colleagues[52] cloned this region from an affected homozygote and resequenced approximately 213 kb of DNA containing and flanking the α-globin cluster, identifying 283 SNPs. The SNP responsible for the mutation was identified when the SNPs were aligned with a tiled microarray analyzed using labeled RNA from the patient's erythroid cells. This configuration revealed a new peak of mRNA expression (located between the ζ and $\psi\zeta$ genes), which coincides with a SNP that creates a GATA-1 binding site. In association studies this SNP is always linked to the phenotype of α-thalassemia. Like the MCS elements, this new GATA site binds erythroid transcription factors in vivo and becomes activated in erythroid cells.

Why should creating a new promoter-like sequence between the α genes and their regulatory elements cause α-thalassemia? Perhaps the most likely explanation is that, because it lies closer to the MCS elements, this new promoter competes with the α-globin promoters and "steals" the activity of the upstream regulatory elements, thus resulting in α-thalassemia. Several lines of evidence suggest that the α-globin promoters may indeed compete for the activity of the upstream regulatory elements, in particular MCS-R2 (HS-40). Firstly it has been noted that although the sequences of the duplicated α genes and their promoters are identical, the gene ($\alpha2$) nearest MCS-R2 is expressed at a higher level than the more distal gene ($\alpha1$). Furthermore, additional duplications of the α genes ($\alpha\alpha\alpha$, $\alpha\alpha\alpha\alpha$ and $\alpha\alpha\alpha\alpha\alpha$) do not lead to a linear increase in α-globin expression[1]; genes located further from MCS-R2 are expressed at progressively lower levels. When one α gene is deleted from the chromosome ($-\alpha$) the remaining α gene appears to recruit more PolII and is expressed at increased levels.[22] It was recently shown that MCS-R2 also regulates expression of another gene (*NME4*) located 300 kb away from this element on chromosome 16.[53] The α-globin genes lie between MCS-R2 and *NME4*. When both α genes are deleted, expression of NME4 increases by a factor of eightfold. Together these findings suggest that promoters may compete for the activity associated with enhancers, and this may provide the explanation for this form of α-thalassemia seen in patients from the south Pacific.

LARGE DELETIONS EXTENDING BEYOND THE α-GLOBIN CLUSTER WITH COMPLEX PHENOTYPES (ATR-16 SYNDROME)

Nearly all patients with large deletions (up to 900 kb) from the end of chromosome 16p (removing one copy of up to 52 genes) appear phenotypically normal apart from the presence of α-thalassemia. However, in 40 patients analyzed to date deletions of

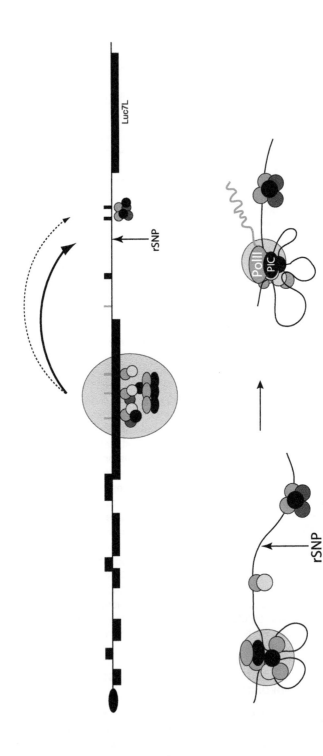

Fig. 5. The key features of the Melanesian form of α-thalassemia. A regulatory SNP (rSNP) located between the ζ- and α_2-globin genes creates a new GATA1 binding site which, in turn, also creates a new promoter. This promoter preferentially interacts with the upstream enhancer elements (*bold curved arrow*) and steals activity from the α genes (*dashed curved arrow*). In the hypothetical looping model (below) the upstream element interacts with the new promoter but not the α genes.

greater than 900 kb have been associated with a variety of developmental abnormalities; such patients are said to have the ATR-16 syndrome.[54] Relating phenotype to genotype is difficult in these cases because of the rather heterogeneous nature of the underlying abnormalities.

Using a combination of conventional cytogenetics, fluorescent in situ hybridization and molecular analysis, at least 3 types of chromosomal rearrangements (translocation, inversion/deletion, and truncation) have now been found in ATR-16 patients. To date, few breakpoints have been fully characterized. However, in some cases telomeric truncations have been documented; in these cases it appears that the affected chromosomes have been broken, truncated, and "healed" by the direct addition of telomeric repeats $(TTAGGG)_n$, as described above for some less extensive 16p deletions in patients with α-thalassemia.

Altogether, 11 cases of ATR-16 have been shown to have pure monosomy for 16p13.3 and deletions of 900 to 1700 kb with various developmental abnormalities (eg, facial dysmorphism, speech delay, and skeletal abnormalities). How might monosomy for 16p13.3 cause such developmental abnormalities? One possibility is that deletion of a large number of genes from one copy of chromosome 16 may unmask mutations in its homologue; the more genes that are deleted the greater the probability of this occurring. However, this is unlikely to be the explanation for most ATR-16 cases because it is estimated that normal individuals only carry a few harmful mutations of this type in the entire genome.[55] A further possibility is that some genes in 16p are imprinted[56] so that deletions could remove the only active copy of the gene. At present there is no evidence for imprinting of the 16p region (reviewed in Ref.[57]), and in the relatively few ATR-16 cases analyzed there appear to be no major clinical differences between patients with deletions of the maternally- or paternally-derived chromosomes. It therefore seems more likely that there are some genes in the 16p region that encode proteins whose effect is critically determined by the amount produced—so-called dosage sensitive genes. Examples of such genes include those encoding proteins that form heterodimers, those required at a critical level for a rate-determining step of a regulatory pathway, and tumor suppressor genes (eg, TSC2). Removal of genes from one copy of 16p13.3 consistently reduces their levels of expression to approximately 50% of normal (Buckle and colleagues, unpublished data, 2008). If the deletion includes one or more dosage-sensitive genes, this could account for the clinical effects seen in ATR-16 patients.

The region lying between 900 and 1700 kb from the 16p telomere, deleted in all patients with the characteristic features of ATR-16 syndrome, contains genes and gene families of known function that have been implicated in a wide range of disorders with few or no features in common with ATR-16. One of these (*SOX8*) was considered as a strong candidate because it is involved in the regulation of embryonic development and is strongly expressed in the brain.[58] However, a recently described Brazilian patient with a deletion that removes both the α-globin locus and *SOX8* was not associated with MR or any dysmorphism.[59] It is clear that further examples of ATR-16 due to monosomy for 16p13.3 must be characterized to identify the gene(s) responsible for the MR and other developmental abnormalities associated with this condition.

The ATR-16 syndrome has served as an important model for improving our general understanding of the molecular basis for mental retardation. The ATR-16 syndrome provided the first examples of mental retardation caused by a cryptic chromosomal translocation and truncation. Further work has shown that such telomeric rearrangements may underlie a significant proportion of unexplained mental retardation.[60] The current challenge is to understand in detail the mechanisms by which monosomy causes developmental abnormalities; the ATR-16 syndrome provides an excellent model for addressing this issue. All deletions currently associated with ATR-16 syndrome are shown in Ref.[20]

TRANS-ACTING MUTATIONS CAUSING α-THALASSEMIA

The regulatory elements (eg, locus control regions, enhancers, promoters, silencers) controlling α- and β-globin gene expression bind many transcription factors and cofactors in common.[11,61] These factors include many of the key transcription factors expressed during erythropoiesis (eg, GATA1, Friend of GATA, SpXKLF proteins, SCL complex, and NF-E2) and general transcription factors (eg, PolII and other components of the preinitiation complex), and therefore it might not be expected that mutations in these genes would cause one cluster to be affected more than another. However, it has been shown either in man or in experimental models that mutations in some erythroid factors (eg, GATA1 and EKLF) cause β-thalassemia by affecting β-globin expression to a greater extent than α-globin expression.[62] Perhaps more surprisingly, mutations in a component (XPD) of a general transcription factor (TFIIH) also cause β-thalassemia.[63] More recently, polymorphisms in the cofactor BCL11A have been shown to exert specific effects on γ- rather than β-globin expression.[64] This finding shows that although they are controlled in similar manners there are many differences in the way that the α- and β-like globin clusters are regulated.

So now we can ask: are there mutations in transcription factors and/or cofactors that predominantly affect α- rather than β-globin expression and cause α-thalassemia? A good starting point is to consider structural and functional differences between the 2 clusters that might provide a logical basis for such different effects. A great deal of work from many groups has shown significant differences between the 2 clusters and, of relevance, it appears these gene loci lie in substantially different chromosomal environments.[65] In contrast to the β cluster, the α cluster lies in an early replicating GC-rich, CpG-rich, repeat-dense, subtelomeric region of chromosome 16 surrounded by widely expressed genes, and is associated with a constitutively open chromatin environment. Could genes (eg, α-globin) lying in such a chromosomal region be targeted by factors that ignore genes like β-globin lying in quite different chromosomal environments?

The authors have previously described 2 syndromes in which mutations in a *trans*-acting factor (called ATRX) give rise to α-thalassemia. The *ATRX* gene was first identified when it was shown that mutations in this X-linked gene caused a form of syndromal mental retardation, with multiple developmental abnormalities and characteristically associated with α-thalassemia (ATR-X syndrome).[66] Some years later it was also shown that acquired mutations in *ATRX* were present in patients who have a rare syndrome in which α-thalassemia is acquired as a secondary mutation in a premalignant hematologic condition called myelodysplastic syndrome (so-called ATMDS syndrome).[67]

To date 128 acquired and/or inherited disease-causing mutations have been found, and these predominantly lie in 2 highly conserved domains of the ATRX protein.[68] At the N-terminus these are located within a globular domain (similar to that found in the de novo methyltransferases, DNMT3 and DNMT3L, the so-called ADD domain) including a plant homeodomain (PHD) that binds the N-terminal tails of histone H3.[69] At the C-terminus there are 7 helicase subdomains that identify ATRX as a member of the SNF2 family of chromatin associated proteins. Many of these proteins remove or slide nucleosomes to allow transcription factors to gain access to their DNA binding sites.[70] ATRX is most closely related to an outlying subgroup (including RAD54) of the SNF2 family, suggesting it may have related but different chromatin-associated functions.

Some clues to the role of ATRX in vivo have come from studying its distribution in the nucleus, the proteins with which it interacts, and the effects of mutations. Using indirect immunofluorescence, ATRX is found at heterochromatic repeats including rDNA repeats and telomeric repeats.[71,72] ATRX also interacts with HP1, a protein widely associated with both interstitial and telomeric heterochromatin. It has also been shown that mutations in *ATRX* are consistently associated with alterations in the pattern of DNA methylation at such repeat sequences.[73] Therefore, the general conclusion from these studies is that ATRX binds to heterochromatic repeat sequences. It has recently been shown that ATRX's role at these sequences may not be to remove or slide nucleosomes but to replace the usual histones (called H3.1) that make up the nucleosomes, with variant histones (called H3.3).[74] Most histones are incorporated into chromatin during replication, but H3.3 is incorporated at regions of nucleosome instability or actively transcribed regions during interphase.[75]

More recently, the genome-wide distribution of the ATRX protein in human erythroid precursors has been established. Nine hundred and seventeen ATRX targets were identified throughout the genome and many dysregulated ATRX targets, like α-globin, were found to be GC-rich, associated with polymorphic tandem repeat sequences, and to lie in subtelomeric chromosomal regions.[76] Furthermore, it has been shown that the larger the tandem repeat the greater the perturbation in gene expression. Therefore it appears that both in heterochromatin and euchromatin, ATRX targets are frequently G- and C-rich and CpG-rich tandemly repeated sequences. Detailed analysis of the α-globin cluster shows that the maximal binding of ATRX is seen at a G-rich tandem repeat in the middle of the globin cluster, clearly explaining why the α-globin genes are targets of ATRX whereas the β-globin genes are not.

How might such repeats interfere with gene expression and why would the presence or absence of ATRX affect this? A common theme shared by telomeres and many of the interstitial targets of ATRX is their potential to form an unusual DNA structure in which 4 strands of DNA interact with each other rather than 2. These structures depend on the presence of G nucleotides within repeat structures to form what is referred to as G-quadruplex DNA.[77] These structures form when DNA becomes single stranded (eg, during transcription) and may destabilize and eject nucleosomes as they do so. Once formed, such structures may stall transcription and subsequent rounds of gene expression unless resolved. It is possible that ATRX is one component of the pathway that resolves such structures and plays a role in replacing ejected nucleosomes with H3.3. In support of this model, it has recently been shown that ATRX binds G4 DNA in vitro.[76]

As a final note, it is interesting that the degree of α-thalassemia seen in patients with ATMDS (acquired *ATRX* mutations) is much greater than in patients with the ATRX syndrome (inherited *ATRX* mutations), even when the same *ATRX* mutation occurs in either condition.[78] This suggests that another component of this pathway resolving tandem repeat structures may frequently be present in patients with the common forms of myelodysplastic syndrome.

SUMMARY

The α-globin cluster provides one of the best models to develop our understanding of how the integration of a transcriptional program and an epigenetic program via a key set of *cis*-acting elements dispersed across a large chromosomal region switch genes on and off at the correct time and place during development and differentiation. In particular, by analyzing the normal cluster, the natural mutants, and experimental models we should gain significant insight into how long-range regulatory elements control gene expression.

There is now sufficient knowledge of the mutations underlying α-thalassemia to develop comprehensive genetic counseling and prenatal diagnosis wherever there is sufficient expertise and resources to support such a program. Further identification of natural mutations of the globin genes should be pursued because these observations continue to elucidate the general principles underlying human molecular genetics.

An important theme that has emerged from analysis of *trans*-acting mutations is that there are pathways that may alter α- but not β-globin expression, and by understanding these in detail it may be possible to manipulate gene expression to redress the imbalance between α- and β-globin expression in β-thalassemia. Preliminary genetic evidence suggests that relatively small changes in globin chain imbalance may have a significant influence on clinical outcome, encouraging the development of pharmacologic agents to target the relevant pathways.

REFERENCES

1. Higgs DR, Vickers MA, Wilkie AO, et al. A review of the molecular genetics of the human alpha-globin gene cluster. Blood 1989;73:1081.
2. Higgs DR, Weatherall DJ. The alpha thalassaemias. Cell Mol Life Sci 2009;66: 1154.
3. Chui DH, Fucharoen S, Chan V. Hemoglobin H disease: not necessarily a benign disorder. Blood 2003;101:791.
4. Lorey F, Charoenkwan P, Witkowska HE, et al. Hb H hydrops foetalis syndrome: a case report and review of literature. Br J Haematol 2001;115:72.
5. Steinberg MH, Forget BG, Higgs DR, et al, editors. Disorders of hemoglobin. 2nd edition. New York: Cambridge University Press; 2008.
6. Thein SL. Genetic modifiers of beta-thalassemia. Haematologica 2005;90:649.
7. Voon HP, Vadolas J. Controlling alpha-globin: a review of alpha-globin expression and its impact on beta-thalassemia. Haematologica 2008;93:1868.
8. Higgs DR, Wood WG. Long-range regulation of alpha globin gene expression during erythropoiesis. Curr Opin Hematol 2008;15:176.
9. Noordermeer D, de Laat W. Joining the loops: beta-globin gene regulation. IUBMB Life 2008;60:824.
10. Anguita E, Hughes J, Heyworth C, et al. Globin gene activation during haemopoiesis is driven by protein complexes nucleated by GATA-1 and GATA-2. EMBO J 2004;23:2841.
11. Vernimmen D, De Gobbi M, Sloane-Stanley JA, et al. Long-range chromosomal interactions regulate the timing of the transition between poised and active gene expression. EMBO J 2007;26:2041.
12. Vernimmen D, Marques-Kranc F, Sharpe JA, et al. Chromosome looping at the human alpha-globin locus is mediated via the major upstream regulatory element (HS -40). Blood 2009;114:4253.
13. Daniels RJ, Peden JF, Lloyd C, et al. Sequence, structure and pathology of the fully annotated terminal 2 Mb of the short arm of human chromosome 16. Hum Mol Genet 2001;10:339.
14. Flint J, Thomas K, Micklem G, et al. The relationship between chromosome structure and function at a human telomeric region. Nat Genet 1997;15:252.
15. Garrick D, De Gobbi M, Samara V, et al. The role of the polycomb complex in silencing alpha-globin gene expression in nonerythroid cells. Blood 2008;112: 3889.

16. Morey L, Helin K. Polycomb group protein-mediated repression of transcription. Trends Biochem Sci 2010;35(6):323–32.
17. Day IN. dbSNP in the detail and copy number complexities. Hum Mutat 2010;31:2.
18. Lupski JR, Stankiewicz P. Genomic disorders: molecular mechanisms for rearrangements and conveyed phenotypes. PLoS Genet 2005;1:e49.
19. Higgs DR, Wainscoat JS, Flint J, et al. Analysis of the human alpha-globin gene cluster reveals a highly informative genetic locus. Proc Natl Acad Sci U S A 1986; 83:5165.
20. Higgs DR. The molecular basis of a thalassemia. In: Steinberg MH, Forget BG, Higgs DR, et al, editors. Disorders of hemoglobin. 2nd edition. Cambridge (UK): Cambridge University Press; 2009. p. 241.
21. Wilkie AO, Higgs DR, Rack KA, et al. Stable length polymorphism of up to 260 kb at the tip of the short arm of human chromosome 16. Cell 1991;64:595.
22. Rugless MJ, Fisher CA, Old JM, et al. A large deletion in the human {alpha}-globin cluster caused by a replication error is associated with an unexpectedly mild phenotype. Hum Mol Genet 2008;17:3084.
23. Buckle VJ, Higgs DR, Wilkie AO, et al. Localisation of human alpha globin to 16p13.3——pter. J Med Genet 1988;25:847.
24. Wainscoat JS, Kanavakis E, Weatherall DJ, et al. Regional localisation of the human alpha-globin genes. Lancet 1981;2:301.
25. Fichera M, Rappazzo G, Spalletta A, et al. Triplicated alpha-globin gene locus with translocation of the whole telomeric end in association with beta-thalassemia trait, results in a severe syndrome. Blood 1994;84:260a.
26. Harteveld CL, Refaldi C, Cassinerio E, et al. Segmental duplications involving the alpha-globin gene cluster are causing beta-thalassemia intermedia phenotypes in beta-thalassemia heterozygous patients. Blood Cells Mol Dis 2008;40(3): 312–6.
27. Wallace HA, Marques-Kranc F, Richardson M, et al. Manipulating the mouse genome to engineer precise functional syntenic replacements with human sequence. Cell 2007;128:197.
28. Hess JF, Schmid CW, Shen CK. A gradient of sequence divergence in the human adult alpha-globin duplication units. Science 1984;226:67.
29. Lauer J, Shen CK, Maniatis T. The chromosomal arrangement of human alpha-like globin genes: sequence homology and alpha-globin gene deletions. Cell 1980; 20:119.
30. Michelson AM, Orkin SH. Boundaries of gene conversion within the duplicated human alpha-globin genes. Concerted evolution by segmental recombination. J Biol Chem 1983;258:15245.
31. Zimmer EA, Martin SL, Beverley SM, et al. Rapid duplication and loss of genes coding for the alpha chains of hemoglobin. Proc Natl Acad Sci U S A 1980;77: 2158.
32. Embury SH, Miller JA, Dozy AM, et al. Two different molecular organizations account for the single alpha-globin gene of the alpha-thalassemia-2 genotype. J Clin Invest 1980;66:1319.
33. Goossens M, Dozy AM, Embury SH, et al. Triplicated alpha-globin loci in humans. Proc Natl Acad Sci U S A 1980;77:518.
34. Trent RJ, Higgs DR, Clegg JB, et al. A new triplicated alpha-globin gene arrangement in man. Br J Haematol 1981;49:149.
35. De Angioletti M, Lacerra G, Castaldo C, et al. Alpha alpha alpha alpha anti-3.7 type II: a new alpha-globin gene rearrangement suggesting that the alpha-globin gene duplication could be caused by intrachromosomal recombination. Hum Genet 1992;89:37.

36. Cook RJ, Hoyer JD, Highsmith WE. Quintuple alpha-globin gene: a novel allele in a Sudanese man. Hemoglobin 2006;30:51.

37. Lam KW, Jeffreys AJ. Processes of de novo duplication of human {alpha}-globin genes. Proc Natl Acad Sci U S A 2007;104:10950.

38. International Human Genome Sequencing Consortium. Finishing the euchromatic sequence of the human genome. Nature 2004;431:931.

39. Nicholls RD, Fischel-Ghodsian N, Higgs DR. Recombination at the human alpha-globin gene cluster: sequence features and topological constraints. Cell 1987;49: 369.

40. Flint J, Craddock CF, Villegas A, et al. Healing of broken human chromosomes by the addition of telomeric repeats. Am J Hum Genet 1994;55:505.

41. Indrak K, Gu YC, Novotny J, et al. A new alpha-thalassemia-2 deletion resulting in microcytosis and hypochromia and in vitro chain imbalance in the heterozygote. Am J Hematol 1993;43:144.

42. Barbour VM, Tufarelli C, Sharpe JA, et al. alpha-thalassemia resulting from a negative chromosomal position effect. Blood 2000;96:800.

43. Tufarelli C, Stanley JA, Garrick D, et al. Transcription of antisense RNA leading to gene silencing and methylation as a novel cause of human genetic disease. Nat Genet 2003;34:157.

44. Ligtenberg MJ, Kuiper RP, Chan TL, et al. Heritable somatic methylation and inactivation of MSH2 in families with Lynch syndrome due to deletion of the 3′exons of TACSTD1. Nat Genet 2009;41:112.

45. Higgs DR, Vernimmen D, Wood B. Long-range regulation of alpha-globin gene expression. Adv Genet 2008;61:143 Chapter 5.

46. Hatton CS, Wilkie AO, Drysdale HC, et al. Alpha-thalassemia caused by a large (62 kb) deletion upstream of the human alpha globin gene cluster. Blood 1990;76:221.

47. Phylipsen M, Prior JF, Lim E, et al. Thalassemia in Western Australia: 11 novel deletions characterized by multiplex ligation-dependent probe amplification. Blood Cells Mol Dis 2010;44:146.

48. Bernet A, Sabatier S, Picketts DJ, et al. Targeted inactivation of the major positive regulatory element (HS-40) of the human alpha-globin gene locus. Blood 1995; 86:1202.

49. Flint J, Rochette J, Craddock CF, et al. Chromosomal stabilisation by a subtelomeric rearrangement involving two closely related Alu elements. Hum Mol Genet 1996;5:1163.

50. Liebhaber SA, Griese EU, Weiss I, et al. Inactivation of human alpha-globin gene expression by a de novo deletion located upstream of the alpha-globin gene cluster. Proc Natl Acad Sci U S A 1990;87:9431.

51. Viprakasit V, Kidd AM, Ayyub H, et al. De novo deletion within the telomeric region flanking the human alpha globin locus as a cause of alpha thalassaemia. Br J Haematol 2003;120:867.

52. De Gobbi M, Viprakasit V, Hughes JR, et al. A regulatory SNP causes a human genetic disease by creating a new transcriptional promoter. Science 2006;312:1215.

53. Lower KM, Hughes JR, De Gobbi M, et al. Adventitious changes in long-range gene expression caused by polymorphic structural variation and promoter competition. Proc Natl Acad Sci U S A 2009;106:21771.

54. Wilkie AO, Buckle VJ, Harris PC, et al. Clinical features and molecular analysis of the alpha thalassemia/mental retardation syndromes. I. Cases due to deletions involving chromosome band 16p13.3. Am J Hum Genet 1990;46:1112.

55. Lupski JR, Reid JG, Gonzaga-Jauregui C, et al. Whole-genome sequencing in a patient with Charcot-Marie-Tooth neuropathy. N Engl J Med 2010;362:1181.

56. Reik W, Walter J. Genomic imprinting: parental influence on the genome. Nat Rev Genet 2001;2:21.
57. Schneider AS, Bischoff FZ, McCaskill C, et al. Comprehensive 4-year follow-up on a case of maternal heterodisomy for chromosome 16. Am J Med Genet 1996;66:204.
58. Pfeifer D, Poulat F, Holinski-Feder E, et al. The SOX8 gene is located within 700 kb of the tip of chromosome 16p and is deleted in a patient with ATR-16 syndrome. Genomics 2000;63:108.
59. Bezerra MA, Araujo AS, Phylipsen M, et al. The deletion of SOX8 is not associated with ATR-16 in an HbH family from Brazil. Br J Haematol 2008;142:324.
60. Flint J, Wilkie AO, Buckle VJ, et al. The detection of subtelomeric chromosomal rearrangements in idiopathic mental retardation. Nat Genet 1995;9:132.
61. Cantor AB, Orkin SH. Transcriptional regulation of erythropoiesis: an affair involving multiple partners. Oncogene 2002;21:3368.
62. Yu C, Niakan KK, Matsushita M, et al. X-linked thrombocytopenia with thalassemia from a mutation in the amino finger of GATA-1 affecting DNA binding rather than FOG-1 interaction. Blood 2002;100:2040.
63. Viprakasit V, Gibbons RJ, Broughton BC, et al. Mutations in the general transcription factor TFIIH result in beta-thalassaemia in individuals with trichothiodystrophy. Hum Mol Genet 2001;10:2797.
64. Sankaran VG, Xu J, Orkin SH. Advances in the understanding of haemoglobin switching. Br J Haematol 2010;149(2):181–94.
65. Higgs DR, Sharpe JA, Wood WG. Understanding alpha globin gene expression: a step towards effective gene therapy. Semin Hematol 1998;35:93.
66. Gibbons RJ, Picketts DJ, Villard L, et al. Mutations in a putative global transcriptional regulator cause X-linked mental retardation with alpha-thalassemia (ATR-X syndrome). Cell 1995;80:837.
67. Gibbons RJ, Pellagatti A, Garrick D, et al. Identification of acquired somatic mutations in the gene encoding chromatin-remodeling factor ATRX in the alpha-thalassemia myelodysplasia syndrome (ATMDS). Nat Genet 2003;34:446.
68. Gibbons RJ, Wada T, Fisher CA, et al. Mutations in the chromatin-associated protein ATRX. Hum Mutat 2008;29:796.
69. Argentaro A, Yang JC, Chapman L, et al. Structural consequences of disease-causing mutations in the ATRX-DNMT3-DNMT3L (ADD) domain of the chromatin-associated protein ATRX. Proc Natl Acad Sci U S A 2007;104:11939.
70. Owen-Hughes T. Colworth memorial lecture. Pathways for remodelling chromatin. Biochem Soc Trans 2003;31:893.
71. McDowell TL, Gibbons RJ, Sutherland H, et al. Localization of a putative transcriptional regulator (ATRX) at pericentromeric heterochromatin and the short arms of acrocentric chromosomes. Proc Natl Acad Sci U S A 1999;96:13983.
72. Wong LH, McGhie JD, Sim M, et al. ATRX interacts with H3.3 in maintaining telomere structural integrity in pluripotent embryonic stem cells. Genome Res 2010;20:351.
73. Gibbons RJ, Bachoo S, Picketts DJ, et al. Mutations in transcriptional regulator ATRX establish the functional significance of a PHD-like domain. Nat Genet 1997;17:146.
74. Goldberg AD, Banaszynski LA, Noh K-M, et al. Distinct factors control histone variant H3.3 localization at specific genomic regions. Cell 2010;140:678.
75. Ahmad K, Henikoff S. Histone H3 variants specify modes of chromatin assembly. Proc Natl Acad Sci U S A 2002;99(Suppl 4):16477.

76. Law MJ, Lower KM, Voon HPJ, et al. A SNF2 protein targets variable number repeats and thereby influences allele-specific expression. Cell 2010, in press.

77. Lipps HJ, Rhodes D. G-quadruplex structures: in vivo evidence and function. Trends Cell Biol 2009;19:414.

78. Steensma DP, Gibbons RJ, Higgs DR. Acquired {alpha} thalassemia in association with myelodysplastic syndrome and other hematologic malignancies. Blood 2005;105:443.

HbE/β-Thalassemia: Basis of Marked Clinical Diversity

Nancy F. Olivieri, MD, FRCP(C)[a,b,]*, Zahra Pakbaz, MD[c], Elliott Vichinsky, MD[d]

KEYWORDS

- Hemoglobin E/β-thalassemia • Diversity • Phenotype
- Genotype • Modifiers

EPIDEMIOLOGY

Worldwide, hemoglobin E (HbE) thalassemia accounts for about one-half of all cases of severe β-thalassemia,[1–7] with the highest frequencies observed in India, Bangladesh, and throughout southeast Asia in regions of Thailand, Laos, and Cambodia.[6–8]

Hemoglobin E β-thalassemia (HbE/β-thalassemia) is causing an increasingly severe public health problem throughout the Indian subcontinent and parts of southeast Asia. Its carrier frequencies are up to 60% in parts of northeast Thailand and Cambodia, it is common for individuals in this region to inherit both HbE and β-thalassemia. In Thailand, 3000 children are born annually with HbE/β-thalassemia and there are more than 100,000 patients in the population.[9] In southern China, gene frequencies are approximately 4% for β-thalassemia and for HbE, resulting in thousands of affected patients.[10] HbE thalassemia accounts for more than half of the cases of severe β-thalassemia in Indonesia, and for about one-third of those in Sri Lanka.

Although, in the past, HbE/β-thalassemia was rarely diagnosed in North America and Europe, it has become the most common form of β-thalassemia identified on state newborn screening programs.[6,7,10–16]

[a] Pediatrics Medicine and Public Health Sciences, University of Toronto, Toronto, Canada
[b] Toronto General Hospital Research Institute, 10th Floor Eaton Wing, Room 226, 200 Elizabeth Street, Toronto M5G 2C4, Canada
[c] Children's Hospital Oakland Research Institute, 5700 Martin Luther King Jr Boulevard, Oakland, CA 94609, USA
[d] Hematology/Oncology, Children's Hospital & Research Center Oakland, 747 52nd Street, Oakland, CA 94609, USA
* Corresponding author. Toronto General Hospital, 10th Floor Eaton Wing Room 226, 200 Elizabeth Street, Toronto M5G 2C4, Canada.
E-mail address: noliv@attglobal.net

Hematol Oncol Clin N Am 24 (2010) 1055–1070
doi:10.1016/j.hoc.2010.08.008
0889-8588/10/$ – see front matter © 2010 Published by Elsevier Inc.

The prevalence of HbE in California parallels the increase in Asian births in that state: the carrier state is observed in 1 in 4 births Cambodian origin and in 1 in 9 babies of Thai/Laotian origin.

There is a widely disparate range of clinical and hematological parameters in affected patients (**Fig. 1**).[8,16–28] Although studies are limited, the natural history of HbE/β-thalassemia may change over time in individuals. The phenotypic variability, the way the later course of the illness cannot be predicted in the first few years of life, and the lack of knowledge of the natural history of the disease combine to make the management of HbE/β-thalassemia particularly challenging.[29]

PATHOPHYSIOLOGY

HbE thalassemia results from coinheritance of a β-thalassemia allele from one parent, and the structural variant, HbE, from the other. HbE results from a $G \rightarrow A$ substitution in codon #26 of the β-globin gene, which, as well as producing a structurally abnormal hemoglobin, activates a cryptic splice site that causes abnormal messenger RNA (mRNA) processing. Because the usual donor site has to compete with this new site, the level of normally spliced mRNA, β^E, is reduced[30] and the abnormally spliced mRNA is nonfunctional because a new stop codon is generated. As a result, HbE is synthesized at a reduced rate, and behaves like a mild form of β-thalassemia.

The pathophysiology of HbE/β-thalassemia is related to many factors including reduced β chain production resulting in globin chain imbalance, ineffective erythropoiesis, apoptosis, oxidative damage, and shortened red cell survival.[31,32] The instability of HbE is a minor factor in the overall pathophysiology of this disorder except during febrile events in which this instability results in accelerated hemolysis.[33]

UNDERSTANDING THE PHENOTYPIC HETEROGENEITY OF HBE/β-THALASSEMIA

The extraordinary clinical heterogeneity of HbE/β-thalassemia is poorly understood. The condition may present as a mild, asymptomatic anemia or a life-threatening

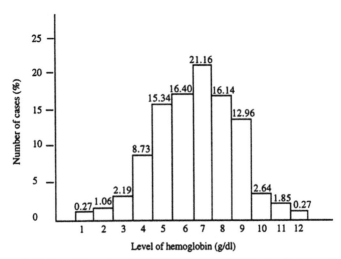

Fig. 1. Hemoglobin levels in patients with E/β-thalassemia (Thailand). (*From* Fucharoen S, Ketvichit P, Pootrakul P, et al. Clinical manifestation of beta-thalassemia/hemoglobin E disease. J Pediatr Hematol Oncol 2000;22(6):553; with permission.)

disorder that may lead to death from anemia in the early first years of life. In an analysis conducted in Sri Lanka, patients with HbE/β-thalassemia would have been expected to account for 40% of the patients affected by thalassemia at any given time but, based on the Hardy-Weinberg distribution, many fewer cases of HbE/β-thalassemia were observed, likely reflecting the mildness of some cases of HbE and its variable clinical course.

The phenotype of HbE/β-thalassemia seems to be unstable. Presently, little is known about the clinical course of older patients. Limited data indicate that patients develop worsening anemia with age.

Longitudinal studies of affected children in Sri Lanka have emphasized the remarkable instability of their phenotypes, particularly in the first 10 years of life, during which there was a variable and changing pattern of anemia, erythroid expansion, and associated growth failure. By contrast, the phenotype became more stable later in development, and it was frequently possible to stop blood transfusion in a proportion of older patients, with no deleterious effects on their further development and function.[24] One of the most important findings identified in the modified natural history study of HbE/β-thalassemia reported from Sri Lanka[24] was that, although about a quarter of patients were not receiving regular blood transfusions, and the rest were maintained on regular or on-demand transfusions, the pretransfusion steady-state hemoglobin concentrations (on average 7.0 g/dL) were not clinically very different from those patients who had never begun a regimen of transfusions (mean 6.1 g/dL). A considerable phenotypic heterogeneity of these patients occurred within a narrow range of hemoglobin values, with the mean difference between the mildest and most severe groups approximately 1 to 2 g/dL.

The lack of a standardized, robust classification of disease severity is a major impairment in understanding the clinical spectrum of the disease and whether it changes with age.

CLINICAL SEVERITY CATEGORIES OF HBE/β-THALASSEMIA

Investigators have attempted to categorize disease severity with the assignment of patients to severe and mild groups, between which putative genetic and environmental factors can be compared.[24,34] Premawardhena and colleagues[24] classified 109 patients with HbE/β-thalassemia aged 1 to 51 years into very mild to very severe groups. About one-quarter of patients were transfusion independent, whereas the remainder had been maintained on regular or intermittent (on demand) transfusion. In an analysis of the patient data, there was little objective difference in the baseline data between the transfused and nontransfused cohorts. In most of the cases, it was unclear whether transfusions were necessary. Therefore, it was decided to stop transfusion in as many patients as possible, and observe the patients closely. This cohort has been prospectively followed for more than 8 years.[24,35]

These patients were classified into 5 groups of severity ranging from mild to severe (**Table 1**).[24,36] Group 1 included those patients who had undergone only minimal transfusion and had normal growth and sexual maturity; group 1 children had adequate growth and all patients rated quality of life as exceeding 5 on the 10-point scale. Group 2 comprised patients similar to those in class 1, except for transfusion history: these patients had a longer history of transfusions. Group 3 comprised patients who had undergone splenectomy and in whom a beneficial response to splenectomy had been observed: in particular, during the 2 years following splenectomy, an improvement in quality of life and an increase in height velocity was observed. Group 4 comprised patients doing poorly without transfusions as shown by poor

Table 1
Clinical, hematological, and genetic findings in patient groups with HbE/β-thalassemia

Class	Patient Group				
	1	2	3	4	5
No.	25	37	14	22	11
Age (y)	4–51 (25.3 ± 16.5)	9–52 (23.2 ± 10.6)	5–16 (10.8 ± 3.0)	5–21 (15.2 ± 3.4)	4–13 (? ± 2.9)
Age diagnosis (y)	1.5–4.8 (15.5 ± 13.4)	0.8–35 (9.9 ± 8.4)	0.4–56 (2.3 ± 2.1)	0.7–8.0 (3.6 ± 2.6)	0.2–4.0 (1.4 ± 0.8)
Maximum liver size (cm)	0–14 (96.0 ± 3.5)	3–18 (9.8 ± 3.5)	6–16 (9.8 ± 1.6)	5–19 (11.1 ± 3.8)	0–12 (7.6 ± 1.7)
Maximum spleen size (cm)	0–18 (8.9 ± 3.2)	6–23 (13.4 ± 3.2)	11–20 (17 ± 38)	5–17 (11.4 ± 3.3)	4–15 (9.9 ± 3.3)
Facial deformity (0–6)	0–2 (0.9 ± 0.7)	0–4 (1.5 ± 1.0)	0–4 (2.0 ± 1.2)	0.5–3.5 (1.92 ± 1.2)	1–3 (1.5 ± 0.9)
Splenectomized (%)	21.0	62.2	100	85	22
Time from splenectomy (y)	2–33 (13.3)	2–19 (7.4)	2–9 (3.1)	1–13 (5.6)	2–7 (4)
History major infection (%)	8.3	18.9	16.7	26.3	11.0
History of malaria (%)	21	37.9	25.0	42.0	11.0
Leg ulcers (%)	33.0	51.3	16.7	15.8	0
Fractures (%)	0	13.9	0	25.0	56
Gallstones (%)	22.0	41.7	9.1	16.7	0
Cholecystectomy (%)	13.0	5.4	0	5.3	0
Hb (g/L)	31–82 (65 ± 12)	36–83 (61 ± 10)	42–71 (58 ± 10)	44–80 (59 ± 12)	40–58 (47 ± 7.0)
Before splenectomy	–	–	3.5–4.3 (3.9)	–	–
After splenectomy	6.5–7.6 (7.0)	5.3–7.2 (6.4)	6.4–8.7 (7.2)	4.1–7.6 (6.1)	4.0–5.5 (4.9 ± ?)

Platelets (10⁹/L)					
Before splenectomy	157–898 (400.5)	223–749 (432)	203–576 (365)	294–474 (392)	287–503 (364.5)
After splenectomy	379–918 (742)	253–1051 (677)	411–948 (690)	303–974 (679)	335–814 (574)
Hb F (g/L)	5.0–38 (20 ± 12)	2.0–37 (17 ± 7.0)	5.0–25 14 ± 5.0)	4.0–27 (15 ± 3.0)	4.0–19 (9.0 ± 4.0)
Hb F (%)	8–60 (32 ± 13)	3–48 (29 ± 10)	10–34 (20 ± 6)	10–42 (26 ± 11)	6–42 (17 ± 8)
β-Thalassemia Mutation (%)					
IVS-1-5 (G→C)	52.0	73.5	74.6	59.1	75.0
IVS-1-1 (G→A)	39.0	26.5	27·3	22·7	13·0
Others	9·0	0	8·1	18·8	12·0
α⁺-Thalassemia (%)	8·0	8·1	7·1	4·5	6
αα/αα (%)	4·7	3·0	0	0	0
Xmn 1 +/+ (no.)	8	5	0	0	0
Xmn 1 −/− (no.)	2	2	2	0	4
ALT (U/L)				5	
HIC (mg iron per gram liver, dry weight)	2.5–26 (9.3)	2.7–42 (14.8)	5.4–52 (16.7)	4.7–30 (15.0)	4.2–28 (16.3)

Abbreviations: ALT, alanine aminotransferase; HIC, hepatic iron concentration.

From Olivieri NF, Muraca GM, O'Donnell A, et al. Studies in haemoglobin E beta-thalassaemia. Br J Haematol 2008;141(3):390; expanded and altered from Premawardhena A, Fisher CA, Olivieri NF, et al. Haemoglobin E beta thalassaemia in Sri Lanka. Lancet 2005;366(9495):1467–70; with permission.

growth, delayed sexual maturation, and quality of life less than 5 on the 10-point scale. Group 5 comprised patients unable to function without transfusions.

FACTORS THAT INFLUENCE THE CLINICAL SEVERITY OF HEMOGLOBIN E/β-THALASSEMIA

There is an increased understanding of the genetic and environmental factors that influence the clinical course and severity of anemia in HbE/β-thalassemia (**Box 1**). These include the type of β-thalassemia mutation coinherited with HbE, the coinheritance of α-thalassemia, and the coinheritance of polymorphisms shown to be associated with increased synthesis of hemoglobin F (HbF).

Inheritance of the β-Thalassemia Allele Trans to HbE Allele

In early studies Thai investigators[27] suggested that patients who coinherit a mild β-thalassemia allele with HbE might have mild disease, whereas those who coinherited severe β^+ or β^0-thalassemia alleles might have more severe disease. More recent studies suggest that the severity of the β mutation is an important, but uncommon, cause of the clinical diversity of HbE/β-thalassemia. In 1993, Winichagoon and colleagues[27] studied the mutations in 90 Thai patients with steady-state hemoglobin concentrations varying from 4.2 to 12.6 g/dL. The same severe β-thalassemia mutation was observed in patients with mild as well as severe anemia. Thirty-six of these patients had a milder clinical phenotype. Nearly half (42%) coinherited a clinical modifying mutation. However, a less severe β-thalassemia mutation was only 1 of several genetic modifiers. Other modifiers included $XmnI$ polymorphism, α^+ thalassemia, and hemoglobin H-Constant Spring.

A more detailed analysis of the effects of the β-thalassemia allele on clinical severity within this population was performed in 2000.[26] A genotype responsible for a mild HbE/β-thalassemia phenotype was documented in 6 out of 88 patients. This mild phenotype resulted from the interaction between HbE and the mutation at nucleotide −28 in the ATA box of the β-globin gene. However, patients with mild disease usually had a severe β-thalassemia mutation. Studies in other HbE/β-thalassemia populations

---

Box 1
Modifying factors responsible for phenotypic diversity in E-B-thalassemia

Genetic Modifiers

β-Thalassemia mutation

Coinheritance of α-thalassemia

Mutations associated with increased HbF synthesis

　Xmnl polymorphism. Single nucleotide polymorphisms (SNPs) within the β gene cluster (chr.11p15). Quantitative trait loci (QTL) with increased F on chromosomes 6q23, 8q, and xp22

　SNPs in the BCL11A gene on chromosome 2p16.1

Polymorphism of the UGT1*1 gene

Serum erythropoietin concentration

Environmental Modifiers

Malaria

Splenectomy

from India and Sri Lanka confirm that the β-thalassemia mutation plays a limited role in the clinical severity of this population.[24,37] Therefore, the β-thalassemia mutation alone does not account for the wide phenotypic variation observed in this population, and other modifying genetic factors must be responsible.[26]

α-Thalassemia

Patients with HbE/β-thalassemia who coinherit a determinant for α-thalassemia should, in theory, have fewer unmatched α-globin chains, leading to the more balanced globin chain synthesis, and resulting in a milder phenotype. Early studies suggested that patients with HbE/β-thalassemia with an α^+-thalassemia allele averaged higher hemoglobins than those without α-thalassemia.[26,38]

Recent studies support the beneficial effect of α-thalassemia on HbE/β-thalassemia but indicate that clinical severity is multifactorial. The effect of coinheritance of different copy numbers of the α-globin genes on the severity of HbE/β-thalassemia was analyzed in 925 Thai patients with HbE/β-thalassemia, aged 2 to 77 years, who showed a wide range of steady-state hemoglobin levels (3.2–12.1 g/dL); 8.8% of the study population had a form of α-thalassemia.[39] Deletional α^+-thalassemia was most often identified ($-\alpha^{3.7}/\alpha\alpha$ (n = 51), $-\alpha^{4.2}/\alpha\alpha$ (n = 8), and $-\alpha^{3.7}/-\alpha^{3.7}$ (n = 1)). Two-thirds of the patients with normal α-globin gene numbers, and about a third (32%) required regular blood transfusions. By contrast, none of the patients with α-thalassemia required regular blood transfusions, although several had received 1 or more transfusions during intercurrent illnesses. The second group of patients with α-thalassemia was further divided into 6 subgroups according to the different α-thalassemia mutations identified. The mean age at presentation of those with α-thalassemia (10.4 ± 9.2 years) was much older than for patients without α-thalassemia (3.7 ± 5.5 years). The data suggested that patients with more severe α-thalassemia mutations may have had a better clinical picture.

Within a longitudinal study of patients with HbE/β-thalassemia in Sri Lanka,[24] the influence of α-thalassemia in 5 groups of patients classified according to clinical severity was analyzed. The restriction of α^+-thalassemia alleles to the groups with the mildest phenotypes suggests an ameliorating effect of α-thalassemia on the severity of HbE/β-thalassemia. However, there are conflicting reports, and mild HbE/β-thalassemia occurs without this mutation.[40] In 148 patients in northeast Thailand (including 103 patients classified as severe and 45 as thalassemia intermedia), there was no evidence that coinheritance of α-thalassemia was a factor modifying the severity of HbE/β-thalassemia.

In summary, coinheritance with α-thalassemia seems to be a major genetic factor modifying the clinical phenotype of HbE/β-thalassemia. Many patients who coinherit α-thalassemia may be diagnosed later in life. The presence of α-thalassemia genes should always be considered in mild cases of HbE/β-thalassemia.

Determinants Associated with Increased HbF Synthesis

Several studies provide evidence supporting polymorphisms that affect HbF synthesis, including *Xmn1* polymorphism, BCL11A, and several other genetic loci.

Xmn1 polymorphism is an important modifying factor in HbF synthesis in normals and in HbE/β-thalassemia. In Chinese β-thalassemia heterozygotes and in healthy Europeans, the *Xmn1* polymorphism accounts for approximately 9% to 13% of the genetic variance of HbF.[41–43] Thai patients with HbE/β-thalassemia and an *Xmn1* +/+ genotype[27] had higher total hemoglobin levels (8.5 g/dL vs <7.0 g/dL) and HbF levels than patients with an *Xmn1* −/− genotype. These findings were consistent with previous findings suggesting that homozygosity for the *Xmn1* polymorphism may be necessary to ameliorate the severity of thalassemia.

In a longitudinal study by Premawardhena and colleagues[24] of patients with HbE/β-thalassemia in Sri Lanka, there was a strong positive correlation between the hemoglobin, fetal hemoglobin concentrations, and homozygosity for the *Xmn1* polymorphism. Patients with the *Xmn1* +/+ genotype were only found in the mild phenotypes. Patients with severe disease presenting at a young age were likely to have *Xmn1* −/−. Others have reported that patients with *Xmn1* −/− were more likely to present at a young age and be transfused compared with patients who were heterozygous (±).[37] Other studies have analyzed the association of several SNPs within the β-globin gene cluster with disease severity.[44] Although SNPs in the locus control region and the δ gene showed severity, the strongest association was with the *Xmn1* polymorphism. Although there are some conflicting data, overall homozygosity for the *Xmn1* polymorphism is one of the most important factors in modifying the severity of thalassemia.[45]

Given the clinical heterogeneity of HbE/β-thalassemia, it is likely that additional genetic factors modifying disease severity await discovery. Association studies are being conducted to elucidate the role of genetic polymorphisms known to influence globin gene expression and erythropoiesis as modifiers of disease severity in this disorder. Other polymorphisms, QTL associated with increased fetal hemoglobin production, have been described on chromosomes 6q23, 8q, and Xp22.[46–48] Recently, 6 SNPs in the BCL11A gene on chromosome 2p16.1 were reported to be associated with F cell numbers in a study of 179 unrelated normal subjects from a British twin registry,[41] and with fetal hemoglobin levels among Sardinians with β-thalassemia. The contribution of the QTL on chromosome 6q23 to the genetic variance of HbF/F cells is estimated to be 19%, and the contribution of BCL11A to be 15%.[41–43]

Sedgewick and colleagues[49] reported that SNPs in BCL11A were associated with fetal hemoglobin production in Thais with either β-thalassemia or HbE trait (as well as in African Americans with sickle cell anemia) and with F cell numbers in Chinese individuals with β-thalassemia trait. Although the studies are limited, it is likely that BCL11a polymorphisms are also important modulators of fetal hemoglobin in HbE/β-thalassemia.

Sripichai and colleagues[50] analyzed 1060 patients with HbE/β-thalassemia for 22 SNPs within 7 genes known to influence globin gene expression and erythropoiesis. These included β-protein 1, erythropoietin (EPO), and transcription factors EKLF, GATA-1, and NF-E2. No statistically significant difference between mild and severe phenotypes was observed for the polymorphisms in the candidate genes. A later genome-wide association study was conducted in 618 patients with HbE/β-thalassemia.[51] Twenty-three SNPs in 3 independent genes/regions identified as being significantly associated with disease severity were studied. The highest association was observed with SNPs in the β-globin gene cluster (chr.11p15); rs2071348 of the HBBP1 gene. The next highest association was identified in the intergenic region between the HBS1L and MYB genes (chr.6q23). The third region was located in the BCL11A gene. The findings in these 3 loci were replicated in an independent cohort of 174 Indonesian patients.[45] These data suggest that several genetic loci act in concert to influence fetal hemoglobin levels of patients with HbE/β-thalassemia, with these 3 reported loci and the α-globin gene locus identified as the best predictors of disease severity.[51]

Other investigators[52] have reported an association of the HBS1L-SNP7 polymorphism in exon 1 of the β-globin gene with HbF levels in 30 selected patients with mild and severe phenotypes of HbE/β-thalassemia, different levels of fetal hemoglobin, and different *XmnI* polymorphisms. Genotyping for a C32T polymorphism identified in a potential E-box binding site of HBS1L in exon 1 was then performed in 455 patients with HbE/β-thalassemia. HBS1L-SNP7 had a slight, but statistically significant, effect in modulating absolute fetal hemoglobin levels among patients with HbE/β-thalassemia and *Xmn1* −/−. The effect of HBS1L-SNP7 was more pronounced among patients with *Xmn1* ±. However, the overall conclusion was that this polymorphism is of minor effect in comparison with the influence of *Xmn1*.

Other Modifying Factors

The α-hemoglobin stabilizing protein gene

The α-hemoglobin stabilizing protein, a chaperone of α-globin, has been suggested as another genetic modifier.[53] However, it was not found to be a modifying factor of clinical severity in Thai patients with β-thalassemia.[54] In patients with HbE/β-thalassemia in Sri Lanka, Premawardhena and colleagues[24] found no difference in the distribution of haplotypes of this gene between patients with mild and severe phenotypes; this has been confirmed by other work.[50]

Bilirubin metabolism

Chronic hyperbilirubinemia, gallstone formation, and gall bladder disease in patients with HbE/β-thalassemia may significantly worsen the phenotype of the disease. There is now clear evidence that the inherited variability in the function of the gene for UDP-glucuronosyltransferase-1 (UGT1*1, the enzyme responsible for hepatic glucuronidation of bilirubin) underlies the chronic hyperbilirubinemia of Gilbert syndrome,[55] some cases of thalassemia trait,[56] as well as the variation in the frequency of gallstones in patients with hereditary spherocytosis.[57] The increased level of bilirubin in these disorders has been related to a polymorphism of the promoter of the UGT1*1 gene.

Premawardhena and colleagues[58] showed that the UGT*1 genotype is also important in the genesis of gallstones in patients with HbE/β-thalassemia. He found significantly higher bilirubin levels in patients with HbE/β-thalassemia and the 7/7 genotype of the *UGTA1A* promoter, compared with those with 6/6 and 6/7 genotypes ($P = .032$ and .0015, respectively). Patients with the 7/7 genotype were also more likely to develop gallstones at more than 15 years of age ($P \geq .0008$).

Coinheritance of other hematologic disorders

Coinheritance of other hematologic abnormalities may contribute to the variation in phenotype in patients with HbE/β-thalassemia. Although pyrimidine 5 nucleotidase-I (P5N-I) deficiency typically presents as mild hemolytic anemia, a family in which the interaction between P5N-I deficiency and homozygous HbE resulted in severe hemolytic anemia has been reported.[59] This individual was shown to have a mutation in the P5N-1 gene[60] affecting expression of the P5N-1 enzyme, believed to be susceptible to free radical damage. Coinheritance of complete P5N-I deficiency and the homozygous HbE state results in a hemolytic phenotype that is more severe than would be expected with either condition alone, raising a possibility that coincidental inhibition of P5N-I activity may contribute to the severe hemolytic phenotype associated with some unstable hemoglobin variants, including HbE.

Variation in iron loading

A common dilemma often encountered in the clinic is whether the poor growth and delayed sexual maturation observed in many patients with HbE/β-thalassemia is a result of chronic anemia, iron overload, or a combination of these. As has been reported in a study in which precise measurements of iron loading were determined systematically, many patients with a clinical history of few transfusions have substantial iron burdens and evidence of end-organ damage that is not evident by screening tests.[61] Further data on gastrointestinal iron overload in the Indian subcontinent and southeast Asia are still awaited. Although some studies have searched for the common hemochromatosis alleles in those regions and found them to be rare,[62–64] Lok and colleagues[65] recently reported several novel mutations in hemojuvelin and hepcidin, and mutations in the SLC40A1 gene, which encodes for ferroportin, in patients originating from countries not normally associated with hemochromatosis, resulting in different presentations of iron overload. These findings suggest that primary iron overload may not be as rare as was previously believed in these geographic areas. Studies to determine the effect of variability in iron loading on the phenotype of HbE/β-thalassemia are urgently needed.

IS ADAPTATION TO ANEMIA A MODIFYING FACTOR IN HBE/β-THALASSEMIA?

HbE/β-thalassemia is characterized by different clinical manifestations at particular stages of development. Whether this reflects developmental changes in adaptation to anemia, or other mechanisms, is presently unclear. Serum EPO concentrations assayed in at least 5 years of observation in patients with HbE/β-thalassemia were significantly correlated with steady-state hemoglobin concentration, with a significant decline in EPO response to anemia observed with age.[24] Age and EPO response to anemia were independent variables. Extended studies of adaptation to anemia in patients with HbE/β-thalassemia led by the same group of investigators in 110 individuals in Sri Lanka[66] again observed a reduced EPO response at different ages for a particular hemoglobin concentration. The effect of age on EPO was independent of the degree of anemia, suggesting that age has a direct effect on the background level of EPO production. A group of patients with HbE/β-thalassemia were then evaluated with respect to the variation in the rate of splenic enlargement, one of the consequences of high levels of EPO production in thalassemia.[67] Serial splenic examinations showed little enlargement over time in older patients who were anemic, but mildly ill. In contrast, more-severe younger patients with the same hemoglobin range as the older, milder patients showed significant progressive splenic enlargement.

The lower level of EPO response in the group of children with mild phenotypes compared with the entire cohort is of particular interest. Although in many cases genetic modifiers that influence the severity of the phenotype in these children have been identified, the reason for milder disease in many is not clear; the possibility that this could be related to inherent differences in EPO response remains to be determined. Because high levels of EPO production in thalassemia result in considerable expansion of the erythroid mass,[68] and because erythropoiesis in severe thalassemia is largely ineffective, the effect of extremely high levels of EPO on increasing the hemoglobin level is limited but, at the same time, is responsible for many disease complications including hepatosplenomegaly and bone deformity.

What is the significance of these findings, if confirmed? First, they may suggest that developmental changes in EPO responsiveness to severe anemia have important implications for the clinical management of HbE/β-thalassemia. The high EPO response in early childhood, and its decline with age, may be partly responsible for some of the phenotypic instability in this disorder during the early years of life.[24] If the EPO response, at a particular hemoglobin level, declines with age, the drive to erythroid expansion will also diminish and, if the magnitude of the EPO response is suppressed by transfusion at times of maximum production, such complications might be avoided. It follows that it should be possible to stop transfusion in a significant number of patients when EPO response declines. In some of the patients described by Premawardhena and colleagues,[24] it was possible to stop transfusion in those aged between 9 and 50 years without any deleterious effect. A program of transient transfusion of this type would save badly needed resources in the developing countries in which this disease is so common.

These findings await confirmation in other populations. Of 2 previous reports of EPO response to anemia in HbE/β-thalassemia,[69,70] one[70] reported a difference in an overall pattern of response between children and adults, but this did not reach statistical significance. In another study of patients with sickle cell anemia, 10 adults seemed to show a less robust increase in serum EPO at approximately the same steady-state hemoglobin concentration than those of children.[71] Although there have been no extensive studies of EPO response at different age groups in patients with HbE/β-thalassemia and profound anemia, longitudinal analysis of individuals with milder forms of anemia of varying causes have yielded inconsistent findings. In some cases, there seem to have been some blunting of response in older patients, whereas in others, the response appeared to be similar across the age range.[72-74]

ENVIRONMENTAL INFLUENCES ON THE PHENOTYPE OF HBE/β-THALASSEMIA
Malaria

One of the major environmental issues in many Asian countries is the high frequency of the transmission of malaria, both *Plasmodium falciparum* and *Plasmodium vivax*. Although the latter was believed to be a mild disorder, recently it has been found that it is much more severe than was previously believed and is causing a major problem in many Asian countries.[75,76] Until recently, malaria of both varieties was a major problem in Sri Lanka, although in recent years the transmission rate has dropped considerably. Between 2002 and 2003, 93 patients with HbE/β-thalassemia were studied and a high proportion of them were positive for antibodies to *P vivax* and *P falciparum*; among the younger patients 28% were positive for *P vivax* using DNA analysis, a particularly sensitive approach to diagnosis of malaria in regions of low transmission.[67] Follow-up studies including age-matched controls indicated that there was a significantly higher level of malarial antibodies, particularly to *P vivax* and in young children, in those with HbE/β-thalassemia compared with the control population. Among those with HbE/β-thalassemia, there was a highly significant increase in antibody levels in those who had been splenectomized, compared with those with intact spleens, although the levels in the latter were still significantly higher than those in the control population. There was a correlation between the clinical phenotype, particularly related to spleen size, and malarial antibody levels. These findings suggest that children with HbE/β-thalassemia may be more prone to *P vivax* malaria in particular, perhaps as a result of their young red cell populations; *P vivax* has a particular propensity for invading younger red cells. If these findings are confirmed in other parts of Asia, it will be extremely important to provide prophylaxis against both forms of malaria for patients with HbE/β-thalassemia. Because this is a complex and potentially expensive approach, it is vital that similar studies be performed, particularly in parts of India and other regions in Asia where there is a high transmission rate of *P vivax*.

RECOMMENDATIONS FOR PRESENT MANAGEMENT OF PATIENTS AND FUTURE STUDIES

Because of the facility of many patients with HbE/β-thalassemia to adapt to low hemoglobin levels, hemoglobin per se may be of limited value in deciding on transfusion. No patient with HbE/β-thalassemia should ever receive regular transfusion without a long period of observation of growth and development, quality of life, and spleen size. By contrast, age of presentation, homozygosity for the *Xmn1* polymorphism, and coexistent α-thalassemia are valuable prognostic indicators.

Several important questions remain. Although some information has been obtained about the clinical course and reasons for the phenotypic heterogeneity of HbE/β-thalassemia, this type of cross-sectional study of different ages suffers from the same difficulties as many studies of the intermediate forms of thalassemia. In particular, because of rapidly changing phenotypes, variable medical interventions, and the ill-understood effects of age on phenotype, it is difficult to accurately characterize disease severity. Hence, although some genetic factors have been defined as possible modifiers, the remarkable phenotypic diversity of this condition is still not well understood. Such understanding would be augmented by a cohort study from birth or, because a significant proportion of patients with this condition present later than the first year of life, in a group of children less than 12 years of age, with phenotypes defined as clearly as possible before any form of medical intervention.

Given what has been learned, what is the optimal management of patients with HbE/β-thalassemia who fail to adapt to anemia? Although Premawardhena and colleagues[24] presented some evidence for benefits on growth and development following splenectomy, it is unclear whether the frequent use of splenectomy is acceptable; morbidity and mortality caused by infection at all ages was significantly higher in splenectomized patients. But because it now seems that marrow expansion and increasing splenomegaly are less marked in older patients, a trial or observational study of transient transfusion during the period of major expansion seems justified.

It is also important to establish the reasons for variable iron loading, and the problems of patients who experience poor growth and sexual retardation in the absence of severe iron loading. Further exploration of individual responses to anemia is required. There are limited data on the environmental factors that may modify the course of this disease; the recrudescence of malaria may be an important factor. It is clear that the costs of thalassemia care represent an important proportion of the future health care budgets of Asia.[77] Hence, consideration of general guidelines for management, including careful consideration of maintaining such patients off transfusions, have been suggested for the management of HbE/β-thalassemia.[36]

REFERENCES

1. Modell B, Darlison M. Global epidemiology of haemoglobin disorders and derived service indicators. Bull World Health Organ 2008;86(6):480–7.
2. Chen S, Eldor A, Barshtein G, et al. Enhanced aggregability of red blood cells of beta-thalassemia major patients. Am J Physiol 1996;270(6 Pt 2):H1951–6.
3. de Silva S, Fisher CA, Premawardhena A, et al. Thalassaemia in Sri Lanka: implications for the future health burden of Asian populations. Sri Lanka Thalassaemia Study Group. Lancet 2000;355(9206):786–91.
4. Premawardhena A, De Silva S, Arambepola M, et al. Thalassemia in Sri Lanka: a progress report. Hum Mol Genet 2004;13(Spec No 2):R203–6.
5. Vichinsky EP. Report of proceedings: 1999 international conference on E-B thalassemia. J Pediatr Hematol Oncol 2000;22(6):550.
6. Weatherall DJ, Clegg JB. Inherited haemoglobin disorders: an increasing global health problem. Bull World Health Organ 2001;79(8):704–12.

7. WHO. Guidelines for the control of haemoglobin disorders. Report of the VIth Annual Meeting of the WHO Working Group on Haemoglobinopathies. Geneva (Switzerland): World Health Organization; 1989. Cagliairi, Sardinia.
8. Weatherall DJ, Clegg JB. The thalassaemia syndromes. 4th edition. Oxford (UK): Blackwell Science Ltd; 2001.
9. Flint J, Harding RM, Boyce AJ, et al. The population genetics of the haemoglobinopathies. In: Higgs DR, Weatherall D, editors. Baillière's clinical haematology; 'Haemoglobinopathies'. London: Baillière Tindall and WB Saunders; 1998. p. 1–51.
10. Angastiniotis M, Modell B. Global epidemiology of hemoglobin disorders. Ann N Y Acad Sci 1998;850:251–69.
11. Lorey F. Asian immigration and public health in California: thalassemia in newborns in California. J Pediatr Hematol Oncol 2000;22(6):564–6.
12. Lorey F, Charoenkwan P, Witkowska HE, et al. Hb H hydrops foetalis syndrome: a case report and review of literature. Br J Haematol 2001;115(1):72–8.
13. Lorey F, Cunningham G, Vichinsky EP, et al. Universal newborn screening for Hb H disease in California. Genet Test 2001;5(2):93–100.
14. Weatherall DJ. The inherited diseases of hemoglobin are an emerging global health burden. Blood 2010;115:4331–6.
15. Weatherall DJ, Clegg JB. Thalassemia–a global public health problem. Nat Med 1996;2(8):847–9.
16. Rees DC, Styles L, Vichinsky EP, et al. The hemoglobin E syndromes. Ann N Y Acad Sci 1998;850:334–43.
17. Agarwal S, Gulati R, Singh K. Hemoglobin E-beta thalassemia in Uttar Pradesh. Indian Pediatr 1997;34(4):287–92.
18. Chernoff AI, Minnich V, Nanakorn S, et al. Studies on hemoglobin E.I. The clinical, hematologic, and genetic characteristics of the hemoglobin E syndromes. J Lab Clin Med 1956;47(3):455–89.
19. Chhotray GP, Dash BP, Ranjit MR, et al. Haemoglobin E/beta-thalassaemia - an experience in the eastern Indian state of Orissa. Acta Haematol 2003;109(4): 214–6.
20. De M, Das SK, Bhattacharya DK, et al. The occurrence of beta-thalassemia mutation and its interaction with hemoglobin E in the eastern India. Int J Hematol 1997; 66(1):31–4.
21. Fucharoen S, Winichagoon P. Hemoglobinopathies in Southeast Asia. Hemoglobin 1987;11(1):65–88.
22. George E, Wong HB. Hb E beta +-thalassaemia in west Malaysia: clinical features in the most common beta-thalassaemia mutation of the Malays [IVS 1-5 (G→C)]. Singapore Med J 1993;34(6):500–3.
23. Piplani S. Hemoglobin E disorders in the North East India. J Assoc Physicians India 2000;48(11):1082–4.
24. Premawardhena A, Fisher CA, Olivieri NF, et al. Haemoglobin E beta thalassaemia in Sri Lanka. Lancet 2005;366(9495):1467–70.
25. Wasi P, Na-Nakorn S, Pootrakul S, et al. Alpha- and beta-thalassemia in Thailand. Ann N Y Acad Sci 1969;165(1):60–82.
26. Winichagoon P, Fucharoen S, Chen P, et al. Genetic factors affecting clinical severity in beta-thalassemia syndromes. J Pediatr Hematol Oncol 2000;22(6): 573–80.
27. Winichagoon P, Thonglairoam V, Fucharoen S, et al. Severity differences in beta-thalassaemia/haemoglobin E syndromes: implication of genetic factors. Br J Haematol 1993;83(4):633–9.

28. Fucharoen S, Ketvichit P, Pootrakul P, et al. Clinical manifestation of beta-thalassemia/hemoglobin E disease. J Pediatr Hematol Oncol 2000;22(6):552–7.

29. Weatherall DJ. Hemoglobin E beta-thalassemia: an increasingly common disease with some diagnostic pitfalls. J Pediatr 1998;132(5):765–7.

30. Orkin SH, Kazazian HH Jr, Antonarakis SE, et al. Abnormal RNA processing due to the exon mutation of beta E-globin gene. Nature 1982;300(5894):768–9.

31. Datta P, Basu S, Chakravarty SB, et al. Enhanced oxidative cross-linking of hemoglobin E with spectrin and loss of erythrocyte membrane asymmetry in hemoglobin Ebeta-thalassemia. Blood Cells Mol Dis 2006;37(2):77–81.

32. Pootrakul P, Sirankapracha P, Hemsorach S, et al. A correlation of erythrokinetics, ineffective erythropoiesis, and erythroid precursor apoptosis in Thai patients with thalassemia. Blood 2000;96(7):2606–12.

33. Jetsrisuparb A, Sanchaisuriya K, Fucharoen G, et al. Development of severe anemia during fever episodes in patients with hemoglobin E trait and hemoglobin H disease combinations. J Pediatr Hematol Oncol 2006;28(4):249–53.

34. Sripichai O, Makarasara W, Munkongdee T, et al. A scoring system for the classification of beta-thalassemia/Hb E disease severity. Am J Hematol 2008;83(6):482–4.

35. Olivieri NF, Brittenham GM. Iron-chelating therapy and the treatment of thalassemia. Blood 1997;89(3):739–61.

36. Olivieri NF, Muraca GM, O'Donnell A, et al. Studies in haemoglobin E beta-thalassaemia. Br J Haematol 2008;141(3):388–97.

37. Panigrahi I, Agarwal S, Gupta T, et al. Hemoglobin E-beta thalassemia: factors affecting phenotype. Indian Pediatr 2005;42(4):357–62.

38. Winichagoon P, Fucharoen S, Weatherall D, et al. Concomitant inheritance of alpha-thalassemia in beta 0-thalassemia/Hb E disease. Am J Hematol 1985;20(3):217–22.

39. Sripichai O, Munkongdee T, Kumkhaek C, et al. Coinheritance of the different copy numbers of alpha-globin gene modifies severity of beta-thalassemia/Hb E disease. Ann Hematol 2008;87(5):375–9.

40. Sharma V, Saxena R. Effect of alpha-gene numbers on phenotype of HbE/beta thalassemia patients. Ann Hematol 2009;88(10):1035–6.

41. Menzel S, Garner C, Gut I, et al. A QTL influencing F cell production maps to a gene encoding a zinc-finger protein on chromosome 2p15. Nat Genet 2007;39(10):1197–9.

42. Gibney GT, Panhuysen CI, So JC, et al. Variation and heritability of Hb F and F-cells among beta-thalassemia heterozygotes in Hong Kong. Am J Hematol 2008;83(6):458–64.

43. Garner C, Tatu T, Reittie JE, et al. Genetic influences on F cells and other hematologic variables: a twin heritability study. Blood 2000;95(1):342–6.

44. Ma Q, Abel K, Sripichai O, et al. Beta-globin gene cluster polymorphisms are strongly associated with severity of HbE/beta(0)-thalassemia. Clin Genet 2007;72(6):497–505.

45. Nuntakarn L, Fucharoen S, Fucharoen G, et al. Molecular, hematological and clinical aspects of thalassemia major and thalassemia intermedia associated with Hb E-beta-thalassemia in Northeast Thailand. Blood Cells Mol Dis 2009;42(1):32–5.

46. Thein SL, Menzel S, Peng X, et al. Intergenic variants of HBS1L-MYB are responsible for a major quantitative trait locus on chromosome 6q23 influencing fetal hemoglobin levels in adults. Proc Natl Acad Sci U S A 2007;104(27):11346–51.

47. Garner C, Menzel S, Martin C, et al. Interaction between two quantitative trait loci affects fetal haemoglobin expression. Ann Hum Genet 2005;69(Pt 6):707–14.

48. Dover GJ, Smith KD, Chang YC, et al. Fetal hemoglobin levels in sickle cell disease and normal individuals are partially controlled by an X-linked gene located at Xp22.2. Blood 1992;80(3):816–24.
49. Sedgewick AE, Timofeev N, Sebastiani P, et al. BCL11A is a major HbF quantitative trait locus in three different populations with beta-hemoglobinopathies. Blood Cells Mol Dis 2008;41(3):255–8.
50. Sripichai O, Whitacre J, Munkongdee T, et al. Genetic analysis of candidate modifier polymorphisms in Hb E-beta 0-thalassemia patients. Ann N Y Acad Sci 2005; 1054:433–8.
51. Nuinoon M, Makarasara W, Mushiroda T, et al. A genome-wide association identified the common genetic variants influence disease severity in beta0-thalassemia/hemoglobin E. Hum Genet 2010;127(3):303–14.
52. Pandit RA, Svasti S, Sripichai O, et al. Association of SNP in exon 1 of HBS1L with hemoglobin F level in beta0-thalassemia/hemoglobin E. Int J Hematol 2008;88(4): 357–61.
53. Kihm AJ, Kong Y, Hong W, et al. An abundant erythroid protein that stabilizes free alpha-haemoglobin. Nature 2002;417(6890):758–63.
54. Viprakasit V, Tanphaichitr VS, Chinchang W, et al. Evaluation of alpha hemoglobin stabilizing protein (AHSP) as a genetic modifier in patients with beta thalassemia. Blood 2004;103(9):3296–9.
55. Bosma PJ, Chowdhury JR, Bakker C, et al. The genetic basis of the reduced expression of bilirubin UDP-glucuronosyltransferase 1 in Gilbert's syndrome. N Engl J Med 1995;333(18):1171–5.
56. Sampietro M, Iolascon A. Molecular pathology of Crigler-Najjar type I and II and Gilbert's syndromes. Haematologica 1999;84(2):150–7.
57. del Giudice EM, Perrotta S, Nobili B, et al. Coinheritance of Gilbert syndrome increases the risk for developing gallstones in patients with hereditary spherocytosis. Blood 1999;94(7):2259–62.
58. Premawardhena A, Fisher CA, Fathiu F, et al. Genetic determinants of jaundice and gallstones in haemoglobin E beta thalassaemia. Lancet 2001;357(9272): 1945–6.
59. Rees DC, Duley J, Simmonds HA, et al. Interaction of hemoglobin E and pyrimidine 5′ nucleotidase deficiency. Blood 1996;88(7):2761–7.
60. Escuredo E, Marinaki AM, Duley JA, et al. The genetic basis of the interaction between pyrimidine 5′ nucleotidase I deficiency and hemoglobin E. Nucleosides Nucleotides Nucleic Acids 2004;23(8–9):1261–3.
61. Olivieri NF, De Silva S, Premawardena A, et al. Iron overload and iron-chelating therapy in hemoglobin E-beta thalassemia. J Pediatr Hematol Oncol 2000; 22(6):593–7.
62. Pointon JJ, Viprakasit V, Miles KL, et al. Hemochromatosis gene (HFE) mutations in South East Asia: a potential for iron overload. Blood Cells Mol Dis 2003;30(3): 302–6.
63. Merryweather-Clarke AT, Pointon JJ, Shearman JD, et al. Global prevalence of putative haemochromatosis mutations. J Med Genet 1997;34(4):275–8.
64. Merryweather-Clarke AT, Pointon JJ, Jouanolle AM, et al. Geography of HFE C282Y and H63D mutations. Genet Test 2000;4(2):183–98.
65. Lok CY, Merryweather-Clarke AT, Viprakasit V, et al. Iron overload in the Asian community. Blood 2009;114(1):20–5.
66. O'Donnell A, Premawardhena A, Arambepola M, et al. Age-related changes in adaptation to severe anemia in childhood in developing countries. Proc Natl Acad Sci U S A 2007;104(22):9440–4.

67. O'Donnell A, Premawardhena A, Arambepola M, et al. Interaction of malaria with a common form of severe thalassemia in an Asian population. Proc Natl Acad Sci U S A 2009;106(44):18716–21.

68. Huebers HA, Beguin Y, Pootrakul P, et al. Intact transferrin receptors in human plasma and their relation to erythropoiesis. Blood 1990;75(1):102–7.

69. Paritpokee N, Wiwanitkit V, Bhokaisawan N, et al. Serum erythropoietin levels in pediatric patients with beta-thalassemia/hemoglobin E. Clin Lab 2002;48(11–12): 631–4.

70. Sukpanichnant S, Opartkiattikul N, Fucharoen S, et al. Difference in pattern of erythropoietin response between beta-thalassemia/hemoglobin E children and adults. Southeast Asian J Trop Med Public Health 1997;28(Suppl 3):134–7.

71. Sherwood JB, Goldwasser E, Chilcote R, et al. Sickle cell anemia patients have low erythropoietin levels for their degree of anemia. Blood 1986;67(1):46–9.

72. Ershler WB, Sheng S, McKelvey J, et al. Serum erythropoietin and aging: a longitudinal analysis. J Am Geriatr Soc 2005;53(8):1360–5.

73. Powers JS, Krantz SB, Collins JC, et al. Erythropoietin response to anemia as a function of age. J Am Geriatr Soc 1991;39(1):30–2.

74. Goodnough LT, Price TH, Parvin CA. The endogenous erythropoietin response and the erythropoietic response to blood loss anemia: the effects of age and gender. J Lab Clin Med 1995;126(1):57–64.

75. Mendis C, Gamage-Mendis AC, De Zoysa AP, et al. Characteristics of malaria transmission in Kataragama, Sri Lanka: a focus for immuno-epidemiological studies. Am J Trop Med Hyg 1990;42(4):298–308.

76. Mendis K, Sina BJ, Marchesini P, et al. The neglected burden of *Plasmodium vivax* malaria. Am J Trop Med Hyg 2001;64(1–2 Suppl):97–106.

77. Weatherall DJ, Kwiatkowski D. Hematologic disorders of children in developing countries. Pediatr Clin North Am 2002;49(6):1149–64.

Protein Quality Control During Erythropoiesis and Hemoglobin Synthesis

Eugene Khandros[a], Mitchell J. Weiss, MD, PhD[b],*

KEYWORDS

• Hemoglobin • Thalassemia • Protein quality control

Hemoglobin synthesis during erythroid maturation is tightly coordinated to maximize the production of functional hemoglobin A ($\alpha_2\beta_2$) and to balance the levels of individual globin subunits, which are unstable and cytotoxic in the absence of their partners. The importance of this homeostasis is illustrated in β-thalassemia, a common inherited anemia in which β-globin gene mutations cause a relative excess of free α-globin, which forms intracellular precipitates and reactive oxygen species.[1] Accumulation of free α chains destroys erythroid precursors by ineffective erythropoiesis and also shortens the life span of mature erythrocytes. The phenotype of β-thalassemia is largely determined by the degree of free α-globin excess and is characterized by minimal symptoms in β-thalassemia minor to severe symptoms in β-thalassemia major. Individuals who are heterozygous for a β-globin null allele (β-thalassemia trait) are usually unaffected despite synthesis of 2-fold excess α-globin, indicating that erythroid precursors are able to neutralize significant amounts of free α-globin. Defining the associated protective mechanisms will provide insights into basic erythroid biology and may also have implications for treating β-thalassemia.

Virtually all cell types detoxify and/or degrade potentially damaging unstable proteins through mechanisms termed protein quality control. Numerous diseases ensue when the levels of unstable proteins exceed tissue capacities for quality control. Excessive protein misfolding, aggregation, and consequent toxicities are linked to the

Work at the authors' laboratory on globin chain metabolism and thalassemia is supported by National Institutes of Health grants 5R01HL087427-04 (M.J.W), 5R01DK061692-08 (M.J.W), and 3T32GM007170-35S1 (E.K.) and by the Cooley's Anemia Foundation.

[a] Cell and Molecular Biology Graduate Group, The Combined Degree Program, University of Pennsylvania School of Medicine, Philadelphia, PA, USA

[b] Division of Hematology, Abramson Research Center, Children's Hospital of Philadelphia, Room 316B, 3615 Civic Center Boulevard, Philadelphia, PA 19104, USA

* Corresponding author.

E-mail address: weissmi@email.chop.edu

Hematol Oncol Clin N Am 24 (2010) 1071–1088
doi:10.1016/j.hoc.2010.08.013
0889-8588/10/$ – see front matter © 2010 Elsevier Inc. All rights reserved.

pathogenesis of numerous diseases affecting the nervous system, heart, pancreas, liver, and other tissues.[2–4] In β-thalassemia, abundant excess α-globin is destabilized by several mechanisms, including deficiency of its natural binding partner β globin and autocatalytic oxidative stress. It is likely that this disease affects erythroid protein quality control mechanisms and vice versa. This article reviews experimental evidence indicating that erythroid cells can mitigate the toxicity of excess α-globin to a certain extent using generally conserved protein quality control pathways. The authors propose that β-thalassemia fits within a broader framework of protein aggregation disorders and that by applying the lessons learned from these nonerythroid diseases, the understanding of β-thalassemia pathogenesis can be extended to devise novel therapies for this common genetic disorder that causes significant morbidity in many areas of the world.[5] Moreover, closer examination of protein quality control using β-thalassemia as a model system could provide new insights into rare protein aggregation disorders affecting other tissues.

GENERAL PRINCIPLES OF PROTEIN QUALITY CONTROL: HOW CELLS HANDLE UNSTABLE PROTEINS

Basic principles of protein quality control are discussed briefly in this article and reviewed more extensively elsewhere.[2–4,6–8] Protein misfolding occurs frequently in all cells by "off-pathway" folding of otherwise normal polypeptides and random biosynthetic errors.[6,8] High protein concentrations and rapid biosynthesis of proteins on polysomes increase nonproductive associations that lead to misfolding and aggregation. These processes are accelerated either during or after protein synthesis by various insults, including destabilizing mutations, deficiency of endogenous binding partners, and environmental stresses such as thermal and oxidant injury (**Table 1**). Several of these factors apply to β-thalassemia and other hemoglobinopathies.

Misfolded and aggregated proteins can be deleterious to the cell not only through loss of protein function but also via toxic gain of function. These proteins can interfere with other normal proteins directly by physical interactions or indirectly by sequestering and monopolizing protein quality control system components that regulate critical cellular functions.[9] Numerous interdependent elements contribute to protein quality control in virtually all cells. These elements include molecular chaperones, the ubiquitin-proteasome system (UPS), and lysosome-autophagy pathways.

Molecular Chaperones

Molecular chaperones represent a diverse and multifunctional class of proteins that bind "client" proteins to facilitate their folding and/or assembly into multisubunit complexes.[7,10,11] Most chaperones, termed "public," recognize a broad range of client proteins, frequently through interactions with hydrophobic surfaces. For example, ubiquitously expressed heat shock protein (Hsp) 70 is estimated to bind up to 15% to 20% of newly synthesized proteins in mammalian cells.[12] Other "private" chaperones perform specialized functions by recognizing more limited repertoires of client proteins. Molecular chaperones participate in protein quality control through several mechanisms. These chaperones promote folding of many newly synthesized proteins and also help to repair proteins that become misfolded during cellular stress. In addition, chaperones irreversibly bind damaged proteins to mitigate their potentially toxic effects, direct their subcellular localization to structures termed aggresomes, and/or facilitate their degradation through lysosome-autophagy or ubiquitin-proteasome proteolytic systems.

Table 1
Causes of protein misfolding and aggregation

Intrinsic Causes

Mutated or incomplete proteins	Coding sequence mutations (missense or nonsense), synthetic errors, premature translation termination, proteolytic cleavage products
Lack of binding partner[a]	Absence of obligate chaperone or multimeric complex partners, excess subunit synthesis
Postsynthetic damage[a]	Oxidative or free radical damage, covalent modifications, denaturation, proteolytic cleavage
Misfolded proteins	Off-pathway folding, an inherent part of protein synthesis and existence

Intracellular Conditions

Thermal stress	Thermal denaturation
Reactive small molecules and free radicals[a]	Oxidation, nitrosylation, glycation, deamidation, oxidative cross-linking
Extremes of ionic strength and pH	Favor multimer dissociation and protein denaturation
Macromolecular crowding[a]	High rates of protein synthesis
Presence of other misfolded or unfolded proteins[a]	Nascent polypeptides (not yet fully folded), misfolded or mutated proteins, depletion of chaperones by other stresses

For further information see Refs.[2–4,6–8]
[a] Factors applicable to β-thalassemia.

The UPS

The UPS for protein degradation was initially recognized and characterized in reticulocytes and is now known to regulate numerous essential functions in all cells.[8,13] For example, the UPS regulates cell growth, division, and differentiation through precisely timed proteolysis of specific substrates. Oxygen-sensitive UPS pathways regulate erythropoietin production to maintain circulating erythrocytes.[14] The UPS also participates in protein quality control by degrading misfolded and otherwise damaged proteins. Proteins are generally marked for degradation by covalent conjugation of polyubiquitin chains, which serve as a recognition signal for the 26S proteasome complex. Ubiquitin is joined to target proteins by the concerted action of E1 ubiquitin-activating enzymes, E2 ubiquitin-conjugating enzymes, and E3 ubiquitin-protein ligases, with the E3-ligase complex providing substrate specificity. E3 ubiquitin ligases recognize substrates on their own or through interactions with chaperones and other adapter proteins, allowing for multiple layers of regulation and specificity for both normal and damaged proteins.

Autophagy

Autophagy refers to numerous processes in which cytoplasmic proteins or whole organelles are degraded by lysosomes.[4,15,16] Macroautophagy, the most commonly cited and best understood form, is a highly conserved pathway for bulk degradation of cytoplasmic contents, including organelles. During this process, the material to be degraded is enveloped in a double-membrane autophagosome, which fuses with a lysosome to form an autolysosome. Chaperone-mediated autophagy represents direct translocation of chaperone-unfolded proteins into the lysosome for subsequent degradation. Microautophagy is the capture of small amounts of cytoplasmic material through direct invagination of lysosomal membranes. The most well-defined function of autophagy is the maintenance of the amino acid pool during starvation through nonspecific bulk protein degradation. However, recent work illustrates the importance of autophagy in a broad range of cellular functions. For example, during erythropoiesis, mitochondria are removed from reticulocytes through macroautophagy (discussed later). Autophagy-mediated processes also participate in cellular protein quality control by removing misfolded and aggregated proteins, as illustrated in studies of neurodegenerative diseases.[4,15]

Aggresomes

Until recently, protein aggregation was thought to be a passive process induced by association of sticky misfolded polypeptides. However, new studies suggest that formation of aggregates may be a conserved and regulated process whereby abnormal proteins are sequestered into organized structures termed aggresomes to inhibit harmful interactions with normal proteins and facilitate subsequent degradation.[3,17,18]

Aggresomes form when the cell's capacity to remove or repair abnormal proteins is exceeded. These structures were initially described for abnormal membrane-bound proteins, including the cystic fibrosis transmembrane receptor,[19] but subsequently identified in a variety of diseases associated with abnormal cytoplasmic proteins.[20–28] In tissue culture models, aggresome formation is induced by the expression of unstable proteins and/or inhibition of proteasomal degradation pathways.[19] Aggresomes surround centrioles (the microtubule organizing center [MTOC]) and may be enclosed in an intermediate filament cage. Aggresome formation is microtubule-dependent, and the current model holds that microtubule-associated motor proteins actively deliver dispersed protein precipitates to MTOC-associated aggresomes. Aggresomes contain ubiquitinated proteins, molecular chaperones, and multiple components of the ubiquitin-proteasome pathway.

Current studies indicate a central role for aggresomes in protein quality control pathways. Proteasomes and chaperones such as Hsp70 and Hsp90 are present at the MTOC under basal conditions, perhaps to form the basis of an organized protein quality control center.[29,30] Although aggresomes are relatively insoluble, their contents are dynamic. Photobleaching studies demonstrate the capacity for aggresomes to exchange contents with soluble cytoplasmic compartments, perhaps through chaperone-mediated refolding.[31] The presence of proteasomes within aggresomes suggests that they can also serve as a proteolysis center. Aggresomes may also target abnormal proteins for degradation through autophagy. A critical aggresome component, p62/SQSTM, can bind polyubiquitinated proteins and polymerize around them, forming a shell to facilitate fusion with lysosomes.[32–35] Aggresomes can also sequester precipitated proteins that cannot be degraded, perhaps limiting their toxicity.[31] Overall, it seems that the functions of aggresomes and the ultimate fate of their contents depend on the cell type and the nature of the resident abnormal proteins.

PROTEIN QUALITY CONTROL PATHWAYS IN DISEASE

Disorders of protein aggregation have mainly been characterized in the central nervous system, but they also involve numerous other tissues including liver, heart, and pancreas (**Table 2**).[2,4,9,10,15,18] Despite divergent affected cell types and clinical features, several common themes emerge. First, abnormal disease-associated

Table 2
Examples of protein aggregation diseases

Disease	Abnormal Protein	Cell Type	Intracellular Inclusion
Alzheimer Disease	Tau	Neurons	Neurofibrillary tangles
Amyotrophic Lateral Sclerosis (Familial)	Superoxide dismutase 1	Neurons	Bunina bodies
Parkinson's Disease	α-Synuclein	Neurons	Lewy bodies
Huntington's Disease	Huntingtin (polyglutamine expansion)	Neurons	—
X-Linked Spinobulbar Muscular Atrophy (Kennedy Disease)	Androgen receptor (polyglutamine expansion)	Neurons	—
Prion Disease	Prion protein	Neurons	—
α₁-Antitrypsin Deficiency	α₁-Antitrypsin	Hepatocytes	—
Alcoholic Liver Disease	Intermediate filaments	Hepatocytes	Mallory bodies
Wilson Disease	ATP7B	Hepatocytes	—
β-Thalassemia	α Globin	Erythrocytes	—

proteins are generally cleared through autophagy and/or the UPS. Clinical manifestations of cytotoxicity ensue when quality control systems become overloaded as cells age and accumulate excess aggregated protein over time. Second, abnormal proteins are frequently sequestered in aggresome-like structures, named according to the disease. For example, Mallory bodies in alcoholic liver disease and Lewy bodies in Parkinson disease resemble aggresomes morphologically and contain known aggresome components such as p62/SQSTM1.[24,36] Third, diverse aggregation-prone proteins share similar mechanisms of cytotoxicity. One hypothesis is that these aggregates globally inhibit protein quality control systems through numerous potential mechanisms, including sequestration of proteasomes and chaperones, physical clogging of proteasomes, depletion of the free ubiquitin pool, and increased oxidative stress.[9,37–39] The result is misfolding and accumulation of "bystander" proteins and impaired degradation of critical physiologic proteasome substrates such as cell cycle regulators, leading to cellular dysfunction and apoptosis.

One example of a protein aggregation disorder is familial ALS caused by mutations in superoxide dismutase 1 gene, *SOD1*.[40] These mutations cause toxicity not through loss of function but rather by generating a misfolded aggregation-prone protein with enhanced ability to generate reactive oxygen species,[41] analogous to the properties of free α globin in β-thalassemia. Mutant SOD1 proteins are associated with aggresome-like structures[20] and cause global dysfunction of the UPS.[42,43] Overexpression of the chaperone Hsp70 or Dorfin, a ubiquitin ligase that recognizes *SOD1* mutants, partially rescues the toxicity of *SOD1* mutations by stabilizing the abnormal proteins or facilitating their degradation.[44,45] In this way, efforts to define how protein quality control systems intersect with disease pathophysiology have elucidated new pathways for potential therapeutic manipulation.

PROTEIN QUALITY CONTROL SYSTEMS IN ERYTHROPOIESIS

Erythroid maturation presents unique protein quality control challenges, including the high concentration of cytotoxic hemoglobin subunit proteins, oxidative stress associated with iron (both free and heme-bound), and the need to clear unnecessary nonglobin proteins and organelles during terminal maturation. Accordingly, many of the principles and systems of protein quality control can be applied to normal erythroid development and associated diseases, particularly hemoglobinopathies such as β-thalassemia.

Molecular Chaperones

The involvement of molecular chaperone systems in erythroid development is reviewed by Weiss and Dos Santos.[46] Reticulocytes can increase the production of chaperones in response to stress by preferential messenger RNA translation, indicating the importance of protein quality control during late-stage erythroid maturation.[47] Public chaperones such as Hsp70 facilitate erythroid maturation through regulation of key erythroid proteins.[48] α-Hemoglobin stabilizing protein (AHSP) is an erythroid-specific private chaperone that specifically stabilizes free α-globin subunits. Loss of AHSP in mice causes hemolytic anemia with globin precipitates (Heinz bodies) and exacerbates β-thalassemia.[49–51] Other important globin chaperones, both private and public, are likely to play additional important roles in erythropoiesis.

Ubiquitin-Mediated Proteolysis

The UPS was initially described in reticulocytes, a relatively simple anucleate cell that degrades multiple proteins as part of normal maturation.[52–54] More recent studies have explored the role of proteasome-dependent protein degradation during erythropoiesis.[55,56] Activated erythropoietin receptors may be cleared in part by proteasomal degradation.[57] Cytoskeletal proteins actin and tubulin are degraded by the UPS in reticulocytes,[55] and pharmacologic proteasome inhibition interferes with numerous aspects of erythroid maturation in vitro, including enucleation.[56] General understanding of the UPS and its components is expanding rapidly, and future studies will likely identify additional roles for targeted proteolysis in globin homeostasis and erythroid maturation.

Autophagy

Maturing erythroid cells eliminate not only soluble proteins but also organelles. Reticulocytes degrade mitochondria and ribosomes by autophagy.[58–61] Targeted deletions of murine genes encoding macroautophagy pathway components, including *Nix*,[62,63] *Ulk1*,[64] and *Atg7*,[65] interfere to varying degrees with physiologic degradation of mitochondria during reticulocyte maturation. Morphologic studies described later in this review illustrate lysosomal engulfment of α-globin inclusions in β-thalassemic erythroblasts, although the overall importance of autophagic pathways in degrading excess α-globin is not known.

PROTEOLYTIC CONTROL OF GLOBIN CHAIN BALANCE

The synthesis and subsequent fate of nascent globin chains have been analyzed extensively through pulse-labeling studies in normal and thalassemic erythroid precursors.[66–71] Normally, globin chain synthesis is relatively balanced, with some studies revealing a slight excess of α chains in a soluble pool.[72,73] The per-cell globin chain synthetic rates are highest in the basophilic erythroblast stage and decrease as the cells mature,[74–76] but globin synthesis and accumulation continues through the late stages, with reticulocytes producing as much as 7% to 20% of the total hemoglobin content.[77] β-Thalassemic erythroid precursors contain a larger pool of excess free α chains that are initially competent to form hemoglobin tetramers but are unstable in the absence of their binding partner.[69,78–80] These early studies provided first evidence linking α-globin excess to the pathophysiology of β-thalassemia.[81–83] Analysis of the erythroid precursors in β-thalassemia trait and intermedia at different stages of maturation provided further insights into globin chain metabolism. In these studies, the α to β chain ratio increased during successive stages of maturation, with the highest amounts of α-globin excess found in circulating reticulocytes. Prolonged labeling experiments showed that in bone marrow erythroblasts, β chains accumulate at a constant rate but nascent α chain levels stabilize over time, so that the α to β chain ratio decreased. This effect was highest in the earlier maturation stages. These data indicate that β-thalassemic erythroid precursors, particularly at early developmental states, degrade excess α-globin to prevent its accumulation. This protective mechanism becomes less effective during the course of maturation as globin chains accumulate and the capacity to remove excess α chains becomes overwhelmed.

Subsequent experiments characterized the proteolytic degradation of α-globin. Hanash and colleagues[84] mixed reticulocyte and normoblast lysates to show that earlier erythroid precursors have a greater capacity to degrade excess α chains. This activity was specific for α-globin and blocked by proteolysis inhibitors.[85–87] Moreover, α-globin proteolysis was higher in erythroid precursors of patients with β-thalassemia than in those of patients with other anemias or causes of reticulocytosis. Early experiments describing the UPS in reticulocyte lysates used denatured globins or globin chains rendered unstable by incorporation of amino acid analogues.[52,53,88] These experiments indicate that erythroid precursors have the capacity to degrade excess or structurally unstable globins.

Studies by Shaeffer[89,90] focused on the role of the UPS in α-globin degradation. Pulse-chase labeling of intact β-thalassemia reticulocytes showed that they degrade endogenous α-globin but not β-globin, in an ATP-dependent manner. Biochemical studies showed that β-thalassemia reticulocyte lysates can ubiquitinate added α-globin at several sites to facilitate its degradation by proteasomes.[90–94] Moreover, mono- or polyubiquitination of α-globin was required for its proteasomal degradation.[94] Further work has shown that free α, β, and γ globin chains can be ubiquitinated and degraded using in vitro reconstituted systems and that this process can occur cotranslationally or shortly after the release of the nascent chains from ribosomes.[95]

One implication of this research is that the differences in proteolytic capacity for α-globin may account for some of the phenotypic heterogeneity in β-thalassemia and for the interspecies differences in the manifestations of β-globin gene mutations. In humans, a 50% reduction in β-globin synthesis usually results in the asymptomatic β-thalassemia trait. In mice, a similar reduction in the β-globin gene dosage causes a more severe phenotype that resembles β-thalassemia intermedia.[96,97] Rouyer-Fessard and colleagues[98,99] have suggested that this interspecies difference may be due in part to reduced capacity for degrading unstable toxic α-globin in mouse erythroblasts.

Accumulation of free β-globin chains in α-thalassemia also poses protein quality control problems for erythroid precursors. For example, pulse-chase labeling of reticulocytes from a patient with α-thalassemia showed normalization of globin chain accumulation through preferential degradation of β-globin, similar to what is seen with α chains in β-thalassemia.[100] However, free β-like globin chains are more stable and soluble than α-globin, partly due to formation of homotetramers. Compared to β-thalassemia, α-thalassemia is associated with fewer globin precipitates in erythroid precursors and reduced ineffective erythropoiesis. However, severe forms of α-thalassemia are characterized by extensive hemoglobin H (HbH) (β_4) inclusions in circulating erythrocytes, causing shortened half-life and anemia. Further comparative studies are required to better define the similarities and differences in how protein quality control pathways handle excess free α and β-globin chains.

Together, numerous studies over many years have indicated that the UPS can degrade unstable globins as a protective mechanism against hemoglobinopathies, particularly β-thalassemia. Additional proteolytic systems may complement this UPS function. For example, oxidant-damaged hemoglobin can be degraded by intact reticulocytes and extracts in ATP- and ubiquitin-independent pathways, possibly through a cytosolic protease.[101,102] This activity seems to be retained in mature erythrocytes.

UNSTABLE GLOBIN AGGREGATION

Inclusion bodies have long been considered a hallmark of the thalassemias. In β-thalassemia, small intracellular aggregates appear in the early normoblast stage and coalesce into large inclusions by the late normoblast and reticulocyte stages.[103,104] The size and frequency of the inclusions correlate with disease severity.[103,104] The inclusions, initially described as stroma-bound globins, were found to contain as much as 10% of all α-globin synthesized in splenectomized patients with β-thalassemia major.[105–107] Labeling studies showed that in β-thalassemia, aggregation-prone α-globin enters the insoluble stromal fraction rapidly after synthesis[67,78,87,108] and may be removed subsequently by ATP-dependent proteolytic pathways.

Klemes and colleagues[88] used unstable valine analogues to label rabbit reticulocytes and found that the resultant abnormal globins formed high–molecular weight non–membrane-bound structures that were insoluble in mild detergents but soluble in harsher ionic detergents. These aggregates increased in molecular weight and decreased in solubility with longer amino acid analogue treatment and after ATP depletion. In pulse-chase studies, the insoluble fraction was subject to ATP-dependent degradation. In β-thalassemic reticulocytes, a similar ATP-dependent turnover of the stromal α-globin fraction was seen in parallel with the removal of soluble α-globin.[89] It is not clear whether this turnover is mediated by cytosolic proteases or membrane/stroma-associated systems, because other studies showed that a proteolytic activity for α-globin also exists in purified stromal fractions.[87,108] Most likely, soluble α chains are degraded by soluble proteasomal components, whereas the insoluble α chains are degraded by a combination of stroma-associated proteasomal and lysosomal pathways.

Wickramasinghe and colleagues[109,110] demonstrated that β-thalassemic erythroblasts contain electron-dense inclusions beginning at early polychromatic stages, which increase in size and frequency during subsequent maturation. These inclusions also occur to a lesser extent in β-thalassemia trait.[111] Remarkably, the α-globin inclusions in β-thalassemia share numerous properties with classical aggresomes discovered years later in studies of other protein precipitation disorders (**Fig. 1**), including cytoplasmic juxtanuclear localization in association with centrioles.[109,111,112] Immunoelectron microscopy confirmed that the β-thalassemic inclusions contain α-globin (but not β-globin) and also ubiquitin, consistent with the presence of ubiquitinated α-globin chains targeted for degradation by the UPS.[113,114] Ultrastructural studies also revealed β-thalassemic α-globin inclusions in autophagic vacuoles, suggesting elimination by macroautophagy.[109,111] Similar inclusions containing both α and β-globins were found in patients with dominantly inherited β-thalassemia caused by mutations that destabilize β-globin chains.[115,116] Ultrastructural studies of α-thalassemia-1 trait and HbH disease showed that excess β-globin chains form similar inclusions, which accumulate according to the degree of chain imbalance.[117,118]

A Perinuclear α globin inclusions

C Autophagosome formation

B Pericentriolar localization

D Association with ubiquitin

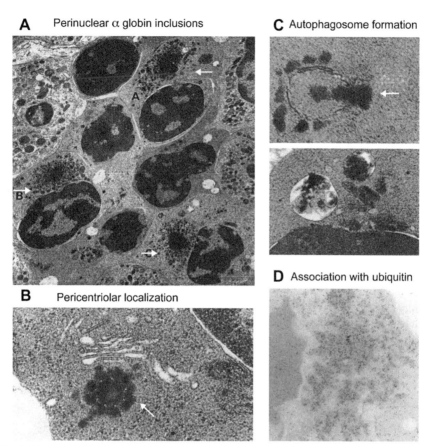

Fig. 1. Electron microscopy reveals aggresome-like α-globin inclusions in β-thalassemia. (*A*) Several late polychromatic erythroblasts, labeled A, B, and C, with intracytoplasmic perinuclear α-chain precipitates (*arrows*). (*B*) Precipitation of α-chains around the centriole of an erythroblast. The arrow indicates microtubule triplets in centriole cross section. (*C*) (*Top*) Autophagosome membrane formation partially enclosing precipitated α chains (*arrow*) and (*bottom*) 2 autophagic vacuoles containing electron-dense material, probably precipitated α chains (*D*) Immunogold staining for ubiquitin within α-globin precipitates of a β-thalassemic erythroblast. (*Adapted from* Wickramasinghe SN, Bush V. Observations on the ultrastructure of erythropoietic cells and reticulum cells in the bone marrow of patients with homozygous beta-thalassaemia. Br J Haematol 1975;30(4):396; with permission [A]; Wickramasinghe SN, Hughes M. Precipitation of alpha-chains on the centrioles of erythroblasts in beta-thalassaemia. Br J Haematol 1982;52(4):682; with permission [B]; Wickramasinghe SN, Hughes M. Ultrastructural studies of erythropoiesis in beta-thalassaemia trait. Br J Haematol 1980;46(3):402; with permission [C]; Wickramasinghe SN, Lee MJ. Evidence that the ubiquitin proteolytic pathway is involved in the degradation of precipitated globin chains in thalassaemia. Br J Haematol 1998;101(2):246; with permission[D].)

Similar-appearing aggregates containing globin and nonglobin proteins are also reported in patients with congenital dyserythropoietic anemia.[114,119,120] Together, these studies indicate that pathologic erythroid precursors sequester unstable globin chains and possibly other abnormal proteins into aggresome-like structures resembling those observed in other protein aggregation disorders affecting various tissues.

PUTTING IT ALL TOGETHER

Many of the pioneering studies to understand globin chain maintenance in β-thalassemia and other hemoglobinopathies were performed when the knowledge of protein quality control was in its infancy. For example, studies of Wickramasinghe and colleagues[109,111–113] indicated that precipitated α-globin accumulates in aggresomes years before this structure was appreciated or defined (see **Fig. 1**). Now, it seems that erythroid cells compartmentalize and metabolize unstable globins, at least in part, through generally conserved pathways, including the UPS and autophagy, which are studied most extensively in other protein aggregation disorders. How protein quality control likely modulates β-thalassemia is illustrated in **Fig. 2**. Early-stage β-thalassemic erythroblasts neutralize low level excess α-globin reasonably well via proteolytic systems and/or chaperones. As total globin levels increase during maturation, accumulated free α-globin becomes compartmentalized into aggresome-like structures, which are modeled and eliminated via the UPS and autophagy. Ultimately, in severe forms of the disease, α-globin precipitation and aggregation overwhelms compensatory detoxification mechanisms, resulting in cellular toxicities associated with ineffective erythropoiesis (**Fig. 3**). Damage from unstable α-globin may arise directly from its toxicity and indirectly via its ability to inhibit protein quality control systems that are essential for various aspects of erythroid maturation. Although erythroid protein quality control systems are not fully defined, they almost certainly contain both generally expressed components, such as ubiquitous proteases and public chaperones, as well as cell type–restricted molecules, such as AHSP.

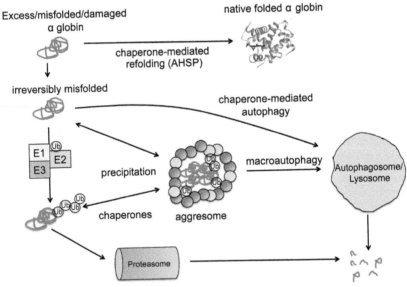

Fig. 2. Model for repair or elimination of free α-globin by cellular protein quality control systems. Misfolded free α-globin may be stabilized by interactions with molecular chaperones, perhaps AHSP and/or generalized public chaperones. Irreversibly damaged protein may be removed either by chaperone-mediated autophagy or UPS pathways. E1 ubiquitin-activating enzymes, E2 ubiquitin-conjugating enzymes, and E3 ubiquitin ligases mediate conjugation of polyubiquitin (Ub) chains to α-globin, targeting it for proteasomal degradation via the UPS. In addition, insoluble α-globin (± Ub) can be shuttled to aggresomes, which are subsequently cleared by macroautophagy.

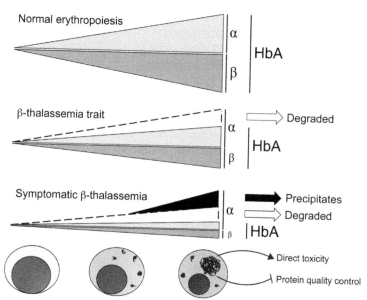

Fig. 3. Overloading of degradation systems leads to accumulation of α-globin in β-thalassemia. During normal erythropoiesis, α- and β-globin subunits are synthesized almost equally and join to form hemoglobin (Hb) A ($\alpha_2\beta_2$) tetramers. In β-thalassemia trait, excess α chains are synthesized but removed by protein quality control systems and there is minimal pathology. In β-thalassemia, free α-globin is degraded in early erythroid precursors to balance globin synthesis. As cellular maturation proceeds, free α chain levels overwhelm compensatory mechanisms, resulting in accumulation of toxic precipitates. Precipitated α-globin can damage the cell either directly or indirectly by interfering with the functions of protein quality control systems.

FUTURE DIRECTIONS

The authors speculate that many general lessons learned from various protein misfolding and aggregation diseases can be applied to better understand β-thalassemia pathogenesis and discover new treatments. Recent technological advances such as the development of animal disease models and high-throughput screening systems should allow closer examination of β-thalassemia, address questions arising from earlier work, and better define the mechanisms of α-globin metabolism. Mouse models of β-thalassemia major and intermedia[96,97] and methods for culture of human erythroid progenitors from patients with β-thalassemia[121] may be used for genetic and pharmacologic dissection of pathways required for α-globin detoxification in vivo. Mice with targeted deletions of key aggresome components[33,122] and critical autophagy pathway genes[63–65] can be bred to β-thalassemia mouse models to determine the genetic interactions. In addition, short hairpin RNA approaches to disrupt these pathways can be used to study cultured human or mice erythroblasts. For example, it should be possible to configure high-throughput screens using small inhibitory RNAs to identify specific E3 ubiquitin ligases and other quality control components that regulate free α-globin in erythroid cells. The UPS and aggresome formation pathways can also be manipulated in thalassemia using pharmacologic inhibitors or enhancers that are either in clinical use for other disorders (such as proteasome inhibitor bortezomib in multiple myeloma) or under development.[18,123–125]

High-resolution immunofluorescence microscopy can confirm whether α-globin inclusions found in β-thalassemic erythroblasts are bona fide aggresomes. Insoluble protein aggregate samples obtained from patients with thalassemia can also be studied by mass spectrometry to identify constituent proteins with presumed roles in α-globin quality control. This proteomic approach has yielded useful information in other unstable protein disorders.[126] For example, mass spectroscopy of Mallory bodies in alcoholic liver disease showed them to contain aggresome-associated intermediate filaments and p62/SQSTM, a critical aggresome component.[35] In addition to identifying known aggresome components, mass spectroscopy of β-thalassemic aggregates might identify new α-globin–specific chaperones or ubiquitin ligases.

As discussed earlier, excessive protein misfolding and aggregation can damage cells by inhibiting protein quality control systems. This pathophysiology may be particularly important in β-thalassemia because erythroid precursors must degrade numerous proteins and organelles to undergo normal maturation. This hypothesis can be tested using newly developed in vivo fluorescent reporters that provide information about UPS activity.[127] Proteomic approaches can define whether UPS substrates accumulate in erythroid precursors. It may also be informative to determine whether some β-thalassemia phenotypes can be recapitulated by overexpression of nonglobin aggregation-prone proteins in erythroid precursors.

In summary, protein quality control pathways are becoming increasingly appreciated as important modifiers of human disease and are likely to function during normal erythropoiesis and in β-thalassemia. In parallel, new technologies are rapidly enhancing the ability to study and manipulate how cells handle unstable proteins. With these new tools and perspectives in hand, it should be possible to initiate new studies to better understand and eventually treat β-thalassemia.

ACKNOWLEDGMENTS

The authors thank Stephen Liebhaber and Vijay Sankaran for helpful critiques of the article.

REFERENCES

1. Weatherall DJ, Clegg JB. The thalassaemia syndromes. 4th edition. Oxford, Malden (MA): Blackwell Science; 2001.
2. Aigelsreiter A, Janig E, Stumptner C, et al. How a cell deals with abnormal proteins. Pathogenetic mechanisms in protein aggregation diseases. Pathobiology 2007;74(3):145–58.
3. Garcia-Mata R, Gao YS, Sztul E. Hassles with taking out the garbage: aggravating aggresomes. Traffic 2002;3(6):388–96.
4. Ding WX, Yin XM. Sorting, recognition and activation of the misfolded protein degradation pathways through macroautophagy and the proteasome. Autophagy 2008;4(2):141–50.
5. Angastiniotis M, Modell B. Global epidemiology of hemoglobin disorders. Ann N Y Acad Sci 1998;850:251–69.
6. Hartl FU, Hayer-Hartl M. Converging concepts of protein folding in vitro and in vivo. Nat Struct Mol Biol 2009;16(6):574–81.
7. McClellan AJ, Tam S, Kaganovich D, et al. Protein quality control: chaperones culling corrupt conformations. Nat Cell Biol 2005;7(8):736–41.
8. Goldberg AL. Protein degradation and protection against misfolded or damaged proteins. Nature 2003;426(6968):895–9.

9. Dantuma N, Lindsten K. Stressing the ubiquitin/proteasome system. Cardiovasc Res 2010;85(2):263–71.
10. Barral JM, Broadley SA, Schaffar G, et al. Roles of molecular chaperones in protein misfolding diseases. Semin Cell Dev Biol 2004;15(1):17–29.
11. Broadley SA, Hartl FU. The role of molecular chaperones in human misfolding diseases. FEBS Lett 2009;583(16):2647–53.
12. Thulasiraman V, Yang CF, Frydman J. In vivo newly translated polypeptides are sequestered in a protected folding environment. EMBO J 1999;18(1): 85–95.
13. Pickart CM. Mechanisms underlying ubiquitination. Annu Rev Biochem 2001;70: 503–33.
14. Jaakkola P, Mole DR, Tian YM, et al. Targeting of HIF-alpha to the von Hippel-Lindau ubiquitylation complex by O2-regulated prolyl hydroxylation. Science 2001;292(5516):468–72.
15. Jaeger PA, Wyss-Coray T. All-you-can-eat: autophagy in neurodegeneration and neuroprotection. Mol Neurodegeneration 2009;4:16.
16. Mizushima N, Yoshimori T, Levine B. Methods in mammalian autophagy research. Cell 2010;140(3):313–26.
17. Kopito RR. Aggresomes, inclusion bodies and protein aggregation. Trends Cell Biol 2000;10(12):524–30.
18. Olzmann JA, Li L, Chin LS. Aggresome formation and neurodegenerative diseases: therapeutic implications. Curr Med Chem 2008;15(1):47–60.
19. Johnston JA, Ward CL, Kopito RR. Aggresomes: a cellular response to misfolded proteins. J Cell Biol 1998;143(7):1883–98.
20. Johnston JA, Dalton MJ, Gurney ME, et al. Formation of high molecular weight complexes of mutant Cu, Zn-superoxide dismutase in a mouse model for familial amyotrophic lateral sclerosis. Proc Natl Acad Sci U S A 2000;97(23): 12571–6.
21. García-Mata R, Bebök Z, Sorscher EJ, et al. Characterization and dynamics of aggresome formation by a cytosolic GFP-chimera. J Cell Biol 1999;146(6): 1239–54.
22. Junn E, Lee SS, Suhr UT, et al. Parkin accumulation in aggresomes due to proteasome impairment. J Biol Chem 2002;277(49):47870–7.
23. Ma J, Lindquist S. Wild-type PrP and a mutant associated with prion disease are subject to retrograde transport and proteasome degradation. Proc Natl Acad Sci U S A 2001;98(26):14955–60.
24. McNaught KS, Shashidharan P, Perl DP, et al. Aggresome-related biogenesis of Lewy bodies. Eur J Neurosci 2002;16(11):2136–48.
25. Mukai H, Isagawa T, Goyama E, et al. Formation of morphologically similar globular aggregates from diverse aggregation-prone proteins in mammalian cells. Proc Natl Acad Sci U S A 2005;102(31):10887–92.
26. Salomons FA, Menéndez-Benito V, Böttcher C, et al. Selective accumulation of aggregation-prone proteasome substrates in response to proteotoxic stress. Mol Cell Biol 2009;29(7):1774–85.
27. Tanaka M, Kim YM, Lee G, et al. Aggresomes formed by alpha-synuclein and synphilin-1 are cytoprotective. J Biol Chem 2004;279(6):4625–31.
28. Waelter S, Boeddrich A, Lurz R, et al. Accumulation of mutant huntingtin fragments in aggresome-like inclusion bodies as a result of insufficient protein degradation. Mol Biol Cell 2001;12(5):1393–407.
29. Wigley WC, Fabunmi RP, Lee MG, et al. Dynamic association of proteasomal machinery with the centrosome. J Cell Biol 1999;145(3):481–90.

30. Wojcik C, Schroeter D, Wilk S, et al. Ubiquitin-mediated proteolysis centers in HeLa cells: indication from studies of an inhibitor of the chymotrypsin-like activity of the proteasome. Eur J Cell Biol 1996;71(3):311–8.

31. Kaganovich D, Kopito R, Frydman J. Misfolded proteins partition between two distinct quality control compartments. Nature 2008;454(7208):1088–95.

32. Bjørkøy G, Lamark T, Brech A, et al. p62/SQSTM1 forms protein aggregates degraded by autophagy and has a protective effect on huntingtin-induced cell death. J Cell Biol 2005;171(4):603–14.

33. Komatsu M, Waguri S, Koike M, et al. Homeostatic levels of p62 control cytoplasmic inclusion body formation in autophagy-deficient mice. Cell 2007; 131(6):1149–63.

34. Pankiv S, Clausen TH, Lamark T, et al. p62/SQSTM1 binds directly to Atg8/LC3 to facilitate degradation of ubiquitinated protein aggregates by autophagy. J Biol Chem 2007;282(33):24131–45.

35. Zatloukal K, Stumptner C, Fuchsbichler A, et al. p62 Is a common component of cytoplasmic inclusions in protein aggregation diseases. Am J Pathol 2002; 160(1):255–63.

36. Riley NE, Li J, Worrall S, et al. The Mallory body as an aggresome: in vitro studies. Exp Mol Pathol 2002;72(1):17–23.

37. Bence NF, Sampat RM, Kopito RR. Impairment of the ubiquitin-proteasome system by protein aggregation. Science 2001;292(5521):1552–5.

38. Bennett EJ, Shaler TA, Woodman B, et al. Global changes to the ubiquitin system in Huntington's disease. Nature 2007;448(7154):704–8.

39. Bennett EJ, Bence NF, Jayakumar R, et al. Global impairment of the ubiquitin-proteasome system by nuclear or cytoplasmic protein aggregates precedes inclusion body formation. Mol Cell 2005;17(3):351–65.

40. Rosen DR, Siddique T, Patterson D, et al. Mutations in Cu/Zn superoxide dismutase gene are associated with familial amyotrophic lateral sclerosis. Nature 1993;362(6415):59–62.

41. Cleveland DW, Liu J. Oxidation versus aggregation – how do SOD1 mutants cause ALS? Nat Med 2000;6(12):1320–1.

42. Cheroni C, Marino M, Tortarolo M, et al. Functional alterations of the ubiquitin-proteasome system in motor neurons of a mouse model of familial amyotrophic lateral sclerosis. Hum Mol Genet 2009;18(1):82–96.

43. Urushitani M, Kurisu J, Tsukita K, et al. Proteasomal inhibition by misfolded mutant superoxide dismutase 1 induces selective motor neuron death in familial amyotrophic lateral sclerosis. J Neurochem 2002;83(5):1030–42.

44. Niwa JI, Ishigaki S, Hishikawa N, et al. Dorfin ubiquitylates mutant SOD1 and prevents mutant SOD1-mediated neurotoxicity. J Biol Chem 2002;277(39): 36793–8.

45. Bruening W, Roy J, Giasson B, et al. Up-regulation of protein chaperones preserves viability of cells expressing toxic Cu/Zn-superoxide dismutase mutants associated with amyotrophic lateral sclerosis. J Neurochem 1999;72(2):693–9.

46. Weiss MJ, Dos Santos CO. Chaperoning erythropoiesis. Blood 2009;113(10): 2136–44.

47. Banerji SS, Theodorakis NG, Morimoto RI. Heat shock-induced translational control of HSP70 and globin synthesis in chicken reticulocytes. Mol Cell Biol 1984;4(11):2437–48.

48. Ribeil JA, Zermati Y, Vandekerckhove J, et al. Hsp70 regulates erythropoiesis by preventing caspase-3-mediated cleavage of GATA-1. Nature 2007;445(7123): 102–5.

49. Kihm AJ, Kong Y, Hong W, et al. An abundant erythroid protein that stabilizes free alpha-haemoglobin. Nature 2002;417(6890):758–63.
50. Yu X, Kong Y, Dore LC, et al. An erythroid chaperone that facilitates folding of alpha-globin subunits for hemoglobin synthesis. J Clin Invest 2007;117(7): 1856–65.
51. Kong Y, Zhou S, Kihm AJ, et al. Loss of alpha-hemoglobin-stabilizing protein impairs erythropoiesis and exacerbates beta-thalassemia. J Clin Invest 2004; 114(10):1457–66.
52. Ciehanover A, Hod Y, Hershko A. A heat-stable polypeptide component of an ATP-dependent proteolytic system from reticulocytes. Biochem Biophys Res Commun 1978;81(4):1100–5.
53. Etlinger JD, Goldberg AL. A soluble ATP-dependent proteolytic system responsible for the degradation of abnormal proteins in reticulocytes. Proc Natl Acad Sci U S A 1977;74(1):54–8.
54. Hershko A, Heller H, Elias S, et al. Components of ubiquitin-protein ligase system. Resolution, affinity purification, and role in protein breakdown. J Biol Chem 1983;258(13):8206–14.
55. Liu J, Guo X, Mohandas N, et al. Membrane remodeling during reticulocyte maturation. Blood 2010;115(10):2021–7.
56. Chen CY, Pajak L, Tamburlin J, et al. The effect of proteasome inhibitors on mammalian erythroid terminal differentiation. Exp Hematol 2002;30(7):634–9.
57. Walrafen P, Verdier F, Kadri Z, et al. Both proteasomes and lysosomes degrade the activated erythropoietin receptor. Blood 2005;105(2):600–8.
58. Gronowicz G, Swift H, Steck TL. Maturation of the reticulocyte in vitro. J Cell Sci 1984;71:177–97.
59. Heynen MJ, Tricot G, Verwilghen RL. Autophagy of mitochondria in rat bone marrow erythroid cells. Relation to nuclear extrusion. Cell Tissue Res 1985; 239(1):235–9.
60. Kent G, Minick OT, Volini FI, et al. Autophagic vacuoles in human red cells. Am J Pathol 1966;48(5):831–57.
61. Takano-Ohmuro H, Mukaida M, Kominami E, et al. Autophagy in embryonic erythroid cells: its role in maturation. Eur J Cell Biol 2000;79(10):759–64.
62. Sandoval H, Thiagarajan P, Dasgupta SK, et al. Essential role for Nix in autophagic maturation of erythroid cells. Nature 2008;454(7201):232–5.
63. Schweers RL, Zhang J, Randall MS, et al. NIX is required for programmed mitochondrial clearance during reticulocyte maturation. Proc Natl Acad Sci U S A 2007;104(49):19500–5.
64. Kundu M, Lindsten T, Yang CY, et al. Ulk1 plays a critical role in the autophagic clearance of mitochondria and ribosomes during reticulocyte maturation. Blood 2008;112(4):1493–502.
65. Zhang J, Randall MS, Loyd MR, et al. Mitochondrial clearance is regulated by Atg7-dependent and -independent mechanisms during reticulocyte maturation. Blood 2009;114(1):157–64.
66. Bank A, O'Donnell JV. Intracellular loss of free alpha chains in beta thalassemia. Nature 1969;222(5190):295–6.
67. Bargellesi A, Pontremoli S, Menini C, et al. Excess of alpha-globin synthesis in homozygous beta-thalassemia and its removal from the red blood cell cytoplasm. Eur J Biochem 1968;3(3):364–8.
68. Chalevelakis G, Clegg JB, Weatherall DJ. Imbalanced globin chain synthesis in heterozygous beta-thalassemic bone marrow. Proc Natl Acad Sci U S A 1975; 72(10):3853–7.

69. Clegg JB, Weatherall DJ. Haemoglobin synthesis during erythroid maturation in β-thalassaemia. Nature New Biol 1972;240(101):190–2.

70. Kan YW, Nathan DG, Lodish HF. Equal synthesis of α- and β-globin chains in erythroid precursors in heterozygous β-thalassemia. J Clin Invest 1972;51(7):1906–9.

71. Wood WG, Stamatoyannopoulos G. Globin synthesis in fractionated normoblasts of beta-thalassemia heterozygotes. J Clin Invest 1975;55(3):567–78.

72. Shaeffer JR. Evidence for soluble alpha-chains as intermediates in hemoglobin synthesis in the rabbit reticulocyte. Biochem Biophys Res Commun 1967;28(4):647–52.

73. Gill FM, Schwartz E. Free alpha-globin pool in human bone marrow. J Clin Invest 1973;52(12):3057–63.

74. Borsook H, Lingrel JB, Scaro JL, et al. Synthesis of haemoglobin in relation to the maturation of erythroid cells. Nature 1962;196:347–50.

75. Casale GP, Khairallah EA, Grasso JA. An analysis of hemoglobin synthesis in erythropoietic cells. Dev Biol 1980;80(1):107–19.

76. Nathan DG, Piomelli S, Gardner FH. The synthesis of heme and globin in the maturing human erythroid cell. J Clin Invest 1961;40:940–6.

77. Skadberg O, Brun A, Sandberg S. Human reticulocytes isolated from peripheral blood: maturation time and hemoglobin synthesis. Lab Hematol 2003;9(4):198–206.

78. Bank A. Hemoglobin synthesis in beta-thalassemia: the properties of the free alpha-chains. J Clin Invest 1968;47(4):860–6.

79. Bargellesi A, Pontremoli S, Menini C, et al. Kinetic evidence for the existence of alpha-globin pool in beta-thalassemic reticulocytes. Eur J Biochem 1968;7(1):73–7.

80. Conconi F, Bargellesi A, Pontremoli S. Excess of alpha-globin synthesis in homozygous beta-thalassemia. Its cytoplasmic molecular forms. Eur J Biochem 1968;5(3):409–14.

81. Nathan DG, Stossel TB, Gunn RB, et al. Influence of hemoglobin precipitation on erythrocyte metabolism in alpha and beta thalassemia. J Clin Invest 1969;48(1):33–41.

82. Rachmilewitz EA, Peisach J, Blumberg WE. Studies on the stability of oxyhemoglobin A and its constituent chains and their derivatives. J Biol Chem 1971;246(10):3356–66.

83. Bank A, Braverman AS, O'Donnell JV, et al. Absolute rates of globin chain synthesis in thalassemia. Blood 1968;31(2):226–33.

84. Hanash SM, Rucknagel DL. Proteolytic activity in erythrocyte precursors. Proc Natl Acad Sci U S A 1978;75(7):3427–31.

85. Braverman AS, Lester D. Evidence for increased proteolysis in intact beta thalassemia erythroid cells. Hemoglobin 1981;5(6):549–64.

86. Loukopoulos D, Karoulias A, Fessas P. Proteolysis in thalassemia: studies with protease inhibitors. Ann N Y Acad Sci 1980;344:323–35.

87. Vettore L, De Matteis MC, Di Iorio EE, et al. Erythrocytic proteases: preferential degradation of alpha hemoglobin chains. Acta Haematol 1983;70(1):35–42.

88. Klemes Y, Etlinger JD, Goldberg AL. Properties of abnormal proteins degraded rapidly in reticulocytes. Intracellular aggregation of the globin molecules prior to hydrolysis. J Biol Chem 1981;256(16):8436–44.

89. Shaeffer JR. Turnover of excess hemoglobin alpha chains in beta-thalassemic cells is ATP-dependent. J Biol Chem 1983;258(21):13172–7.

90. Shaeffer JR. ATP-dependent proteolysis of hemoglobin alpha chains in beta-thalassemic hemolysates is ubiquitin-dependent. J Biol Chem 1988;263(27): 13663–9.

91. Shaeffer JR. Monoubiquitinated alpha globin is an intermediate in the ATP-dependent proteolysis of alpha globin. J Biol Chem 1994;269(35):22205–10.

92. Shaeffer JR. Heterogeneity in the structure of the ubiquitin conjugates of human alpha globin. J Biol Chem 1994;269(47):29530–6.

93. Shaeffer JR, Cohen RE. Ubiquitin aldehyde increases adenosine triphosphate-dependent proteolysis of hemoglobin alpha-subunits in beta-thalassemic hemo-lysates. Blood 1997;90(3):1300–8.

94. Shaeffer JR, Kania MA. Degradation of monoubiquitinated alpha-globin by 26S proteasomes. Biochemistry 1995;34(12):4015–21.

95. Adachi K, Lakka V, Zhao Y, et al. Ubiquitylation of nascent globin chains in a cell-free system. J Biol Chem 2004;279(40):41767–74.

96. Ciavatta DJ, Ryan TM, Farmer SC, et al. Mouse model of human beta zero thal-assemia: targeted deletion of the mouse beta maj- and beta min-globin genes in embryonic stem cells. Proc Natl Acad Sci U S A 1995;92(20):9259–63.

97. Yang B, Kirby S, Lewis J, et al. A mouse model for beta 0-thalassemia. Proc Natl Acad Sci U S A 1995;92(25):11608–12.

98. Rouyer-Fessard P, Leroy-Viard K, Domenget C, et al. Mouse beta thalassemia, a model for the membrane defects of erythrocytes in the human disease. J Biol Chem 1990;265(33):20247–51.

99. Rouyer-Fessard P, Scott MD, Leroy-Viard K, et al. Fate of alpha-hemoglobin chains and erythrocyte defects in beta-thalassemia. Ann N Y Acad Sci 1990; 612:106–17.

100. Sancar GB, Cedeno MM, Rieder RF. Rapid destruction of newly synthesized excess beta-globin chains in HbH disease. Blood 1981;57(5):967–71.

101. Fagan JM, Waxman L. The ATP-independent pathway in red blood cells that degrades oxidant-damaged hemoglobin. J Biol Chem 1992;267(32):23015–22.

102. Fagan JM, Waxman L, Goldberg AL. Red blood cells contain a pathway for the degradation of oxidant-damaged hemoglobin that does not require ATP or ubiq-uitin. J Biol Chem 1986;261(13):5705–13.

103. Fessas P. Inclusions of hemoglobin erythroblasts and erythrocytes of thalas-semia. Blood 1963;21:21–32.

104. Yataganas X, Fessas P. The pattern of hemoglobin precipitation in thalassemia and its significance. Ann N Y Acad Sci 1969;165(1):270–87.

105. Braverman AS, Schwartzberg L, Berkowitz R. Soluble and stroma-bound globin chains in mild and severe beta thalassemia. Hemoglobin 1982;6(4):347–67.

106. Fessas P, Loukopoulos D, Kaltsoya A. Peptide analysis of the inclusions of erythroid cells in beta-thalassemia. Biochim Biophys Acta 1966;124(2):430–2.

107. Fessas P, Loukopoulos D, Thorell B. Absorption spectra of inclusion bodies in beta-thalassemia. Blood 1965;25:105–9.

108. Ballas SK, Burka ER, Gill FM. Abnormal red cell membrane proteolytic activity in severe heterozygous beta-thalassemia. J Lab Clin Med 1982;99(2):263–74.

109. Wickramasinghe SN, Bush V. Observations on the ultrastructure of erythropoi-etic cells and reticulum cells in the bone marrow of patients with homozygous beta-thalassaemia. Br J Haematol 1975;30(4):395–9.

110. Polliack A, Rachmilewitz EA. Ultrastructural studies in beta-thalassaemia major. Br J Haematol 1973;24(3):319–26.

111. Wickramasinghe SN, Hughes M. Ultrastructural studies of erythropoiesis in beta-thalassaemia trait. Br J Haematol 1980;46(3):401–7.

112. Wickramasinghe SN, Hughes M. Precipitation of alpha-chains on the centrioles of erythroblasts in beta-thalassaemia. Br J Haematol 1982;52(4):681–2.

113. Wickramasinghe SN, Lee MJ. Evidence that the ubiquitin proteolytic pathway is involved in the degradation of precipitated globin chains in thalassaemia. Br J Haematol 1998;101(2):245–50.

114. Wickramasinghe SN, Lee MJ, Furukawa T, et al. Composition of the intra-erythroblastic precipitates in thalassaemia and congenital dyserythropoietic anaemia (CDA): identification of a new type of CDA with intra-erythroblastic precipitates not reacting with monoclonal antibodies to alpha- and beta-globin chains. Br J Haematol 1996;93(3):576–85.

115. Ho PJ, Wickramasinghe SN, Rees DC, et al. Erythroblastic inclusions in dominantly inherited beta thalassemias. Blood 1997;89(1):322–8.

116. Beris P, Miescher PA, Diaz-Chico JC, et al. Inclusion body beta-thalassemia trait in a Swiss family is caused by an abnormal hemoglobin (Geneva) with an altered and extended beta chain carboxy-terminus due to a modification in codon beta 114. Blood 1988;72(2):801–5.

117. Wickramasinghe SN, Hughes M, Fucharoen S, et al. The fate of excess beta-globin chains within erythropoietic cells in alpha-thalassaemia 2 trait, alpha-thalassaemia 1 trait, haemoglobin H disease and haemoglobin Q-H disease: an electron microscope study. Br J Haematol 1984;56(3):473–82.

118. Wickramasinghe SN, Hughes M, Hollan SR, et al. Electron microscope and high resolution autoradiographic studies of the erythroblasts in haemoglobin H disease. Br J Haematol 1980;45(3):401–4.

119. Antonelou MH, Papassideri IS, Karababa FJ, et al. Ultrastructural characterization of the erythroid cells in a novel case of congenital anemia. Blood Cells Mol Dis 2003;30(1):30–42.

120. Iolascon A, Martire B, Lee MJ, et al. Transfusion-dependent congenital dyserythropoietic anaemia with intraerythroblastic inclusions of a non-globin protein. Eur J Haematol 2000;65(2):140–3.

121. Salvatori F, Breveglieri G, Zuccato C, et al. Production of beta-globin and adult hemoglobin following G418 treatment of erythroid precursor cells from homozygous beta(0)39 thalassemia patients. Am J Hematol 2009;84(11):720–8.

122. Zhang Y, Kwon S, Yamaguchi T, et al. Mice lacking histone deacetylase 6 have hyperacetylated tubulin but are viable and develop normally. Mol Cell Biol 2008; 28(5):1688–701.

123. Hideshima T, Bradner JE, Wong J, et al. Small-molecule inhibition of proteasome and aggresome function induces synergistic antitumor activity in multiple myeloma. Proc Natl Acad Sci U S A 2005;102(24):8567–72.

124. Colland F. The therapeutic potential of deubiquitinating enzyme inhibitors. Biochem Soc Trans 2010;38(Pt 1):137–43.

125. Testa U. Proteasome inhibitors in cancer therapy. Curr Drug Targets 2009; 10(10):968–81.

126. Schessl J, Zou Y, McGrath MJ, et al. Proteomic identification of FHL1 as the protein mutated in human reducing body myopathy. J Clin Invest 2008;118(3): 904–12.

127. Lindsten K, Menéndez-Benito V, Masucci MG, et al. A transgenic mouse model of the ubiquitin/proteasome system. Nat Biotechnol 2003;21(8):897–902.

Anemia, Ineffective Erythropoiesis, and Hepcidin: Interacting Factors in Abnormal Iron Metabolism Leading to Iron Overload in β-Thalassemia

Sara Gardenghi, PhD[a], Robert W. Grady, PhD[b],
Stefano Rivella, PhD[c],*

KEYWORDS

- β-Thalassemia • Ineffective erythropoiesis • Iron overload
- Splenomegaly • Hepcidin • Jak2

β-THALASSEMIA
Genetic Causes, Consequences and Pleiotropic Effects

As discussed in more detail in the overview by Sankaran and Nathan elsewhere in this issue, β-thalassemia is an inherited disorder characterized by mutations in the gene encoding β-globin that lead to the quantitative reduction or, in the most severe cases, the total absence of β-globin synthesis in human erythroid cells. As a consequence, α-globin chains accumulate in excess, forming aggregates that impair erythroid cell maturation, which ultimately leads to a chronic hemolytic anemia and ineffective

This work was supported by the Cooley's Anemia Foundation (CAF), the Associazione Veneta Lotta alla Talassemia (AVLT) (S.G.), and by grants from the Carlo and Micol Schejola Foundation, the Children's Cancer and Blood Foundation and NIH-R21DK065169 (S.R.), R01DK55463 (R.W.G.).
The authors declare no conflict of interest.
[a] Hematology-Oncology, Department of Pediatrics, Weill Cornell Medical College, 515 East 71st Street, Room S724, Mailbox 284, New York, NY 10021, USA
[b] Hematology-Oncology, Department of Pediatrics, Weill Cornell Medical College, 515 East 71st Street, Room S703, Mailbox 284, New York, NY 10021, USA
[c] Hematology-Oncology, Department of Pediatrics, Weill Cornell Medical College, 515 East 71st Street, Room S702, Mailbox 284, New York, NY 10021, USA
* Corresponding author.
E-mail address: str2010@med.cornell.edu

Hematol Oncol Clin N Am 24 (2010) 1089–1107
doi:10.1016/j.hoc.2010.08.003
0889-8588/10/$ – see front matter. Published by Elsevier Inc.

erythropoiesis (IE) (**Fig. 1**). The severity of the clinical manifestations in β-thalassemia varies widely, ranging from patients that are almost asymptomatic to individuals who suffer from severe anemia and require regular blood transfusion to sustain life.[1–6] In general, the clinical severity of the disease correlates with the size of the free α-chain pool and the degree of imbalance between the production of α- and β-like globin chains.

The α/β globin chain imbalance is responsible for the hemolysis of red blood cells (RBCs) and for the premature death (apoptosis) of erythroid precursors in the bone marrow and at extramedullary sites (see **Fig. 1**). The α-globin chain aggregates form inclusion bodies responsible for oxidative stress and membrane damage within RBCs and immature developing erythroblasts. These events are followed by the premature death of many late erythroid precursors in the bone marrow and spleen. Together, these phenomena are designated as IE. The anemia and resulting hypoxia lead to a dramatic increase in serum erythropoietin (Epo) levels in an attempt to compensate for the reduced oxygen-carrying capacity. The marked increase in Epo stimulation, if it is not inhibited by proper transfusion therapy, can lead to uncontrolled expansion of erythroid precursors in the marrow as well as in other sites, such as the spleen and liver, leading to extramedullary hematopoiesis (EMH) (see **Fig. 1**).

The defect in hemoglobin synthesis that occurs in β-thalassemia leads to the development of pleiotropic effects on different body compartments. For example, one of the consequences of IE and EMH is splenomegaly (see **Fig. 1**). The abnormal and damaged RBCs that are produced in β-thalassemia are sequestered by the reticulo-endothelial system in the spleen, causing its enlargement. This enlargement leads to increased sequestration of RBCs, including transfused RBCs, in the spleen, with worsening of the anemia and an increase in transfusion requirement. Increased Epo synthesis is also reflected in marrow expansion, leading to bone marrow hyperplasia, bone deformities, and osteopenia (see **Fig. 1**), which contribute to increased morbidity as the disease progresses.[7]

However, iron overload is the principal and multifaceted complication of β-thalassemia. Physiologically, it is caused by an increased absorption of iron from the gastrointestinal (GI) tract as a consequence of IE, and is greatly aggravated by chronic transfusion therapy. Thus, transfusion-independent individuals with thalassemia

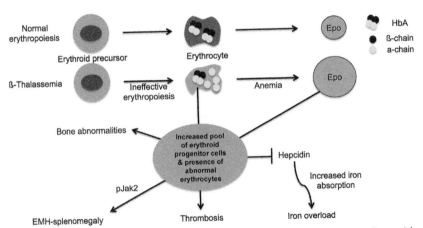

Fig. 1. Consequences of IE and abnormal erythrocyte production. Lines ending with an arrow indicate activation. Lines ending with a line indicate repression.

intermedia have a slower progression of iron overload and generally develop complications later in life compared with patients with thalassemia major who are chronically transfused (see **Fig. 1**). A remarkable variability of tissue iron distribution has been observed in β-thalassemia; liver, heart, and endocrine glands are the organs most severely affected.[5] Accumulation of iron at these sites (siderosis) leads to oxidative damage as a result of the generation of reactive oxygen species (ROS). Death from cardiac failure is the most common clinical consequence of iron excess. Pathologic analysis of cardiac tissue has shown that this occurs initially by hypertrophy and dilatation followed by degeneration of myocardial fibers and fibrosis. Endocrine problems are also related to iron overload (see **Fig. 1**). These problems include hypogonadism, which leads to disturbances of growth and sexual maturation, as well as hypothyroidism, hypoparathyroidism, and diabetes mellitus, which are seen in variable numbers of patients. Therefore, effective iron chelation therapy is a critical component in the management of thalassemia.[8–10] For more than 3 decades, deferoxamine (Desferal) was the chelator of choice.[11] Although this drug is capable of placing all patients into net negative iron balance, it has a disadvantage because it must be infused subcutaneously for 8 to 12 hours, 5 to 7 days a week for the duration of life. Not surprisingly, adherence to such a regimen is generally poor. More recently, 2 orally effective iron chelators, Exjade (deferasirox) and deferiprone (Ferriprox), have been developed to overcome this limitation.[11] Iron overload and chelation therapy are discussed in greater detail elsewhere in this issue in the article by Porter and Shah.

The only definitive cure for thalassemia is the transplant of hematopoietic stem cells (HSC) from cord blood or the bone marrow. This topic is discussed in detail elsewhere in this issue in the article by Gaziev and Lucarelli, as well as that by Kanathezhath and Walters. Splenectomy is another facet in the management of β-thalassemia. However, removal of the spleen can lead to further problems such as an increased risk of infections, pulmonary hypertension, and thrombosis,[12–14] and is usually considered only in the most severe cases of splenomegaly. New approaches to treat/cure the disease are being developed, such as gene therapy, discussed in the article by Bank elsewhere in this issue, or the use of induced pluripotent stem cells as alternatives to the use of HSC.[15,16]

Mouse Models of β-Thalassemia

The use of mouse models of β-thalassemia has been of fundamental importance in clarifying the molecular mechanisms responsible for disease. The 2 available mouse models of β-thalassemia intermedia are th1/th1 and th3/+. In the th1/th1 mouse, the deletion removes the β^{major} gene in the homozygous state,[17] producing hemoglobin levels in the range of 9 to 10 g/dL.[17–19] In the th3/+ mouse model, the deletion removes both the β^{minor} and β^{major} genes in the heterozygous state.[20,21] These mice have hemoglobin levels in the range of 8 to 9 g/dL.[19–21] Both models have a degree of disease severity (hepatosplenomegaly, anemia, aberrant erythrocyte morphology) comparable with that of patients affected by transfusion-independent β-thalassemia intermedia. Their IE is characterized by a modest reduction in RBCs and an increase in reticulocytes.[22] Homozygous (th3/th3) mice that completely lack any adult β-globin chain synthesis die late in gestation,[20] precluding their use as a model for β-thalassemia major. To overcome this limitation, th3/th3 mice are generated by transplantation of hematopoietic fetal liver cells (HFLCs) into lethally irradiated syngeneic adult recipients, the HFLCs being harvested from th3/th3 embryos at 14.5 days of gestation.[22] These mice exhibit severe anemia (3–4 g/dL) 6 to 8 weeks after transplant as well as low RBC levels and reticulocyte counts, together with massive splenomegaly and extensive EMH.[22]

IE

The Epo/EpoR/Jak2/Stat5 Pathway and its Potential Effect(s) on Iron Intake in Erythroid Cells

The hallmark of β-thalassemia is IE that stems from a lack of or reduced synthesis of β-globin, which leads to an excess of α-globin chains that aggregate and precipitate, adhering to the membrane of erythroid precursors. These α-globin aggregates cause cellular and membrane damage, apoptosis of the erythroid precursors in the bone marrow and generation of mature red cells that are abnormal and accumulate in limited numbers. Moreover, the production of red cells, EMH, and the anemia can change significantly over time. Therefore, β-thalassemia serves as a good example of the dynamic balance between expansion of the erythroid pool and production of red cells, and of the many factors that can alter this relationship with critical effects. When pathologic levels of damaged erythrocytes are trapped in the spleen they cause splenomegaly, anemia, and hypoxia. Anemia and hypoxia, in turn, stimulate Epo synthesis, which increases the number of erythroid precursors and abnormal mature red cells in circulation. This situation exacerbates the trapping of erythrocytes in the spleen, thereby worsening the splenomegaly. Moreover, increased erythropoiesis augments iron absorption. Iron overload can increase the formation of ROS, causing damage to many organs and further aggravating the anemia. Blood transfusion is an effective method for ameliorating the anemia and the consequences of IE. But good adherence to iron chelation therapy is necessary to prevent the detrimental effects of iron overload.

Epo is a 34-kDa renal glycoprotein that functions as the main regulator of erythro-poiesis, both under basal and stress conditions. Epo binds to its specific receptor, the erythropoietin receptor (EpoR), at the surface of erythroid cells. EpoR is expressed by the earliest erythroid progenitors at the burst-forming unit-erythroid (BFU-E) stage.[23–25] The Epo/EpoR signaling pathway begins with dimerization of the receptor and activation of the tyrosine-Janus kinase 2 (Jak2),[26–29] which preassembles at a conserved site in the cytoplasmic domain of the EpoR. Jak2 catalyzes transfer of the γ-phosphate group of ATP to the hydroxyl groups of specific tyrosine residues in signal transduction molecules and mediates signaling downstream of cytokine receptors after ligand-induced autophosphorylation of itself and of tyrosine residues of the receptor. In particular, Jak2 mediates the phosphorylation of tyrosine residues localized in a conserved cytoplasmic domain of the EpoR. The resulting phosphory-lated tyrosine residues of the EpoR function as a scaffold or docking sites for the assembly of signal transduction factors containing Src-homology 2 (SH2) domains. The main downstream effectors of Jak2 are a family of transcription factors known as signal transducers and activators of transcription (Stat). In erythroid cells, the main target is Stat5, which, on phosphorylation, translocates to the nucleus as a dimer to drive expression of target genes. The ultimate effect of Jak2 and Stat5 activation is to induce multiple signaling pathways designed to regulate erythroid proliferation and differentiation, and to protect the cells from apoptosis.[28,30,31]

Polycythemia vera (PV), essential thombocytosis, and primary myelofibrosis are classified as myeloproliferative disorders, a subgroup of myeloid malignancies.[32] These are clonal stem cell diseases characterized by an expansion of morphologically mature cells of the granulocyte, erythroid, megakaryocyte, or monocyte lineage. Several studies have described a close association between an activating JAK2 muta-tion (Val 617 to Phe; JAK2V617F) and these disorders.[33] This mutation is believed to prevent the pseudokinase domain from inhibiting the kinase domain, resulting in a constitutively active state of the protein. Thus, JAK2V617F confers constitutive kinase activation. In erythroid cells this leads to STAT5 phosphorylation and Epo-independent erythroid colony formation.[34]

Mice lacking Stat5 expression (Stat5$^{-/-}$) have shown early lethality associated with microcytic anemia and enhanced apoptosis of early erythroblasts.[35–37] Although the anemia in these mice correlates with loss of expression of the antiapoptotic Bcl-X$_L$ gene and enhanced apoptosis,[38] additional analyses indicate that Stat5$^{-/-}$ mice have a significant decrease in expression of the iron transporter transferrin receptor-1 (Tfr1).[38,39] Therefore, it is possible that erythroid cells might express higher levels of Tfr1 under conditions of constitutive activation or upregulation of Jak2. Potential consequences of Jak2 modulation of iron intake in β-thalassemic red cells are discussed in the next section.

New Studies on Jak2 and IE in β-Thalassemia

Original ferrokinetic studies and analysis of erythroid precursors in β-thalassemia indicated that many of these cells die in the marrow and extramedullary sites,[40–43] and suggested that the relative excess of α chains triggering apoptosis was responsible for IE. However, several recent observations suggest that the balance between proliferation and differentiation in some of the erythroid precursors might be different under normal conditions and those of IE.[44] These results and those of new studies in mice (discussed later) suggest that the mechanism(s) and various factors associated with the process known as IE have not yet been completely elucidated.

The splenomegaly exhibited by th3/+ mice[44] is similar to that observed in patients affected by β-thalassemia intermedia (transfusion independent). Studies on th3/+ mice have shown that their spleen fills with erythroid precursors and sequesters abnormal/damaged erythrocytes, likely contributing to lowering of the hemoglobin level over time.[44] Similar observations have been confirmed in splenic specimens from patients with thalassemia intermedia.[15,44,45] However, analysis of the erythroid precursors in both the bone marrow and spleen in these animals indicated that a large number of these cells were actively proliferating, whereas the proportion of cells undergoing apoptosis, although higher than in normal mice, was modest.[44] Compared with wild-type animals, th3/+ mice have a higher number of erythroid cells associated with the expression of cell cycle-promoting genes such as EpoR, Jak2 (see **Fig. 1**), Cyclin-A, Cdk2, and Ki-67, together with increased levels of the Bcl-X$_L$ protein.[44] These cells also differentiate less than the corresponding normal cells in vitro. Based on this observation, we can speculate that thalassemic patients may increase the number of erythroid precursors in their spleen and liver over time, this being one factor leading to hepatosplenomegaly. In turn, this factor also exacerbates the anemia in β-thalassemia.[15,44,45]

The increase of Epo levels in response to anemia and hypoxia has already been discussed. Based on the observations made earlier, it is reasonable to expect that increased Epo levels could also activate the EpoR/Jak2 pathway, leading to a physiologic gain of function of Jak2. Under these circumstances, the persistent phosphorylation of Jak2 might lead to an increased number of erythroid progenitor cells. Therefore, suppression of Jak2 activity might modulate IE. Based on this model, we showed that use of a Jak2 inhibitor has a beneficial effect in limiting IE, splenomegaly, and the number of erythroid progenitor cells in β-thalassemia.[44] In particular, limiting the number of erythroid progenitors might have a beneficial effect on iron metabolism, because it has been suggested that these cells are the most plausible source of the erythroid factor, whose function is to increase iron absorption by repressing hepcidin expression, as shown in **Figs. 1** and **2** and further discussed later. Therefore, future

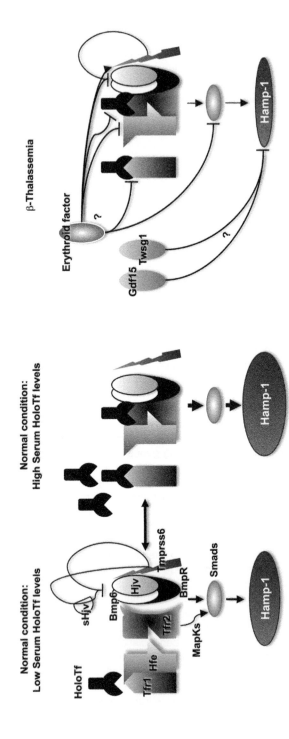

Fig. 2. Potential pathways controlling iron absorption in β-thalassemia. Lines ending with an arrow indicate activation. Lines ending with a line indicate repression.

studies need to address whether the use of Jak2 inhibitors could also limit iron absorption in β-thalassemia.

Activation of the Epo/EpoR/Jak2 pathway is not likely to be the only cause for the limited erythroid differentiation observed in β-thalassemia. For example, in the absence of other erythroid defects, mutations responsible for the constitutive activation of Jak2 lead to the development of PV rather than IE.[46] Therefore, it is possible to predict that other factors and/or abnormal physiologic conditions present in β-thalassemia interfere with erythroid cell differentiation. Among the possible factors acting together with Jak2, iron overload, ROS, the unbalanced synthesis of globin chains and/or heme can be considered.[45] Iron is essential for all cells but is toxic in excess. We recently focused on the potential role of iron and heme in modulating IE. Our hypothesis was that thalassemic erythroid cells accumulate an excess of toxic heme associated with free α chains, leading to the formation of ROS, which has been associated with red cell hemolysis and altered differentiation.[47,48] Our preliminary data suggest that this is the case and that if the hemoglobin content per cell (mean corpuscular hemoglobin [MCH]) and the overall amount of heme are reduced in thalassemic erythroid cells, both ROS and the accumulation of α-chains on red cell plasma membranes are reduced, ameliorating not only the quality and life span of the RBCs but also the anemia and IE (Gardenghi and colleagues, unpublished data, 2010). The amelioration of IE was associated with decreased splenomegaly and a better balance between erythroid precursors and mature RBCs. Based on these preliminary observations, we speculate that ROS play a role in modulating the balance between proliferation and differentiation of the erythroid cells. Additional studies point to the role of ROS in cell differentiation in erythropoiesis, stem cells, and cancer, supporting this hypothesis.[49,50]

Serum iron is bound to transferrin and enters erythroid cells primarily via receptor-mediated endocytosis of the transferrin/Tfr1 complex. Tfr1 is essential for developing erythrocytes. Reduced Tfr1 expression is associated with anemia. *Stat5-null* mice are severely anemic and die perinatally. Two studies have associated Stat5 with iron homeostasis,[38,39] showing that ablation of Stat5 leads to a dramatic reduction in both the mRNA and protein levels of iron regulatory protein 2 (IRP-2) and *Tfr1*. Both genes have been shown to be direct transcriptional targets of Stat5, establishing a clear link between EpoR/Jak2/Stat5 signaling and iron metabolism. As we proposed previously, reduced iron intake in erythroid cells limits the formation of toxic α-chain/heme aggregates and ROS formation, having a beneficial effect on IE. This finding has been supported indirectly by the work of Ginzburg and colleagues.[51] In their studies, iron delivery to erythroid cells in mice affected by β-thalassemia intermedia was modulated by administration of apo-transferrin. This finding was associated with reduction of splenomegaly and IE, improvement in hemoglobin levels, and an increased number of RBCs. The hemoglobin content per cell (MCH) was also decreased, as was the formation of membrane-bound α-chain aggregates. These data reinforce the notion that decreasing iron availability, either by decreasing iron absorption or transferrin saturation, is beneficial to abnormal erythroid cells. Therefore, based on the association between Jak2 and Tfr1, Jak2 inhibitors might also ameliorate IE by decreasing expression of Tfr1, iron intake, formation of toxic α-chain/heme aggregates, and ROS. In conclusion, use of Jak2 inhibitors in β-thalassemia might also be beneficial because of their role in controlling iron metabolism in erythroid cells.

IRON METABOLISM
Hepcidin and Regulation of Iron Absorption

Erythropoiesis and iron metabolism are closely interconnected. The iron used by the body is obtained by recycling that present in senescent RBCs or absorbed from the diet at the level of the proximal intestine. More than two-thirds of the iron content of the body is incorporated into hemoglobin in developing erythroid precursors and mature RBCs.[52] Hepcidin (HAMP/Hamp),[53,54] a cysteine-rich 25-amino acid peptide synthesized in the liver from an 84-amino acid prepropeptide, plays a major role in iron homeostasis. Hepcidin was originally isolated from blood ultra filtrate and urine.[53,54] Its target is ferroportin, which is the only known iron exporter on enterocytes, hepatocytes, and macrophages. Hepcidin binds ferroportin, promoting its internalization and degradation,[55,56] thereby negatively regulating iron absorption and iron recycling within the body. Hepcidin is upregulated in response to iron overload[57] and inflammation,[58–61] and downregulated by erythropoietic stimuli such as anemia, hypoxia, or EPO synthesis/administration.[58,62,63] In all these scenarios, hepcidin acts primarily on ferroportin, controlling iron egress from enterocytes and macrophages, and modulating dietary iron absorption as well as erythropoiesis.

In the last few years, many studies have characterized proteins that contribute to hepcidin regulation. **Fig. 2** is a nonexhaustive representation of the proteins and pathways involved in hepcidin regulation. Hepatic cells can take up holo transferrin (holoTf) through Tfr1 by receptor-mediated endocytosis. The same region of Tfr1 that binds holoTf is also recognized by Hfe (see **Fig. 2**).[64,65] HFE is an atypical HLA class I protein. Mutations in *HFE* cause hemochromatosis, which is a disorder characterized by excess total body iron as a result of hyperabsorption from the diet.[66] When the concentration of holoTf in the serum increases, both holoTf and Hfe bind to Tfr2, which is a protein homologous to Tfr1, although the relative affinity of Tfr2 for holoTf and Hfe is reduced compared with that of Tfr1.[67–69] The Hfe/Tfr2 complex then interacts with a second protein complex to signal upregulation of hepcidin. This second complex of proteins involves the association of bone morphogenetic protein-6 (Bmp6) ligand with a complex of type I and type II serine threonine kinase receptors and the hemojuvelin (Hjv) coreceptor yielding the hepcidin signaling or iron sensor complex (see **Fig. 2**).[68,70–74] The resulting complex propagates the signal through phosphorylation of cytoplasmic effectors Smad1, Smad5, and Smad8. Once phosphorylated, Smad1/5/8 form heteromeric complexes with the common mediator Smad4 and translocate to the nucleus where they modulate transcription of target genes, including hepcidin.[73,75] Moreover, it has been shown that Tfr2 can be activated by its ligand holoTf, leading to stimulation of the extracellular signal regulated kinase (Erk)/mitogen activated protein kinase (MapK) pathway, and induction of hepcidin.[76,77] Even in this case, Erk activation by holoTf provokes increased levels of phospho-Smad1/5/8.

Mutations in some of these proteins (Hamp, Hfe, Hjv, Tfr2, Bmp6) have clearly been associated with conditions that lead to iron overload because they impair hepcidin expression, either directly or indirectly.[78,79] In contrast, mutations in TMPRSS6, a type II transmembrane serine protease, are associated with a condition termed iron-refractory iron-deficiency anemia, in which hepcidin expression is increased and both patients and mice suffer from iron deficiency and severe anemia.[80,81] Several studies indicate that Tmprss6 targets and degrades Hjv, preventing its assembly in the iron sensor complex, profoundly impairing the Bmp6/Smad pathway (see **Fig. 2**).[82] A soluble form(s) of Hjv (sHjv) might also act as a decoy for some of the proteins in the complex, limiting its assembly.[83] Moreover, it has been shown that mice deficient in Tmprss6 have decreased iron stores and decreased Bmp6 mRNA, but markedly increased mRNA for Id1, another target gene of Bmp6 signaling. Id1, whose promoter is strongly activated by Bmp6 in a Smad-dependent manner, encodes a negative inhibitor of basic helix-loop-helix (bHLH) proteins. Mice deficient in both Tmprss6 and Hjv showed decreased hepatic levels of hepcidin and Id1 mRNA, whereas

Bmp6 mRNA was markedly increased.[84] These mice suffer from systemic iron overload similar to mice deficient in Hjv alone.[85] Such findings suggest that regulation of hepcidin expression and maintenance of systemic iron homeostasis by Tmprss6 requires downregulation of Bmp6/Smad signaling and expression of Id1.

As mentioned previously, hepcidin synthesis is downregulated by erythropoietic stimuli such as anemia, hypoxia, and Epo synthesis/administration,[58,62,63] thereby increasing the GI absorption of iron and its release from stores. It has been postulated that an erythroid regulator modulates these responses by acting, directly or indirectly, on the synthesis of hepcidin (see **Fig. 2**). The existence of an erythroid factor is supported by studies in which the serum of patients affected by β-thalassemia or Hfe-related hemochromatosis were compared in terms of their ability to induce the expression of hepcidin and other genes related to iron metabolism in hepatic cells. Sera from β-thalassemia major and intermedia patients downregulated hepcidin expression, whereas sera from those affected by hemochromatosis had no effect on hepcidin.[86] Although it has been suggested that hypoxia and Epo suppress hepcidin expression, there is considerable evidence indicating that the erythropoietic regulator must involve a soluble factor from the hematopoietic bone marrow. For instance, inhibitors of erythropoiesis can be administered after phlebotomy to disassociate the effects of anemia, hypoxia, and Epo from those of increased erythropoiesis. Phlebotomized mice develop anemia, tissue hypoxia, increased levels of Epo and erythropoiesis, and decreased levels of hepatic hepcidin mRNA. When erythropoietic inhibitors were administered, hepcidin mRNA rose dramatically, even although the mice were anemic, hypoxic, and exhibited increased Epo levels.[87] If this scenario is correct, it is reasonable to predict that the mediator is a factor secreted by erythroid cells, most likely immature and proliferating erythroid cells. Therefore, we propose that this factor should be more abundant under conditions in which the number of erythroid progenitors is increased, such as after recovery from acute anemia or when IE is present (see **Figs. 1** and **2**). Because erythropoiesis is the most important process using iron in the body, we also speculate that the erythroid regulator operates efficiently in controlling iron metabolism. The function of the erythroid regulator should be to maintain production of erythrocytes irrespective of the iron balance of the body. However, as we do not know yet how this factor works, we can only speculate that it might operate by targeting one or more components of the iron sensor complex, the mediators activated by this complex, or the hepcidin promoter, as shown in **Fig. 2**.

The Role of Hepcidin in β-Thalassemia

Studies have shown that the rate of iron absorption from the GI tract in patients affected by β-thalassemia is approximately 3 to 4 times greater than that in healthy individuals.[88] But how does the increased iron absorption affect tissue iron distribution and ultimately erythropoiesis in β-thalassemia? Ferrokinetic studies showed that when donor serum labeled with ^{59}Fe was injected into healthy subjects, 75% to 90% of the iron was incorporated into newly formed red cells within 7 to 10 days. However, when ^{59}Fe was injected into thalassemic patients, only 15% to 20% of it was found in circulating erythrocytes.[40] It was hypothesized that the remaining iron was sequestered in those organs in which erythroid precursors are subject to premature destruction, such as the bone marrow in humans, and the bone marrow and spleen in mice.

Numerous studies have shown that altered hepcidin expression is responsible for the increased iron absorption observed in β-thalassemia.[89–91] In particular, the correlation between IE, iron distribution, and the expression of hepcidin have been investigated in mice affected by thalassemia intermedia and major, models characterized by different degrees of anemia and IE.[19,89] The major conclusion is that the pattern of iron distribution in β-thalassemia is dictated by the degree of IE. Where severe anemia exists, hepcidin levels are low, and iron overload occurs rapidly, involving predominantly liver parenchymal cells. On the other hand, when the anemia is milder, iron accumulates progressively in splenic macrophages and Kupffer cells in the liver. When thalassemia major mice were transfused, their anemia and IE improved, whereas iron deposition in the liver was reduced. Analyses using human specimens indicated that urinary hepcidin levels were lower in β-thalassemic patients than those that would be predicted by their iron burden, whereas transfusion therapy led to an increase in the hepcidin levels.[92–96]

In mice affected by β-thalassemia intermedia, it has been observed that they exhibit low hepcidin levels during the first months of life.[16,89,91,97–99] As these animals age and iron overload worsens, the level of hepcidin increases, indicating that hepcidin is still partially responsive to iron overload when IE is moderate.[16,89,98] In contrast, the extreme degree of IE in mice affected by thalassemia major limited hepcidin from sensing the iron burden and kept its expression low. Altogether these observations indicate that the relative levels of IE and iron overload mediate the synthesis of hepcidin in β-thalassemia.

Two erythroid regulators have been proposed called growth differentiation factor 15 (GDF15) and twisted gastrulation protein homolog 1 (TWSG1).[100,101] They are members of the transforming growth factor β (TGF-β) superfamily of proteins known to control proliferation, differentiation, and apoptosis in numerous cell types. Both GDF15 and TWSG1 are increased in the serum of β-thalassemic patients and suppress hepcidin expression in vitro.[101] Comparing normal and thalassemic erythroid cells differentiating in vitro, GDF15 was isolated during the final stages of erythroid differentiation.[101] This finding suggests that GDF15 is secreted by erythroid precursors undergoing cell death. GDF15 is not increased after stem cell transplantation in patients with hematopoietic malignancies or in patients with iron deficiency secondary to blood donation, conditions in which apoptosis of erythroid cells is not observed.[102,103] These findings confirm that GDF15 is not produced by proliferating erythroid precursors but rather by apoptotic erythroid cells, as in β-thalassemia or refractory anemia with ring-sideroblasts.[104] Therefore, GDF15 may limit hepcidin synthesis when erythroid precursors undergo cell death.[44] In contrast to GDF15, the highest levels of TWSG1 were detected at early stages of erythroblast differentiation, before hemoglobinization of the cells.[100] Future studies will determine whether TWSG1 is an erythroid factor present only in sera of thalassemic patients or whether it is associated with many other conditions characterized by increased erythropoiesis and hepcidin suppression.

QUESTIONS AND POTENTIAL NOVEL THERAPIES
Administration of Jak2 Inhibitors, and Potential Effects Following Reduced Iron Intake by Erythroid Cells

Previously, we discussed how Jak2 might influence IE, splenomegaly, and anemia in β-thalassemia. One obvious consequence of these observations has been to investigate whether Jak2 inhibitors might have beneficial effects in reducing/preventing splenomegaly and ameliorating the clinical phenotype of this disease. Our preclinical data obtained by using Jak2 inhibitors in mice affected by β-thalassemia intermedia support the notion that patients might benefit from using such compounds.[44] Many patients with thalassemia intermedia develop splenomegaly and the need for transfusion therapy, most of them eventually requiring splenectomy. However, because the V617F mutation is localized in a region away from the ATP-binding site of JAK2, the

ATP-competitive inhibitors of JAK2 kinase (ATP analogs) presently used in clinical trials are not likely to discriminate between the wild-type and mutant enzyme. Therefore, their use could decrease RBC synthesis and worsen anemia. With these facts in mind, we tested the effect of administering a Jak2 inhibitor to thalassemic mice in association with blood transfusion. Our preliminary data indicate that the combined use of a Jak2 inhibitor and blood transfusion is superior to either treatment alone in ameliorating splenomegaly and IE (Melchiori and colleagues, unpublished data, 2010). Thus, Jak2 inhibitors might be used temporarily to reduce the spleen size and, in the presence of blood transfusions, to treat or prevent worsening of the anemia. The ultimate goal would be to prevent or delay the need for splenectomy and indirectly to improve the management of the anemia, thereby reducing the need for blood transfusions. Moreover, future studies should investigate whether Jak2 inhibitors, through their potential modulation of Tfr1 synthesis, can also modify iron uptake into forming thalassemic erythroid cells, limiting the formation of α-chain/heme aggregates and ameliorating the phenotype of the erythroid cells.

Administration of Hepcidin Agonists or Activators of Hepcidin Expression

As a result of hepcidin deficiency, patients with β-thalassemia intermedia develop iron overload in a manner similar to those with hereditary hemochromatosis. Accordingly, abnormal iron absorption in these patients might be prevented by administration or upregulation of hepcidin (Gardenghi and colleagues, unpublished data, 2010).[105] In β-thalassemia major, transfusions rather than dietary iron absorption are the predominant cause of iron overload. In affected individuals, hepcidin levels are higher because IE is suppressed by transfusion therapy. Moreover, hepcidin production is stimulated by the additional iron load derived from the transfusion of red cells. However, hepcidin concentrations decrease in the intervals between transfusions, as the effect of each transfusion is lost.[92,93,101] Thus, although intestinal iron absorption contributes less to the total iron load in these patients, hepcidin therapy may be effective when endogenous hepcidin decreases and intestinal iron uptake increases. The potential benefits of hepcidin therapy are already supported by a few studies using mouse models of hemochromatosis.[65,106] Based on these assumptions and observations, we are further investigating whether or not modulation of hepcidin could be beneficial in β-thalassemia. For this purpose we are using mice affected by β-thalassemia intermedia genetically altered to overexpress hepcidin.

Our preliminary data indicate that hepcidin-mediated iron restriction may not only ameliorate iron overload in mice affected by β-thalassemia intermedia but also improve their erythropoiesis. We hypothesize that amelioration of erythropoiesis in these mice is caused by decreased α-chain/heme aggregates and ROS formation. Alpha-chain/heme aggregates can precipitate and lodge in red cell plasma membranes, affecting the properties and lifespan of RBCs. Therefore, reduction of these aggregates might improve the phenotype of the thalassemic red cells and increase their life span, with positive feedback on IE (**Fig. 3**). Moreover, these aggregates are also likely to cause the formation of ROS in erythroid cells. ROS levels are increased in red cells derived from patients with β-thalassemia. As a result, glutathione levels are lower than in normal red cells.[107] ROS likely exacerbate the anemia, further decreasing the already shortened survival of mature RBCs in the circulation.[47,108] Excessive ROS formation in maturing erythroid cells might also affect the cell cycle and worsen IE. The Forkhead Box O (FoxO) family of transcription factors plays an essential role in the regulation of oxidative stress in hematopoietic stem and erythroid cells.[109] In FoxO3 null mice, red cell survival is reduced and is associated with enhanced mitotic arrest of intermediate erythroid progenitor cells, resulting in

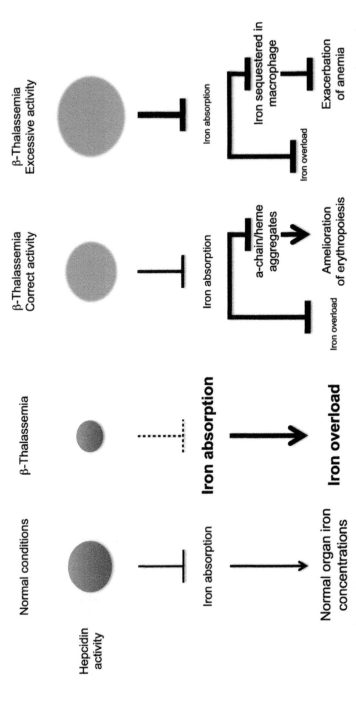

Fig. 3. Potential effects of hepcidin agonists or activators on iron absorption under normal and β-thalassemic conditions. Lines ending with an arrow indicate activation. Lines ending with a line indicate repression.

a decreased rate of erythroid maturation.[48] This finding raises the interesting possibility that ROS levels regulate not only RBC survival but also the maturation process of erythroid progenitor cells, modulating IE. Therefore, using hepcidin as a tool to reduce iron absorption might be a novel and exciting approach to controlling IE and managing β-thalassemia.

The studies undertaken to evaluate the effect of overexpressing hepcidin on iron overload and erythropoiesis have used genetic models and have not explored the feasibility of using hepcidin or its agonists as drugs. Development of such compounds determines their potential to prevent iron overload or reverse its toxic effects based on a dose-response relationship. However, because ferroportin is localized on macrophages as well, the administration or upregulation of hepcidin in thalassemia may also affect iron recycling and its availability for erythropoiesis, ultimately worsening anemia (see **Fig. 3**). For this reason, preclinical studies must address the effect of these drugs on both iron overload and erythropoiesis. Because the levels of hepcidin are low in thalassemia and body iron is in excess, hepcidin therapy may be feasible depending on the level of hepcidin achieved (see **Fig. 3**). Further study in mouse models of thalassemia followed by rigorous clinical trials in patients will address these issues.

SUMMARY

- Patients with β-thalassemia develop secondary effects such as splenomegaly and iron overload.
- IE is the hallmark of β-thalassemia, characterized by the premature death of erythroid precursors in the bone marrow and extramedullary sites.
- Erythrocytes trapped in the spleen are the cause of splenomegaly, anemia, and hypoxia, which lead to increased Epo production.
- Splenomegaly eventually contributes to worsening of the anemia, necessitating splenectomy.
- Because of increased Epo expression, the Epo/EpoR/Jak2/Stat5 pathway, which regulates erythropoiesis, is overactive in β-thalassemia, contributing to EMH and splenomegaly.
- Jak2 inhibitors, used in combination with transfusion therapy, represent an alternative approach aimed at modulating IE and preventing splenomegaly/splenectomy.
- Inhibition of Jak2 activity might also modulate the number of erythroid progenitor cells in β-thalassemia. These cells are the most plausible source of the erythroid factor, the proposed function of which is to increase iron absorption by suppressing hepcidin expression. Therefore, reducing Jak2 activity might have a beneficial effect on iron metabolism as well.
- The only effective treatment of iron overload is chelation therapy.
- Decreased expression of hepcidin is the cause of increased iron absorption in β-thalassemia.
- Alternative therapies to prevent iron overload include upregulation of hepcidin expression and the direct administration of hepcidin agonists.

REFERENCES

1. Cooley TB, Lee P. A series of cases of splenomegaly in children with anemia and peculiar bone changes. Trans Am Pediatr Soc 1925;37:29.
2. Weatherall DJ. Single gene disorders or complex traits: lessons from the thalassaemias and other monogenic diseases. BMJ 2000;321(7269):1117–20.

3. Weatherall DJ. Phenotype-genotype relationships in monogenic disease: lessons from the thalassaemias. Nat Rev Genet 2001;2(4):245–55.

4. Forget BG. Molecular mechanisms of β thalassemia. In: Steinberg MH, Forget BG, Higgs DR, et al, editors. Disorders of hemoglobin: genetics, pathophysiology and clinical management. Cambridge (UK): Cambridge University Press; 2001. p. 252–76.

5. Steinberg MH, Forget BG, Higgs DR, et al. Disorders of hemoglobin: genetics, pathophysiology and clinical management. 2nd edition. Cambridge (UK): Cambridge University Press; 2009. p. 1–826.

6. Cao A, Pintus L, Lecca U, et al. Control of homozygous beta-thalassemia by carrier screening and antenatal diagnosis in Sardinians. Clin Genet 1984; 26(1):12–22.

7. Vichinsky EP. The morbidity of bone disease in thalassemia. Ann N Y Acad Sci 1998;850:344–8.

8. Wonke B. Clinical management of beta-thalassemia major. Semin Hematol 2001; 38(4):350–9.

9. Cohen AR, Galanello R, Pennell DJ, et al. Thalassemia. Hematology Am Soc Hematol Educ Program 2004;14–34.

10. Piomelli S. The management of patients with Cooley's anemia: transfusions and splenectomy. Semin Hematol 1995;32(4):262–8.

11. Giardina PJ, Grady RW. Chelation therapy in beta-thalassemia: an optimistic update. Semin Hematol 2001;38(4):360–6.

12. Crary SE, Buchanan GR. Vascular complications after splenectomy for hematologic disorders. Blood 2009;114(14):2861–8.

13. Eldor A, Rachmilewitz EA. The hypercoagulable state in thalassemia. Blood 2002;99(1):36–43.

14. Taher A, Mehio G, Isma'eel H, et al. Stroke in thalassemia: a dilemma. Am J Hematol 2008;83(4):343.

15. Rivella S, Rachmilewitz E. Future alternative therapies for beta-thalassemia. Expert Rev Hematol 2009;2(6):685.

16. Breda L, Gambari R, Rivella S. Gene therapy in thalassemia and hemoglobinopathies. Mediterranean Journal of Hematology and Infectious Diseases 2009; 1(1):e2009008.

17. Skow LC, Burkhart BA, Johnson FM, et al. A mouse model for beta-thalassemia. Cell 1983;34(3):1043–52.

18. Curcio MJ, Kantoff P, Schafer MP, et al. Compensatory increase in levels of beta minor globin in murine beta-thalassemia is under translational control. J Biol Chem 1986;261(34):16126–32.

19. De Franceschi L, Daraio F, Filippini A, et al. Liver expression of hepcidin and other iron genes in two mouse models of beta-thalassemia. Haematologica 2006;91(10):1336–42.

20. Yang B, Kirby S, Lewis J, et al. A mouse model for beta 0-thalassemia. Proc Natl Acad Sci U S A 1995;92(25):11608–12.

21. Ciavatta DJ, Ryan TM, Farmer SC, et al. Mouse model of human beta zero thalassemia: targeted deletion of the mouse beta maj- and beta min-globin genes in embryonic stem cells. Proc Natl Acad Sci U S A 1995;92(20): 9259–63.

22. Rivella S, May C, Chadburn A, et al. A novel murine model of Cooley anemia and its rescue by lentiviral-mediated human beta -globin gene transfer. Blood 2003; 101(8):2932–9.

23. Wu H, Liu X, Jaenisch R, et al. Generation of committed erythroid BFU-E and CFU-E progenitors does not require erythropoietin or the erythropoietin receptor. Cell 1995;83(1):59–67.
24. D'Andrea A, Fasman G, Wong G, et al. Erythropoietin receptor: cloning strategy and structural features. Int J Cell Cloning 1990;8(Suppl 1):173–80.
25. D'Andrea AD, Lodish HF, Wong GG. Expression cloning of the murine erythropoietin receptor. Cell 1989;57(2):277–85.
26. Li K, Miller C, Hegde S, et al. Roles for an Epo receptor Tyr-343 Stat5 pathway in proliferative co-signaling with kit. J Biol Chem 2003;278(42):40702–9.
27. Menon MP, Fang J, Wojchowski DM. Core erythropoietin receptor signals for late erythroblast development. Blood 2006;107(7):2662–72.
28. Menon MP, Karur V, Bogacheva O, et al. Signals for stress erythropoiesis are integrated via an erythropoietin receptor-phosphotyrosine-343-Stat5 axis. J Clin Invest 2006;116(3):683–94.
29. von Lindern M, Zauner W, Mellitzer G, et al. The glucocorticoid receptor cooperates with the erythropoietin receptor and c-Kit to enhance and sustain proliferation of erythroid progenitors in vitro. Blood 1999;94(2):550–9.
30. Fang J, Menon M, Kapelle W, et al. EPO modulation of cell-cycle regulatory genes, and cell division, in primary bone marrow erythroblasts. Blood 2007;110(7):2361–70.
31. Socolovsky M, Murrell M, Liu Y, et al. Negative autoregulation by FAS mediates robust fetal erythropoiesis. PLoS Biol 2007;5(10):e252.
32. James C. The JAK2V617F mutation in polycythemia vera and other myeloproliferative disorders: one mutation for three diseases? Hematology Am Soc Hematol Educ Program 2008;69–75.
33. Levine RL. Mechanisms of mutations in myeloproliferative neoplasms. Best Pract Res Clin Haematol 2009;22(4):489–94.
34. Garcon L, Rivat C, James C, et al. Constitutive activation of STAT5 and Bcl-xL overexpression can induce endogenous erythroid colony formation in human primary cells. Blood 2006;108(5):1551–4.
35. Socolovsky M, Nam H, Fleming MD, et al. Ineffective erythropoiesis in Stat5a(-/-) 5b(-/-) mice due to decreased survival of early erythroblasts. Blood 2001;98(12):3261–73.
36. Socolovsky M, Fallon AE, Wang S, et al. Fetal anemia and apoptosis of red cell progenitors in Stat5a-/-5b-/- mice: a direct role for Stat5 in Bcl-X(L) induction. Cell 1999;98(2):181–91.
37. Dolznig H, Grebien F, Deiner EM, et al. Erythroid progenitor renewal versus differentiation: genetic evidence for cell autonomous, essential functions of EpoR, Stat5 and the GR. Oncogene 2006;25(20):2890–900.
38. Kerenyi MA, Grebien F, Gehart H, et al. Stat5 regulates cellular iron uptake of erythroid cells via IRP-2 and TfR-1. Blood 2008;112(9):3878–88.
39. Zhu BM, McLaughlin SK, Na R, et al. Hematopoietic-specific Stat5-null mice display microcytic hypochromic anemia associated with reduced transferrin receptor gene expression. Blood 2008;112(5):2071–80.
40. Finch CA, Deubelbeiss K, Cook JD, et al. Ferrokinetics in man. Medicine 1970;49(1):17–53.
41. Centis F, Tabellini L, Lucarelli G, et al. The importance of erythroid expansion in determining the extent of apoptosis in erythroid precursors in patients with beta-thalassemia major. Blood 2000;96(10):3624–9.

42. Mathias LA, Fisher TC, Zeng L, et al. Ineffective erythropoiesis in beta-thalassemia major is due to apoptosis at the polychromatophilic normoblast stage. Exp Hematol 2000;28(12):1343–53.

43. Yuan J, Angelucci E, Lucarelli G, et al. Accelerated programmed cell death (apoptosis) in erythroid precursors of patients with severe beta-thalassemia (Cooley's anemia). Blood 1993;82(2):374–7.

44. Libani IV, Guy EC, Melchiori L, et al. Decreased differentiation of erythroid cells exacerbates ineffective erythropoiesis in {beta}-thalassemia. Blood 2008; 112(3):875–85.

45. Rivella S. Ineffective erythropoiesis and thalassemias. Curr Opin Hematol 2009; 16(3):187–94.

46. Wang YL, Vandris K, Jones A, et al. JAK2 mutations are present in all cases of polycythemia vera. Leukemia 2008;22(6):1289.

47. Fibach E, Rachmilewitz E. The role of oxidative stress in hemolytic anemia. Curr Mol Med 2008;8(7):609–19.

48. Marinkovic D, Zhang X, Yalcin S, et al. Foxo3 is required for the regulation of oxidative stress in erythropoiesis. J Clin Invest 2007;117(8):2133–44.

49. Callens C, Coulon S, Naudin J, et al. Targeting iron homeostasis induces cellular differentiation and synergizes with differentiating agents in acute myeloid leukemia. J Exp Med 2010;207(4):731–50.

50. Abdel-Wahab O, Levine RL. Metabolism and the leukemic stem cell. J Exp Med 2010;207(4):677–80.

51. Li H, Rybicki AC, Suzuka SM, et al. Transferrin therapy ameliorates disease in beta-thalassemic mice. Nat Med 2010;16(2):177–82.

52. Andrews NC. Disorders of iron metabolism. N Engl J Med 1999;341(26): 1986–95.

53. Krause A, Neitz S, Magert HJ, et al. LEAP-1, a novel highly disulfide-bonded human peptide, exhibits antimicrobial activity. FEBS Lett 2000;480(2–3):147–50.

54. Park CH, Valore EV, Waring AJ, et al. Hepcidin, a urinary antimicrobial peptide synthesized in the liver. J Biol Chem 2001;276(11):7806–10.

55. Nemeth E, Tuttle MS, Powelson J, et al. Hepcidin regulates cellular iron efflux by binding to ferroportin and inducing its internalization. Science 2004;306(5704): 2090–3.

56. Nemeth E, Preza GC, Jung CL, et al. The N-terminus of hepcidin is essential for its interaction with ferroportin: structure-function study. Blood 2006;107(1):328–33.

57. Pigeon C, Ilyin G, Courselaud B, et al. A new mouse liver-specific gene, encoding a protein homologous to human antimicrobial peptide hepcidin, is overexpressed during iron overload. J Biol Chem 2001;276(11):7811–9.

58. Nicolas G, Chauvet C, Viatte L, et al. The gene encoding the iron regulatory peptide hepcidin is regulated by anemia, hypoxia, and inflammation. J Clin Invest 2002;110(7):1037–44.

59. Nemeth E, Rivera S, Gabayan V, et al. IL-6 mediates hypoferremia of inflammation by inducing the synthesis of the iron regulatory hormone hepcidin. J Clin Invest 2004;113(9):1271–6.

60. Nemeth E, Valore EV, Territo M, et al. Hepcidin, a putative mediator of anemia of inflammation, is a type II acute-phase protein. Blood 2003;101(7):2461–3.

61. Wrighting DM, Andrews NC. Interleukin-6 induces hepcidin expression through STAT3. Blood 2006;108(9):3204–9.

62. Nicolas G, Viatte L, Bennoun M, et al. Hepcidin, a new iron regulatory peptide. Blood Cells Mol Dis 2002;29(3):327–35.

63. Vokurka M, Krijt J, Sulc K, et al. Hepcidin mRNA levels in mouse liver respond to inhibition of erythropoiesis. Physiol Res 2006;55(6):667–74.

64. Lebron JA, West AP Jr, Bjorkman PJ. The hemochromatosis protein HFE competes with transferrin for binding to the transferrin receptor. J Mol Biol 1999;294(1):239–45.

65. Schmidt PJ, Toran PT, Giannetti AM, et al. The transferrin receptor modulates Hfe-dependent regulation of hepcidin expression. Cell Metab 2008;7(3):205–14.

66. Feder JN, Gnirke A, Thomas W, et al. A novel MHC class I-like gene is mutated in patients with hereditary haemochromatosis. Nat Genet 1996; 13(4):399–408.

67. Kawabata H, Yang R, Hirama T, et al. Molecular cloning of transferrin receptor 2. A new member of the transferrin receptor-like family. J Biol Chem 1999;274(30): 20826–32.

68. Goswami T, Andrews NC. Hereditary hemochromatosis protein, HFE, interaction with transferrin receptor 2 suggests a molecular mechanism for mammalian iron sensing. J Biol Chem 2006;281(39):28494–8.

69. Gao J, Chen J, Kramer M, et al. Interaction of the hereditary hemochromatosis protein HFE with transferrin receptor 2 is required for transferrin-induced hepcidin expression. Cell Metab 2009;9(3):217–27.

70. Wang RH, Li C, Xu X, et al. A role of SMAD4 in iron metabolism through the positive regulation of hepcidin expression. Cell Metab 2005;2(6):399–409.

71. Babitt JL, Huang FW, Wrighting DM, et al. Bone morphogenetic protein signaling by hemojuvelin regulates hepcidin expression. Nat Genet 2006; 38(5):531–9.

72. Babitt JL, Huang FW, Xia Y, et al. Modulation of bone morphogenetic protein signaling in vivo regulates systemic iron balance. J Clin Invest 2007;117(7): 1933–9.

73. Kautz L, Meynard D, Monnier A, et al. Iron regulates phosphorylation of Smad1/ 5/8 and gene expression of Bmp6, Smad7, Id1, and Atoh8 in the mouse liver. Blood 2008;112(4):1503–9.

74. Xia Y, Babitt JL, Sidis Y, et al. Hemojuvelin regulates hepcidin expression via a selective subset of BMP ligands and receptors independently of neogenin. Blood 2008;111(10):5195–204.

75. Meynard D, Kautz L, Darnaud V, et al. Lack of the bone morphogenetic protein BMP6 induces massive iron overload. Nat Genet 2009;41(4):478–81.

76. Ramey G, Deschemin JC, Vaulont S. Cross-talk between the mitogen activated protein kinase and bone morphogenetic protein/hemojuvelin pathways is required for the induction of hepcidin by holotransferrin in primary mouse hepatocytes. Haematologica 2009;94(6):765–72.

77. Calzolari A, Raggi C, Deaglio S, et al. TfR2 localizes in lipid raft domains and is released in exosomes to activate signal transduction along the MAPK pathway. J Cell Sci 2006;119(Pt 21):4486–98.

78. Andrews NC. Forging a field: the golden age of iron biology. Blood 2008;112(2): 219–30.

79. Nemeth E, Ganz T. The role of hepcidin in iron metabolism. Acta Haematol 2009;122(2–3):78–86.

80. Finberg KE, Heeney MM, Campagna DR, et al. Mutations in TMPRSS6 cause iron-refractory iron deficiency anemia (IRIDA). Nat Genet 2008;40(5):569–71.

81. Du X, She E, Gelbart T, et al. The serine protease TMPRSS6 is required to sense iron deficiency. Science 2008;320(5879):1088–92.

82. Silvestri L, Pagani A, Nai A, et al. The serine protease matriptase-2 (TMPRSS6) inhibits hepcidin activation by cleaving membrane hemojuvelin. Cell Metab 2008;8(6):502–11.

83. Lin L, Goldberg YP, Ganz T. Competitive regulation of hepcidin mRNA by soluble and cell-associated hemojuvelin. Blood 2005;106(8):2884–9.

84. Finberg KE, Whittlesey RL, Fleming MD, et al. Downregulation of Bmp/Smad signaling by Tmprss6 is required for maintenance of systemic iron homeostasis. Blood 2010;115(18):3817–26.

85. Huang FW, Pinkus JL, Pinkus GS, et al. A mouse model of juvenile hemochromatosis. J Clin Invest 2005;115(8):2187–91.

86. Adamsky K, Weizer O, Amariglio N, et al. Decreased hepcidin mRNA expression in thalassemic mice. Br J Haematol 2004;124(1):123–4.

87. Pak M, Lopez MA, Gabayan V, et al. Suppression of hepcidin during anemia requires erythropoietic activity. Blood 2006;108(12):3730–5.

88. Fiorelli G, Fargion S, Piperno A, et al. Iron metabolism in thalassemia intermedia. Haematologica 1990;75(Suppl 5):89–95.

89. Gardenghi S, Marongiu MF, Ramos P, et al. Ineffective erythropoiesis in {beta}-thalassemia is characterized by increased iron absorption mediated by down-regulation of hepcidin and up-regulation of ferroportin. Blood 2007;109(11):5027–35.

90. Weizer-Stern O, Adamsky K, Amariglio N, et al. Downregulation of hepcidin and haemojuvelin expression in the hepatocyte cell-line HepG2 induced by thalassaemic sera. Br J Haematol 2006;135(1):129–38.

91. Weizer-Stern O, Adamsky K, Amariglio N, et al. mRNA expression of iron regulatory genes in beta-thalassemia intermedia and beta-thalassemia major mouse models. Am J Hematol 2006;81(7):479–83.

92. Origa R, Galanello R, Ganz T, et al. Liver iron concentrations and urinary hepcidin in beta-thalassemia. Haematologica 2007;92(5):583–8.

93. Kearney SL, Nemeth E, Neufeld EJ, et al. Urinary hepcidin in congenital chronic anemias. Pediatr Blood Cancer 2007;48(1):57–63.

94. Papanikolaou G, Tzilianos M, Christakis JI, et al. Hepcidin in iron overload disorders. Blood 2005;105(10):4103–5.

95. Kattamis A, Papassotiriou I, Palaiologou D, et al. The effects of erythropoetic activity and iron burden on hepcidin expression in patients with thalassemia major. Haematologica 2006;91(6):809–12.

96. Jenkins ZA, Hagar W, Bowlus CL, et al. Iron homeostasis during transfusional iron overload in beta-thalassemia and sickle cell disease: changes in iron regulatory protein, hepcidin, and ferritin expression. Pediatr Hematol Oncol 2007; 24(4):237–43.

97. Adamsky K, Weizer O, Amariglio N, et al. Decreased hepcidin mRNA expression in thalassemic mice. Br J Haematol 2004;124(1):123–4.

98. Rechavi G, Rivella S. Regulation of iron absorption in hemoglobinopathies. Curr Mol Med 2008;8(7):646–62.

99. de Franceschi L, Turrini F, Honczarenko M, et al. In vivo reduction of erythrocyte oxidant stress in a murine model of beta-thalassemia. Haematologica 2004; 89(11):1287–98.

100. Tanno T, Porayette P, Sripichai O, et al. Identification of TWSG1 as a second novel erythroid regulator of hepcidin expression in murine and human cells. Blood 2009;114(1):181–6.

101. Tanno T, Bhanu NV, Oneal PA, et al. High levels of GDF15 in thalassemia suppress expression of the iron regulatory protein hepcidin. Nat Med 2007; 13(9):1096–101.

102. Kanda J, Mizumoto C, Kawabata H, et al. Serum hepcidin level and erythropoietic activity after hematopoietic stem cell transplantation. Haematologica 2008; 93(10):1550–4.
103. Tanno T, Rabel A, Lee YT, et al. Expression of growth differentiation factor 15 is not elevated in individuals with iron deficiency secondary to volunteer blood donation. Transfusion 2010;50(7):1532–5.
104. Ramirez JM, Schaad O, Durual S, et al. Growth differentiation factor 15 production is necessary for normal erythroid differentiation and is increased in refractory anaemia with ring-sideroblasts. Br J Haematol 2009;144(2):251–62.
105. Gardenghi S, Ramos P, Follenzi A, et al. Hepcidin and Hfe in iron overload in beta-thalassemia. Ann N Y Acad Sci 2010;1202:221–5.
106. Nicolas G, Viatte L, Lou DQ, et al. Constitutive hepcidin expression prevents iron overload in a mouse model of hemochromatosis. Nat Genet 2003;34(1):97–101.
107. Ghoti H, Amer J, Winder A, et al. Oxidative stress in red blood cells, platelets and polymorphonuclear leukocytes from patients with myelodysplastic syndrome. Eur J Haematol 2007;79(6):463–7.
108. Shinar E, Rachmilewitz EA. Oxidative denaturation of red blood cells in thalassemia. Semin Hematol 1990;27(1):70–82.
109. Greer EL, Brunet A. FOXO transcription factors at the interface between longevity and tumor suppression. Oncogene 2005;24(50):7410–25.

Iron Overload in Thalassemia and Related Conditions: Therapeutic Goals and Assessment of Response to Chelation Therapies

John B. Porter, MD[a,b,*], Farrukh T. Shah, MD[a,b]

KEYWORDS

- Chelation • Iron • Deferiprone • Deferoxamine • Deferasirox
- Thalassemia • Sickle

FACTORS CONTRIBUTING TO IRON OVERLOAD AND ITS DISTRIBUTION

With regular blood transfusion, iron stores increase to many times the norm unless chelation treatment is given. Approximately 200 mg of iron is present in a unit (420 mL) of donated blood, or approximately 1.08 mg of iron per 1 mL of pure red blood cells (ie, hematocrit 1.0).[1] Mean transfusional loading in thalassemia major (TM) is 0.4 mg/kg/d,[2] but this varies. In 20% of patients, this is less than 0.35 mg/kg/d, approximately 60% receive 0.3 to 0.55 mg/kg/d, and a further 20% receive greater than 0.5 mg/kg/d.[2] This transfusional loading is less in sickle cell disease (SCD; 0.22 mg/kg/d)[3] than in TM and is further decreased by approximately 60% when using manual exchanges, whereas neutral iron balance can be achieved with automated exchanges.[4] In myelodysplastic syndromes (MDS), the average rate of iron loading (0.28 mg/kg/d) is less on average than TM.[5] Iron loading may worsen from increased iron absorption caused by increased rates of ineffective erythropoiesis. Thus, iron absorption in thalassemia intermedia (TI) can be up to 5 to 10 times normal, or 0.1 mg/kg/d.[6,7] Splenectomy seems to increase the rate of gastrointestinal hyperabsorption

Dr Porter receives research support and has served of advisory boards for Novartis.
Dr Shah has served on Novartis advisory boards and received Swedish Orphan lecture fees.
[a] Red Cell Disorders Unit, University College London Hospital, 250 Euston Road, London NW1 2PG, UK
[b] Red Cell Disorders Unit, Whittington Hospital, Magdala Avenue, London N19 5NF, UK
* Corresponding author. Department of Haematology, University College London, UCL Cancer Institute, Paul O'Gorman Building, 72 Huntley Street, WC1E 6BT UK.
E-mail address: j.porter@ucl.ac.uk

in TI[8] and other conditions, such as pyruvate kinase deficiency,[9] but interestingly patients with hyposplenic SCD do not hyperabsorb iron.

Tissue iron uptake, in the absence of iron overload, is determined by the distribution of transferrin receptors and by transferrin saturation. However, once transferrin becomes saturated, and with the appearance of plasma iron species that are not bound to transferrin (so-called plasma nontransferrin bound iron [NTBI]), the pattern of tissue iron uptake differs considerably and uptake is mediated through different pathways, such as calcium[10] and zinc channels.[11]

The pattern of tissue iron distribution resulting from transfusional iron overload is best described in TM, in which without chelation therapy, death from iron-induced cardiac failure was usual from the second decade.[12] Postmortem examination in the prechelation era showed high concentrations in liver, heart, and endocrine glands, little in striated muscle, and none in the brain and nervous tissue.[13] Cardiac iron overloading occurred after approximately 70 to 100 units of blood (containing 14–20 g iron) across a range of diagnoses, including MDS.[14,15] Although cirrhosis has been found in approximately 50% of patients with TM at postmortem, particularly when chronic hepatitis is present, this has historically been an uncommon cause of death, because cardiac disease typically develops first. However, as patients live longer with improved chelation, cirrhosis and hepatocellular carcinoma[16] are likely to increase. Hypogonadism historically occurred in more than half of patients older than 12 years old,[17] leading to disturbances of growth and sexual maturation.

In patients with multitransfused SCD, liver disease is common with cirrhosis in nearly half of the patients who died with severe liver siderosis.[18] By contrast, extrahepatic iron distribution may be delayed in transfused SCD, with MRI showing a lower incidence of myocardial iron deposition,[19,20] although cardiac iron may be visible postmortem.[18] Lower rates of endocrine complications at matched levels of iron loading to those of patients with TM have also been noted.[21,22] Possible mechanisms for the lower extrahepatic iron distribution in SCD include lower transfusion rates, less ineffective erythropoiesis, higher plasma hepcidin values,[23] chronic inflammation, and lower NTBI[24] values at matched levels of body iron to those of TM.

GOALS OF CHELATION THERAPY

The primary objective is to maintain body iron at safe levels at all times. Iron stored as ferritin or hemosiderin is not chelated directly at clinically useful rates, so that once accumulated, iron removal is slow and inefficient, relying on the tiny fraction of labile iron that is available for chelation at any moment, either from the breakdown of red cells in macrophages or from the turnover of tissue iron stores in lysosomes. Ideally, chelation therapy therefore should begin before clinically significant iron loading develops. Ample evidence shows that the age at which chelation is started in TM is a key factor in survival,[17,25,26] although this is often not accounted for in the retrospective analysis of survival data.

In practice, chelation with deferoxamine (DFO) has traditionally been started only after 2 to 3 years of transfusion or when ferritin exceeds 1000 g/L, for fear of the unwanted effects of overchelation at low levels of body iron (see later discussion). Whether chelation can be safely started earlier with other iron chelators remains to be seen, but this would be desirable. What constitutes safe levels of body iron burden is debated. It may differ depending on the underlying diagnosis and the chelation therapy being used. Preventing the primary accumulation of iron overload in hepatocytes should avoid secondary distribution of iron to endocrine organs and the heart.

The small fraction of body iron that is available in a chelatable form results in only a small proportion of the chelator binding iron before it is excreted or metabolized. Once iron overload has developed, it may take years to reduce body storage iron to safe levels even with the most intensive treatment. Furthermore, iron is removed much more slowly from the heart than from the liver.[27,28] Consequently, body iron levels that are safe for preventing iron distribution to tissues outside the liver may differ from those that are safe once distribution to these tissues has occurred. Increasing the doses of chelators in an attempt to accelerate iron removal presents a risk for increasing toxicity by chelating iron that is needed for normal tissue metabolism. Therefore, although the slow process of decreasing tissue iron to safe levels is being achieved, a second goal is to make the iron as safe as possible by binding the toxic iron pools responsible for causing tissue damage. Plasma NTBI and labile iron rebound rapidly after a chelator ceases to be present in plasma, so that in principle the continuous presence of chelator is desirable.[29] Continuous chelation therapy also has the potential to minimize the uptake of NTBI species (including labile plasma iron [LPI]) into organs such as heart and endocrine tissues. Whatever the regime, poor adherence decreases exposure to chelation and hence the detoxification of iron. Many studies have shown that adherence has a major influence on outcome with DFO treatment,[25,30] and this is clearly also important regarding response to oral chelation.[31]

An issue that recently has come into sharper focus is how low the target body iron should be to achieve the optimal balance between iron-induced toxicity and the risk of toxicity from the chelation regime itself. Although the tolerability of DFO clearly decreases as body iron levels fall, this is far from clear with other chelation regimes. Whether toxicity from deferiprone (DFP), with or without DFO, or from deferasirox (DFX) increases at low levels of iron loading is unclear. Evidence suggests that lower levels of iron load can be achieved with these regimes without increasing the risk of these toxicities,[32,33] and this is likely to impact increasingly on perceived therapeutic goals and guidelines in future.

MEASURES OF IRON OVERLOAD AND RESPONSE TO CHELATION THERAPY

Liver Iron Concentration

Body iron stores are predicted from the liver iron concentration (LIC) using the formula: total body iron stores in mg/kg $= 10.6 \times$ the LIC (in mg/g dry weight).[34] Normal LIC values are up to 1.8 mg/g dry weight, and levels up to 7 mg/g dry weight are seen in some nonthalassemic populations without apparent adverse effects.[35] In unchelated patients, high LIC values predict an increased risk of myocardial iron deposition,[14,15] but once chelation therapy has been initiated, this simple relationship no longer exists.[27] Despite this, high LIC values (>15–20 mg/g dry weight) have been linked to worsening prognosis,[25,36] liver fibrosis progression,[37] and liver function abnormalities.[15] Measurement of LIC has historically required a liver biopsy of adequate size (>1 mg/g dry weight, >4 mg wet weight, or approximately a 2.5-cm core length). MRI techniques are now available,[38,39] relying on the general principle that tissue iron exerts a paramagnetic effect on surrounding tissues, affecting the relaxation time of molecules excited by the application of a magnetic field. One method (R2, Ferriscan) is available in a standardized and validated format that is predictive over a clinically useful range, is registered in the European Union and United States, and can use widely available MRI equipment with little extra training of local staff.[38]

Serum Ferritin

Serum ferritin broadly correlates with body iron stores, but in TM, variation in body iron stores accounts for only 57% of the variability in plasma ferritin.[40] This variability is partly because inflammation increases serum ferritin independently of the body iron levels and partly because the distribution of liver iron between macrophages (Kupffer cells) and hepatocytes in the liver has a major impact on plasma ferritin. A sudden increase in serum ferritin should prompt a search for hepatitis, other infections, or inflammatory conditions. Unlike tissue ferritin, serum ferritin is predominantly iron-free and is secreted by macrophages proportionally to their iron content up to values of approximately 3000 µg/L.[41] Greater than this value, iron-rich ferritin tends to leak from hepatocytes, so that responses to treatment may occur at a different rate than at values lower than 3000 µg/L.[42] The relationship between serum ferritin and iron stores is similar in TM and SCD,[40] provided serum values are taken several weeks away from a vaso-occlusive sickle crisis,[43] but in TI, serum ferritin tends to underestimate the degree of iron overloading.[44] The relationship between serum ferritin and body iron stores may also vary with the chelator being used[45] and with the duration of chelation therapy.[46] Despite these caveats, control of serum ferritin lower than 2500 µg/L (with DFO) on a long-term basis is associated with a significantly lower risk of cardiac disease and death.[17,26,30,36,47,48] Maintenance of an even lower serum ferritin of 1000 µg/L may be associated with additional advantages.[17]

Monitoring of the Heart

With the development of MRI techniques for estimating myocardial iron, the factors influencing myocardial iron deposition and removal are being increasingly studied. However, the extent to which the rate of iron loading, age of starting iron loading, the underlying cause of iron loading, and the type of chelation therapy on myocardial iron loading are still incompletely understood. In TM, the risk of developing clinically relevant left ventricular (LV) dysfunction increases as the T2* falls below the lower limit found in healthy adults of approximately 20 ms. However, tissue iron correlates inversely with T2* but linearly with 1/T2* (R2*), and this latter function clearly shows a linear continuum of increasing left ventricular risk as heart iron rises, rather than a stepwise increase of risk T2* of 20 ms (**Fig. 1**). Prospective studies have shown that the risk of developing heart failure in the next 12 months rises particularly in patients with T2* values less than 10 ms.[49]

Plasma NTBI and LPI

NTBI is a heterogeneous collection of plasma species unbound to transferrin, some of which are bound to citrate and plasma proteins.[50] Various assays for NTBI provide variable reference ranges but generally correlate with each other. An assay measuring a redox-labile subfraction (the component capable of accelerating oxidation of a flurophore, termed *LPI assay*)[51] is suitable for measurements in the presence of chelators. NTBI broadly correlates with transferrin saturation,[29] as does LPI.[52] Weak correlations with serum ferritin and LIC[53] have also been noted, and possible correlations with cardiac iron loading.[54,55] More recently, clear correlations of LPI with the transfusional iron loading rate have been observed (Porter and colleagues in preparation). LPI values also decline immediately after a single dose of chelator, and progressively with chelation treatments.[53,56]

Response Rate

Nonresponder is a term that has recently begun to be used in the field of chelation.[57] The term must be used with caution because it implies a fundamental difference between a responder and a nonresponder, which may not necessarily be the case. In this article, the term *responder* refers to any patient who shows an improving trend

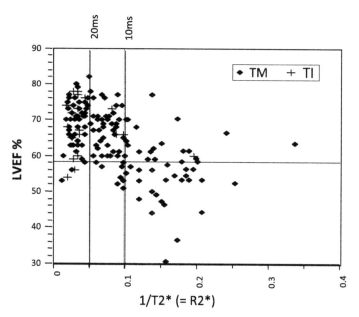

Shah F, MD Thesis University London, 2008

Fig. 1. The relationship between left ventricular ejection fraction and 1/T2* or R2* is shown for patients with thalassemia major (TM, *diamonds*) or thalassemia intermedia (TI, *crosses*). It can be seen that the relationship is broadly linear and continuous (with no inflection point at a given R2*). A high proportion of patients show decreased LVEF when R2* is greater than 0.1 Hz (T2*<10 ms), whereas for R2* values less than 0.05 Hz (T2* 20 ms), all but 4 patients have LVEF>60%.

in the specified variable of interest (ferritin, LIC, myocardial T2* [mT2*]). The term *response* could also be applied to the attainment of certain desirable thresholds for a given variable (eg, ferritin <2500 μg/L). However, the term *responder* in this article refers to patients showing improvement rather than reaching a given threshold. In principle, the reasons for nonresponse may relate to the dose prescribed, adherence of patients to treatment, the blood transfusion rate in an individual, or the underlying pharmacology of the chelation regime itself. The latter includes factors such as variability in absorption and metabolism. Changes or lack of changes in ferritin values, although broadly reflecting trends in body iron, can be misleading.[46] A more robust way to measure response is to assess changes in total body iron, calculated based on changes in LIC, over a measured period. However, if only mean population changes are given, it does not inform the clinician about the proportion of patients likely to respond. Fortunately, recent randomized studies have provided some data on iron balance response rates (see later discussion), but these data are only available in prospective studies for mT2* response rates with DFX (70%),[58] because larger studies with other chelation regimes have only reported mean values with DFP monotherapy or DFP with DFO, with individual responses being confined to small numbers of patients.[59,60]

CHELATION REGIMES TO CONTROL IRON OVERLOAD
DFO

Chemistry and pharmacology
DFO is a hexadentate chelator binding iron at a 1:1 molar ratio, thus preventing its participation in toxic reactions. In addition to its relatively high molecular weight, the

drug is highly hydrophilic, which retards its entry into most cell types except hepato-cytes, which seems to have a facilitated uptake mechanism.[61] The iron complex of DFO is highly stable, with good iron scavenging properties at low concentrations of iron or chelator. When DFO is infused subcutaneously at 40 to 50 mg/kg/d, steady-state plasma concentrations are typically no more that 10 μM.[29,62] Because of the short half-life, levels of the iron-free drug fall to negligible values within a few minutes of stopping infusion, although this takes longer after subcutaneous infusion.[61] Metabolism of the iron-free drug, but not the iron complex, occurs within hepatocytes, so that an increase in metabolites indicates a decrease in the availability of chelatable iron.[61,63] With 24-hour infusion regimes, the duration of protection from NTBI and labile plasma iron is continuous, but plasma levels still rarely exceed 10 μM at conventional doses, and NTBI is incompletely removed.[61,64] In contrast, the LPI subfraction of NTBI is effectively removed when chelator is present in plasma.[51,65]

Iron balance and LIC

Early formal iron balance studies suggested that daily 12-hour infusions at 30 mg/kg could achieve iron balance in TM, particularly if oral ascorbic acid was supplemented at the equivalent of 2 to 3 mg/kg/d.[66] In practice most patients are prescribed DFO approximately five times a week, and under these conditions higher doses are likely to be necessary, but this has only recently been examined systematically (response rates are discussed later). Prospective randomized studies have shown that the percentage of patients experiencing negative iron balance depends on the transfu-sional loading rate and the dose given (**Tables 1** and **2**).[2] At typical rates of transfu-sional ion loading (0.3–0.5 mg/kg/d), negative balance was achieved in 75% of patients prescribed 35 to 49 mg/kg/d given subcutaneously 5 days per week, whereas at doses of 50 mg/kg/d or greater, response rates increased to 86%. At higher trans-fusional loading rates ($\geq$0.5 mg/kg/d), response was seen in only half of the patients

Table 1
Percentage of patients in negative iron balance (response rate for LIC or negative iron balance) over 1 year of treatment with DFO subcutaneously 5 d/wk at the doses shown

Dose mg/kg	Low Transfusion <0.3 mg/kg/d	Medium Transfusion 0.3–0.5 mg/kg/d	High Transfusion >0.5 mg/kg/d
35 to 49	76	75	52
$\geq$50	100	86	89

Data from Cohen AR, Glimm E, Porter JB, et al. Effect of transfusional iron intake on response to chelation therapy in beta-thalassemia major. Blood 2008;111:583–7.

Table 2
Impact of transfusion rates on the percentage of patients in negative iron balance (responders) over 1 year of treatment with DFX once daily at the doses shown

Dose mg/kg	Low Transfusion <0.3 mg/kg/d	Medium Transfusion 0.3–0.5 mg/kg/d	High Transfusion >0.5 mg/kg/d
10	29	14	0
20	76	55	47
30	96	83	82

Data from Cohen AR, Glimm E, Porter JB, et al. Effect of transfusional iron intake on response to chelation therapy in beta-thalassemia major. Blood 2008;111:583–7.

prescribed 35 to 49 mg/kg/d given subcutaneously 5 days per week, but this increased to 89% at doses on 50 mg/kg or greater.[2]

Effect on serum ferritin

Dose-dependent reductions with DFO have been recognized for several decades, and the impact of ferritin control on survival are discussed earlier. In general, the trend in serum ferritin often reveals more about compliance and trends in iron balance than do body iron levels at any given time. The impact of dose on ferritin decrements has been shown in large-scale trials.[67] These studies have shown only mean changes, and therefore the percentage of patients experiencing response is unclear.

Effects on the heart

Progressive decreases in cardiac mortality since DFO infusions were first introduced in the late 1970s, together with the reversal of cardiac failure using continuous intravenous DFO,[68,69] argue persuasively for the clinical beneficial effects. DFO also removes myocardial iron. At very high levels of myocardial iron (T2* values $\leq$5 ms), a 58% improvement in mT2* was seen over 1 year of intravenous therapy.[27] Improvement in heart function preceded these changes in T2*, suggesting that a beneficial effect of DFO on labile iron pools was independent of the slower improvement in T2*. With continued infusions, improvement usually continues but may take up to 5 years to normalize.[70] Subcutaneous DFO at standard doses given 5 days per week also improved myocardial iron significantly in patients with mild to moderate myocardial iron loading (10–20 ms) in the context of randomized clinical trials over 1 year.[71] Although both studies used the same methodology, gave similar treatment regimes, and had similar patient baseline characteristics, the change in T2* with DFO differed considerably, being 1.1% change in one study[72] and 2.2% in the second.[73] This finding illustrates the variability that can result from patient selection in different clinics, even when baseline measures of iron load seem comparable.

Tolerability and unwanted effects

Although toxic effects and their management have been described in detail elsewhere,[74,75] key principles about DFO toxicity are discussed here. First, most of the toxic effects of DFO are dose-related; effects on growth, skeletal changes, and audiometric and retinopathic effects are more likely at higher doses of the drug. In an adult, these effects are unlikely if the dose does not exceed 50 mg/kg and care is taken to reduce the dose as ferritin levels fall (see later discussion). Retinal effects can present with a loss of visual acuity, field defects, and defects in night or color vision. Doses of 100 mg/kg/d, at which these effects were originally described,[69] are rarely given today. Drug-related ototoxicity is typically symmetric and of a high-frequency sensorineural nature.[76] In patients who develop complications, DFO should be temporarily stopped and reintroduced at lower doses when investigations show improvement.

The second principle is that some adverse effects are more likely when iron stores are low; this is particularly clear for neurotoxic complications, with standard doses associated with coma in patients with rheumatoid arthritis without iron overload,[77] and audiometric and retinopathic effects more likely at lower serum ferritin levels,[76] particularly less than 1000 µg/L.[78] The third principle is that some effects limit the dose that can be prescribed to children: doses greater than 40 mg/kg have been associated with an increased risk of impaired growth and skeletal changes in children. Growth retardation was seen when treatment was started early (<3 y) and at higher doses of treatment.[79,80] Rickets-like bony lesions and genu valgum, in association with metaphyseal changes, particularly in the vertebrae, giving a disproportionately short trunk, can also occur, often with vertebral demineralization and flatness of verte-bral bodies radiographically.[79,81]

Finally, some unwanted effects, such a local skin reactions, allergic reactions, and *Yesinia enterocolitica* infections, are less obviously dose-related. Management of these is discussed elsewhere.[75]

DFP

Chemistry and pharmacology
This 3-hydroxypyridin-4-one bidentate chelator binds to iron in a 3:1 ratio with a stability constant approximately six orders of magnitude higher than DFO. However, the pM of 20-log of the uncoordinated metal (M, iron) concentration calculated at pH of 7.4, 10 μM ligand, and 1 μM iron (III) is lower than that of DFO at 27.6,[82] and therefore the iron complex is less stable and can donate iron to other ligands, as seen in combined therapy with DFO.[64] DFP has a short plasma half-life of 1.5 hours,[83] and is therefore usually given three times daily. After a single dose, peak plasma concentrations reach approximately 100 μM, with rapid inactivation by glucuronidation in the liver.[84] The low pM implies that the drug will tend to redistribute iron at low chelator or iron concentrations. Conse-quently, the drug is well suited to shuttling iron when using combined therapies,[64] and will tend to become less efficient at chelating iron as levels of overload decrease.[85]

Effects on iron balance and LIC
In metabolic balance studies, DFP (75 mg/kg) produced a negative iron balance with daily excretion of 0.53 mg/kg/d[86] and excretion mainly in the urine.[83] Meta-analysis of iron balance based on long-term LIC trends from several studies totaling 143 people[87] show considerable variation among studies, reflecting the heterogeneity of dosing schedules, transfusion rates, baseline LIC values, and follow-up periods (response rates are discussed below). The response rates for negative iron balance (decrements in LIC) have not been directly reported in prospective trials, but information can be gleaned from data within some papers. In general, response rates seem to be lower at higher transfusional loading rates, and fall with time and at lower levels of iron load. In a prospective study, 76% of patients with TM showed an LIC response at a mean of 3 years,[88] but this decreased to 56% after further follow-up.[89] In another prospective study over 2 years using LIC measured using a superconducting quantum interference device (SQUID), 24% overall showed response with negative iron balance over 2 years). When analysis is confined to patients with baseline LIC values greater than 9 mg/g dry weight, this response rate increases to 50%.[85] This article also showed lower response rates at higher transfusional iron-loading rates.

Effects on serum ferritin
The effects on serum ferritin have been examined in several randomized trials using DFO as the comparator (combined total, 235 people).[71,90–92] The relative effects of the two drugs differ considerably among the studies, which may reflect the different doses of drugs used and differences in baseline characteristics of patients both within and between studies. Pooled analysis[87] shows a statistically significant decrease in serum ferritin at 6 months, in favor of DFO. Ferritin response rates (percentage of patients showing decrements in serum ferritin) may show discrepancies from LIC effects and lower response rates at baseline ferritin values of less than 2500 μg/L. In one study,[93] 83% of patients were responders with respect to serum ferritin at 70 mg/kg for a minimum of 1 year, but only 30% of patients were responders with respect to LIC. A similar discrepancy between responses in LIC and serum ferritin were found in another study in which, although a correlation was seen regarding changes in LIC and ferritin, the response rate for ferritin was considerably greater

(58%) than for LIC (24%).[85] It is also clear that the ferritin response is greater at higher baseline values with low response rates when baseline values are less than 2500 µg/L.[94,95] Response rates (percentage of patients showing an improving trend) have not been reported at doses greater than 75 mg/kg.

Effects on the heart

Initial studies with DFP monotherapy showed continued cardiac mortality,[96] but more recent reports show a declining frequency that several authors have attributed to this chelator being used with or without DFO. A retrospective analysis of survival that included seven Italian hospitals[97] included 359 patients treated by DFO and 157 receiving DFP for a median of 4.3 years. The investigators noted 52 cardiac events, including 10 cardiac deaths, among patients treated with DFO, but no cardiac events in a smaller number of patients who received DFP.[17] However this absence of mortality in the DFP patients contrasted with a larger 3-year prospective study of 532 patients, among whom 11 cardiac deaths (2%) were seen.[94]

In a single-center Italian study, 54 DFP-treated patients were compared retrospectively with 75 DFO-treated patients for cardiac complications and survival.[98] Worsening of preexisting cardiac disease or new onset of cardiac abnormalities occurred in 4% of the patients treated with DFP compared with 20% of the patients treated with DFO. However this was not a balanced comparison, because the three patients who died on DFO were 6 to 8 years older than the mean age of those in the DFP group, and five patients in the DFO group had New York Heart Association (NYHA) class II to IV cardiac disease at outset compared with only one in the DFP group. These differences illustrate the influences of center effects and patient selection on outcome, and the need for prospective randomized studies if relative long-term merits of chelating regimes are to be inferred.

A prospective randomized study has provided persuasive evidence for the cardioprotective effects of DFP. This study compared DFP at 92 mg/kg with subcutaneous DFO at 53 mg/kg given 5 days a week in thalassemic patients with mild to moderate cardiac siderosis (T2* 8–20 ms).[71] After 1 year of treatment, although the proportion of patients experiencing response was not given, the average improvement in T2* and increase in left ventricular ejection fraction were significantly greater in those treated with DFP than with DFO.[71]

Tolerability and unwanted effects

Tolerability and unwanted effects have been described in detail elsewhere,[99] but some key principles are discussed. The International Study Group on Oral Chelators found that nausea and other gastrointestinal symptoms, arthralgia, zinc deficiency, and fluctuating liver function tests, especially in patients positive for anti–hepatitis C virus antibodies, were the most frequent complications.[100] No prospective study has compared tolerability of the drug at two doses. However, although the effect of dosing on agranulocytosis and cytopenias in humans is unclear, in animal studies, bone marrow hypoplasia with leucopaenia is dose-related.[101] Systematic tolerability studies in children have not been reported, but a high rate of thrombocytopenia (45%) has been reported in only one study in children younger than 6 years that was reversible on cessation of treatment.[102] Arthropathy may be more common with high levels of iron overload,[103,104] suggesting a possible effect of the iron complex. The duration of observation may also influence the frequency of arthropathy, because in one prospective study it increased from 6% at 1 year to 13% at

4 years.[105] Whether unwanted effects increase at low levels of body iron, as occurs with DFO, is unclear; however, experience with combined DFP and DFO suggests that toxicity may not be increased at low body iron burdens, although this has not been studied prospectively.[32]

DFP and DFO Combinations

Pharmacology
Combined therapy could provide an advantage through several ways. First, chelators could be alternated to provide continuous exposure to chelation; for example, DFO given every night and DFP during the day. This regimen, in principle, can provide 24-hour removal of LPI.[51] These chelators can also be given at the same time, giving the possibility of a drug interaction through a so called shuttle mechanism, in which iron is chelated rapidly by DFP at sites relatively unavailable to DFO and then donated to the more stable DFO molecules. Experimental evidence has shown this effect in animal models of iron overload,[106] and this shuttling effect was recently shown for the removal of NTBI in the plasma compartment of patients with TM.[64] In practice, sequential use of these chelators is more commonly adopted, but with numbers of days of DFO varying from 2 to 5 days per week.[91,107–110]

Effects on liver iron
In a randomized study of 60 patients,[107] the LIC was less than 7 mg/g dry weight at baseline and was on average maintained both with combination and DFO monotherapy. In a prospective randomized study from Turkey, the effect of DFO monotherapy at 40 to 50 mg/kg subcutaneously five times per week was compared with DFO at 75 mg/kg daily or DFP at 75 mg/kg daily plus twice-weekly DFO.[108] The decrease in liver iron was highest in the DFO monotherapy group and lowest in the DFP monotherapy group, with sequential combination treatment showing an intermediate effect. A randomized study in Italian patients compared DFP at 75 mg/kg/d plus DFO five times per week and DFO monotherapy five times a week, and found that the improvement in liver T2* (as a surrogate measure of LIC) was greater in the combination arm.[73] The proportion of patients experiencing response to treatment with a decrease in LIC can be extracted from some articles showing responses in individual patients. In a small randomized study, the LIC response rate at 12 months was 87% with combined therapy compared with only 32% with DFP monotherapy (**Fig. 2**).[108]

Effects on serum ferritin
Several studies have been systematically reviewed with respect to serum ferritin trends.[87] Effects vary among studies; some of the differences may result from the regimes and doses used, whereas others may reflect pretreatment differences in study populations or with treatment compliance. A study of 30 patients in India, randomized to three different treatments, showed the largest decrease with 5 nights of DFO monotherapy, the smallest effect with DFP monotherapy, and an intermediate effect with combined treatment with DFO given 2 nights per week plus DFP 7 days per week.[91] In a larger study involving 60 Sardinian patients,[107] ferritin changes were similar in patients randomized to either combined treatment (2 days of DFO plus 7 days of DFP) or DFO monotherapy. In a randomized study of 65 patients in whom DFO was used 5 days per week in the combination arm, serum ferritin deceased more with combined treatment than with 5 days of DFO monotherapy.[73] Thus, the greatest decrease in serum ferritin (and LIC) values have tended to occur in studies in which DFO is used most frequently in the combination arm.

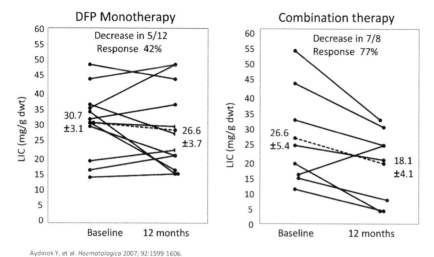

Aydinok Y, et al. *Haematologica* 2007; 92:1599-1606.

Fig. 2. The change in LIC over 1 year with DFP monotherapy, 75 mg/kg (n = 12), or combined with DFO (40–50 mg/kg twice weekly) (n = 8). Solid lines show values for individual patients, and broken line shows mean changes. Negative iron balance is obtained in 42% of patients on monotherapy and in 77% of patients on combined treatment. (Blood consumption 156 ± 45 mL/y and 145 ± 20 mL/y). (*Data from* Aydinok Y, Ulger Z, Nart D, et al. A randomized controlled 1-year study of daily deferiprone plus twice weekly desferrioxamine compared with daily deferiprone monotherapy in patients with thalassemia major. Haematologica 2007;92:1599–606.)

Cardiac effects

In a randomized study of 65 patients with mild to moderate heart iron loading (T2* 8–20 ms), mT2* changes with combined DFP 75 mg/kg given 7 days per week plus DFO given for 5 days were compared with subcutaneous DFO given 5 times per week.[73] T2* improved in both groups but was significantly greater with combined treatment than with DFO monotherapy (6 vs 3 ms). In an observational study, the T2* of the heart improved with combined therapy.[111]

Possible survival benefits have also been claimed. In a retrospective study from Cyprus of 539 patients with thalassemia born after 1960 and followed from 1980 to 2004,[112] 58 deaths occurred, 53% of which were from cardiac causes. A decline in cardiac mortality was seen after 2000, which the authors attributed to the introduction of combined therapy around this time. In a randomized controlled study of 65 patients[73] with baseline left ventricular ejection fraction (LVEF) greater than 56%, changes in LVEF improved by approximately 2.5% in the combination arm and 0.5% in the monotherapy arm. Changes in heart function were also reported in two observational studies with combined treatment. Among 79 patients treated with a variable DFO regime plus DFP at 75 mg/kg given 7 days per week for a variable time, an improvement in LVEF was seen on echocardiograph.[113] In an observational study of 42 patients involving sequential use of treatment over 3 to 4 years (DFP at 75 mg/kg/d plus DFO 2–6 days per week), the left ventricular shortening fraction improved.[111]

Safety and tolerability

Formal safety data on combined treatments are limited. In general, alternating regimes are less likely to be an issue for toxicity compared with regimes in which chelation is simultaneous or overlapping. A meta-analysis of the incidence of agranulocytosis in patients treated with combined regimes suggested that the risk may be increased several-fold compared with DFX monotherapy, although the numbers of evaluable patients were small (Macklin, Investigational New Drug submission to the U.S. Food and Drug Administration, unpublished data, 2004). The increased incidence seemed to occur mostly in regimes in which the drugs were administered simultaneously. The most common adverse events were gastrointestinal symptoms (20%) and transaminitis (18%), with agranulocytosis at 4.2 cases per 100 patient-years.[111] In a recently reported prospective study, one case of agranulocytosis and two of neutropenia were seen at 1 year in the combination arm containing 32 patients.[73] No excess in arthropathy was seen in the combination arm and no new tolerability entities that were not recognized with monotherapy have been reported.

Recent retrospective studies suggest that very low levels of serum ferritin may be obtained with combination treatments when the frequency and dose of DFO is adjusted as serum ferritin values decline.[32]

DFX

Chemistry and pharmacology

DFX is a bis-hydroxyphenyl-triazole (molecular weight, 373), binding iron in a 2:1 ratio. The pM values for ferric iron (22.5) are intermediate between DFO and DFP. The free ligand has a high lipid solubility and protein binding, whereas the iron complex has low lipid solubility.[114] Because of the low water solubility of the free ligand, DFX is administered as a suspension in water or fruit juice. Animal models have shown it has greater efficiency of iron mobilization compared with DFO,[115] with effective myocardial iron mobilization.[116] Clinically, a plasma half-life of 11 to 19 hours supported the use of a once-daily oral dosing.[117,118] Metabolism is predominantly to iron-binding glucuronides in the liver.[119] With once-daily repeat dosing at 20 mg/kg, peak plasma levels reach a mean of 80 μM, with trough values of 20 μM.[120] The response rate, with respect to the proportion of patients showing falling serum ferritin trends, may relate to variability in the absorption of this drug,[57] which is known to be enhanced when given with a fatty meal.[121] The efficiency of chelation (the proportion of administered drug excreted in the iron bound form), which is 27% to 34%, is essentially the same across all diagnoses and doses tested,[5] implying that as iron levels fall, iron will continue to be mobilized at a similar rate.

Iron balance and LIC response

Phase I clinical trials showed that iron excretion was dose-dependent and was almost entirely fecal.[117,118] Excretion averaged 0.13, 0.34, and 0.56 mg/kg/d at doses of 10, 20, and 40 mg/kg/d, respectively, predicting equilibrium or negative iron balance at daily does of 20 mg and greater.[118] Effects on iron balance over 1 year have been evaluated through comparing baseline and end-of-treatment LIC values.[67] In this preregistration study, a conservative dosing system was applied and adapted to initial LICs. Analysis of this and other phase I studies, including those involving patients with MDS[5] and SCD,[122] shows dose linearity with respect to iron excretion so that the doses required to balance iron excretion can be selected based on the transfusional iron intake.[2] At low transfusion rates of less than 0.3 mg/kg/d, 96% of patients had a negative iron balance, and are therefore considered responders when taking 30 mg/kg/d. At higher transfusion rates, 82% of patients had a negative iron balance at the same dose.

Effects on ferritin

A significant correlation has been shown between the serum ferritin trend and LIC trend with DFX across a wide range of diagnoses.[5] However, a lag in ferritin response may occur, possibly reflecting preferential iron removal from hepatocytes compared with macrophages,[123] which are the main source of serum ferritin below levels of 4000 µg/L. The proportion of patients with decreasing ferritin trends increases with duration of treatment. The percentage of patients achieving serum ferritin levels less than 1000 µg/L increases gradually from 14% in year 1 to 37% at 4 to 5 years.[33] In the large-scale 1-year EPIC study involving more than 1700 patients, dosing was adjusted successfully at a median of 24 weeks, based on baseline ferritin, trends in ferritin, and transfusional iron loading rates.[124] Based on these findings, and the theoretical considerations discussed earlier, dose escalation based on ferritin trends would typically be considered only after at least 3 months of treatment. These and other studies reported mean ferritin changes rather than percentage of responders. In preliminary observations of the effects of DFX on mT2* (see later discussion),[125] serum ferritin changes were also examined in a way that allows interpretation of the ferritin response rate at 1 year. In these studies, 87% of patients showed a decease in serum ferritin at 12 months, with doses ranging from 10 to 30 mg/kg/d (**Fig. 3**A).

Effects on the heart

Initial observations of improved cardiac T2* in phase III studies were encouraging, with a significant improvement in mT2* using variable dosing from 10 to 30 mg/kg/d.[125] The proportion of patients responding with improved mT2* at 12 months was approximately 73% (see **Fig. 3**B).[125]

Larger prospective studies with defined dosing regimes followed. In a study of more than 100 patients with established mild to moderate excess of myocardial iron, a significant reduction was seen at 1 year at mean doses of 33 mg/kg/d. Baseline T2* values of 10 to 20 ms increased significantly from 14.6 to 17.4 ms, whereas for patients with baseline T2* values less than 10 ms, the T2* also increased significantly from 7.4 to 8.2 ms over 1 year.[58] The response rate for improvement of mT2* at 1 year was 70% in this study.[58] Experience for up to 2 years now shows further progressive improvement in mT2*, often with normalization of myocardial iron.[126] In 75 patients without preexisting myocardial loading, no new cases developed. These studies have included only patients with normal LVEFs, and no significant changes have been seen, although right ventricular ejection fraction, which is also related to myocardial iron loading,[127] improved significantly.[128]

Tolerability and unwanted effects

More than 3000 patients have been studied in prospective trials of DFX. Most studies were designed to last 1 year, but by now several have been extended up to 5 years, with discontinuation rates generally lower than those seen with long-term DFP administration. DFX is typically well tolerated, with adverse events generally mild and involving transient gastrointestinal events, including abdominal pain, nausea and vomiting, diarrhea, and constipation, in approximately 15% of patients with thalassemia,[67] and somewhat higher numbers of patients with MDS.[124] Skin rashes occur early in approximately 10% of patients and are usually transient.[67] In one study, mild dose-dependent increases in serum creatinine in approximately one-third of patients were seen, occurring within a few weeks of starting or increasing therapy. These increases were not progressive and reversed or stabilized when doses were adjusted. Increased liver enzymes, judged to be related to DFX, occurred in fewer than 1% of patients. Audiometric effects and lens opacities did not differ significantly from the control arm treated with DFO,[67] and no drug-related agranulocytosis was observed. In pediatric patients, growth and development proceeded normally.[129] Follow-up data from the five core phase II/III studies, now at a median of 3.5 years, show no

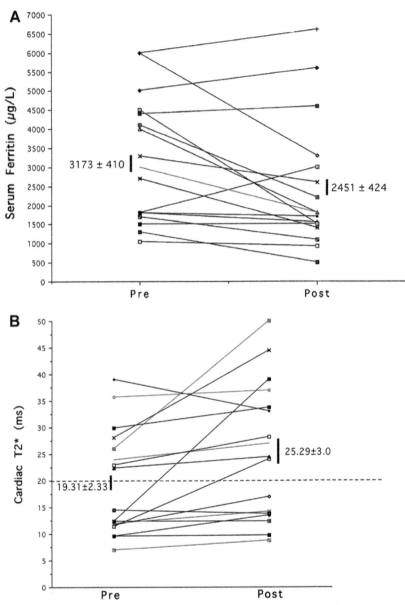

Fig. 3. (A) A total of 17 patients from UCLH included in the deferasirox studies 107 and 108 received once daily dosing at 20–30 mg/kg for 1 year. Mean changes in levels of ferritin and T2* are as previously reported,[125] with a significant drop in mean ferritin level (P = .02). The individual responses are shown, with a decrease in serum ferritin level in 13 of the 17 patients, giving a ferritin response of 77% over 1 year. (B) Mean changes in mT2* are as previously reported,[125] with a significant increase in mean myocardial T2* (P = .01). Of the 17 patients, 14 (82%) showed an increase in mT2* over 1 year.

evidence of new or progressive toxicities.[130] It is too early yet to allow any statements on the impact of DFX on survival. Recommended patient monitoring includes monthly creatinine, urine protein, and liver function tests and annual auditory and ophthalmic examinations. Experience at doses greater than 30 mg/kg/d has been gained in extension phases of the core studies, and with a subset of patients 252 Middle Eastern patients with heavy liver iron loading (mean LIC 19 mg/d dry weight).[131] A clear trend for decreasing serum ferritin after dose escalation was seen without a trend for increasing serum creatinine. Another key principle of tolerability is to establish whether this changes as iron levels fall. Analysis of patients in the extension phases of core studies shows no increase in effects on serum creatinine or gastrointestinal tolerability issues as the proportion of patients with ferritin values less than 1000 μg/L increases.[33] It is wise to decrease dosing gradually as ferritin values fall to less than 1000 μg/L to negotiate a "soft landing." Further work is needed to examine the safety at serum ferritin levels less than 500 μg/L.

SUMMARY AND FUTURE CHALLENGES

The goal of this article was to highlight some key concepts in the management of transfusional iron overload, rather than provide prescriptive management guidelines that are available elsewhere. Despite the large volume of recent publications, only some of variables that contribute to the relative risks of extrahepatic iron loading are understood. Sustained high levels of body iron (determined by serum ferritin or LIC) are clearly risk factors but may be influenced by transfusional loading rates, labile iron pool levels, nutritional and genetic factors, and the underlying hematologic disease itself. Uncertainties also still exist about how far and how quickly total body and tissue iron levels can be safely reduced and normalized. Although good prospective data are now available on trends in LIC, ferritin, and mT2*, these are uneven with respect to predicting the likely response rates to some chelation regimes. Understand how far body iron levels can be reduced without increasing the toxicities for each of the various chelation regimes will be important to understand in the future. This issue is a particular challenge when liver iron and ferritin have been reduced while high levels of myocardial iron remain.

REFERENCES

1. Porter JB. Practical management of iron overload. Br J Haematol 2001;115: 239–52.
2. Cohen AR, Glimm E, Porter JB. Effect of transfusional iron intake on response to chelation therapy in beta-thalassemia major. Blood 2008;111:583–7.
3. Cappellini D, Taher A, Vichinsky E, et al. Efficacy and tolerability of deferasirox at doses >30 mg/kg/day in patients with transfusion-dependent anaemia and iron overload [abstract]. Haematologica 2008;93(Suppl 1):abstract 0845.
4. Kim HC, Dugan NP, Silber JH, et al. Erythrocytapheresis therapy to reduce iron overload in chronically transfused patients with sickle cell disease. Blood 1994; 83:1136–42.
5. Porter J, Galanello R, Saglio G, et al. Relative response of patients with myelodysplastic syndromes and other transfusion-dependent anaemias to deferasirox (ICL670): a 1-yr prospective study. Eur J Haematol 2008;80:168–76.
6. Pippard MJ, Callender ST, Warner GT, et al. Iron absorption and loading in beta-thalassaemia intermedia. Lancet 1979;2:819–21.
7. Pootrakul P, Kitcharoen K, Yansukon P, et al. The effect of erythroid hyperplasia on iron balance. Blood 1988;71:1124–9.

8. Fiorelli G, Fargion S, Piperno A, et al. Iron metabolism in thalassemia intermedia. Haematologica 1990;75(Suppl 5):89–95.

9. Zanella A, Berzuini A, Colombo MB, et al. Iron status in red cell pyruvate kinase deficiency: study of Italian cases. Br J Haematol 1993;83:485–90.

10. Oudit GY, Trivieri MG, Khaper N, et al. Role of L-type Ca2+ channels in iron transport and iron-overload cardiomyopathy. J Mol Med 2006;84:349–64.

11. Liuzzi JP, Aydemir F, Nam H, et al. Zip14 (Slc39a14) mediates non-transferrin-bound iron uptake into cells. Proc Natl Acad Sci U S A 2006;103: 13612–7.

12. Zurlo MG, De Stefano P, Borgna-Pignatti C, et al. Survival and causes of death in thalassaemia major. Lancet 1989;2:27–30.

13. Modell B, Mathews R. Thalassaemia in Britain and Australia. Birth Defects Orig Artic Ser 1976;12:13–29.

14. Buja LM, Roberts WC. Iron in the heart. Etiology and clinical significance. Am J Med 1971;51:209–21.

15. Jensen PD, Jensen FT, Christensen T, et al. Evaluation of myocardial iron by magnetic resonance imaging during iron chelation therapy with deferrioxamine: indication of close relation between myocardial iron content and chelatable iron pool. Blood 2003;101:4632–9.

16. Borgna-Pignatti C, Vergine G, Lombardo T, et al. Hepatocellular carcinoma in the thalassaemia syndromes. Br J Haematol 2004;124:114–7.

17. Borgna-Pignatti C, Rugolotto S, De Stefano P, et al. Survival and complications in patients with thalassemia major treated with transfusion and deferoxamine. Haematologica 2004;89:1187–93.

18. Darbari DS, Kple-Faget P, Kwagyan J, et al. Circumstances of death in adult sickle cell disease patients. Am J Hematol 2006;81:858–63.

19. Westwood MA, Shah F, Anderson LJ, et al. Myocardial tissue characterization and the role of chronic anemia in sickle cell cardiomyopathy. J Magn Reson Imaging 2007;26:564–8.

20. Wood JC, Tyszka JM, Carson S, et al. Myocardial iron loading in transfusion-dependent thalassemia and sickle cell disease. Blood 2004;103:1934–6.

21. Vichinsky E, Butensky E, Fung E, et al. Comparison of organ dysfunction in transfused patients with SCD or beta thalassemia. Am J Hematol 2005;80:70–4.

22. Fung EB, Harmatz PR, Lee PD, et al. Increased prevalence of iron-overload associated endocrinopathy in thalassaemia versus sickle-cell disease. Br J Haematol 2006;135:574–82.

23. Sayani F, Bansal S, Evans P, et al. Disease specific modulation of serum hepcidin: impact of gdf-15 and iron metabolism markers in thalassemia major, thalassemia intermedia and sickle cell disease: a univariate and multivariate analysis. [abstract: 3850]. Blood 2008;112.

24. Walter PB, Fung EB, Killilea DW, et al. Oxidative stress and inflammation in iron-overloaded patients with beta-thalassaemia or sickle cell disease. Br J Haematol 2006;135:254–63.

25. Brittenham GM, Griffith PM, Nienhuis AW, et al. Efficacy of deferoxamine in preventing complications of iron overload in patients with thalassemia major. N Engl J Med 1994;331:567–73.

26. Davis BA, O'Sullivan C, Jarritt PH, et al. Value of sequential monitoring of left ventricular ejection fraction in the management of thalassemia major. Blood 2004;104:263–9.

27. Anderson LJ, Westwood MA, Holden S, et al. Myocardial iron clearance during reversal of siderotic cardiomyopathy with intravenous desferrioxamine:

a prospective study using T2* cardiovascular magnetic resonance. Br J Haematol 2004;127:348–55.

28. Tanner MA, Galanello R, Dessi C, et al. Combined chelation therapy in thalassemia major for the treatment of severe myocardial siderosis with left ventricular dysfunction. J Cardiovasc Magn Reson 2008;10:12.

29. Porter JB, Abeysinghe RD, Marshall L, et al. Kinetics of removal and reappearance of non-transferrin-bound plasma iron with deferoxamine therapy. Blood 1996;88:705–13.

30. Gabutti V, Piga A. Results of long-term iron-chelating therapy. Acta Haematol 1996;95:26–36.

31. Garbowski M, Eleftheriou P, Pennell D, et al. Impact of compliance, ferritin and LIC on long-term trends in myocardial T2* with deferasirox [abstract]. Blood 2008;112:abstract 116.

32. Farmaki K, Tzoumari I, Pappa C, et al. Normalisation of total body iron load with very intensive combined chelation reverses cardiac and endocrine complications of thalassaemia major. Br J Haematol 2010;148:466–75.

33. Porter JB, Piga A, Cohen A, et al. Safety of deferasirox (Exjade(r)) in patients with transfusion-dependent anemias and iron overload who achieve serum ferritin levels <1000 ng/ml during long-term treatment [abstract]. Blood 2008; 112:abstract 5423.

34. Angelucci E, Brittenham GM, McLaren CE, et al. Hepatic iron concentration and total body iron stores in thalassemia major. N Engl J Med 2000;343: 327–31.

35. Cartwright GE, Edwards CQ, Kravitz K, et al. Hereditary hemochromatosis. Phenotypic expression of the disease. N Engl J Med 1979;301:175–9.

36. Telfer PT, Prestcott E, Holden S, et al. Hepatic iron concentration combined with long-term monitoring of serum ferritin to predict complications of iron overload in thalassaemia major. Br J Haematol 2000;110:971–7.

37. Angelucci E, Muretto P, Nicolucci A, et al. Effects of iron overload and hepatitis C virus positivity in determining progression of liver fibrosis in thalassemia following bone marrow transplantation. Blood 2002;100:17–21.

38. St Pierre TG, Clark PR, Chua-Anusorn W, et al. Noninvasive measurement and imaging of liver iron concentrations using proton magnetic resonance. Blood 2005;105:855–61.

39. Gandon Y, Olivie D, Guyader D, et al. Non-invasive assessment of hepatic iron stores by MRI. Lancet 2004;363:357–62.

40. Brittenham GM, Cohen AR, McLaren CE, et al. Hepatic iron stores and plasma ferritin concentration in patients with sickle cell anemia and thalassemia major. Am J Hematol 1993;42:81–5.

41. Worwood M, Cragg SJ, Jacobs A, et al. Binding of serum ferritin to concanavalin A: patients with homozygous beta thalassaemia and transfusional iron overload. Br J Haematol 1980;46:409–16.

42. Davis BA, Porter JB. Long-term outcome of continuous 24-hour deferoxamine infusion via indwelling intravenous catheters in high-risk beta-thalassemia. Blood 2000;95:1229–36.

43. Porter JB, Huehns ER. Transfusion and exchange transfusion in sickle cell anaemias, with particular reference to iron metabolism. Acta Haematol 1987;78:198–205.

44. Origa R, Galanello R, Ganz T, et al. Liver iron concentrations and urinary hepcidin in beta-thalassemia. Haematologica 2007;92:583–8.

45. Fischer R, Engelhardt R. Deferiprone versus desferrioxamine in thalassaemia, and T2* validation and utility. Lancet 2003;361:182–3 [author reply: 3–4].

46. Porter J, Elalfy M, Aydinok Y, et al. Correlations of serum ferritin (sf) and liver iron concentration before and after 1 year of deferasirox treatment. Haematologia 2010;95(Suppl 2):708.
47. Olivieri NF, Nathan DG, MacMillan JH, et al. Survival in medically treated patients with homozygous beta-thalassemia. N Engl J Med 1994;331:574–8.
48. Anderson LJ, Holden S, Davis B, et al. Cardiovascular T2-star (T2*) magnetic resonance for the early diagnosis of myocardial iron overload. Eur Heart J 2001;22:2171–9.
49. Kirk P, Roughton M, Porter JB, et al. Cardiac T2* magnetic resonance for prediction of cardiac complications in thalassemia major. Circulation 2009; 120:1961–8.
50. Evans RW, Rafique R, Zarea A, et al. Nature of non-transferrin-bound iron: studies on iron citrate complexes and thalassemic sera. J Biol Inorg Chem 2008;13:57–74.
51. Cabantchik ZI, Breuer W, Zanninelli G, et al. LPI-labile plasma iron in iron overload. Best Pract Res Clin Haematol 2005;18:277–87.
52. Jacobs EM, Hendriks JC, van Tits BL, et al. Results of an international round robin for the quantification of serum non-transferrin-bound iron: need for defining standardization and a clinically relevant isoform. Anal Biochem 2005; 341:241–50.
53. Daar S, Pathare A, Nick H, et al. Reduction in labile plasma iron during treatment with deferasirox, a once-daily oral iron chelator, in heavily iron-overloaded patients with beta-thalassaemia. Eur J Haematol 2009;82:454–7.
54. Shah FT. The relationship between non transferrin bound iron and iron overload in thalassaemia and sickle syndromes [MD thesis]. University of London; 2008.
55. Piga A, Longo F, Duca L, et al. High nontransferrin bound iron levels and heart disease in thalassemia major. Am J Hematol 2009;84:29–33.
56. Pootrakul P, Breuer W, Sametband M, et al. Labile plasma iron (LPI) as an indicator of chelatable plasma redox activity in iron-overloaded beta-thalassemia/HbE patients treated with an oral chelator. Blood 2004;104:1504–10.
57. Chirnomas D, Smith AL, Braunstein J, et al. Deferasirox pharmacokinetics in patients with adequate versus inadequate response. Blood 2009;114:4009–13.
58. Pennell DJ, Porter JB, Cappellini MD, et al. Efficacy of deferasirox in reducing and preventing cardiac iron overload in beta-thalassemia. Blood 2010;115: 2364–71.
59. Tsironi M, Assimakopoulos G, Polonofi K, et al. Effects of combined deferiprone and deferoxamine chelation therapy on iron load indices in beta-thalassemia. Hemoglobin 2008;32:29–34.
60. Ricchi P, Ammirabile M, Spasiano A, et al. Combined chelation therapy in thalassemia major with deferiprone and desferrioxamine: a retrospective study. Eur J Haematol 2010;85(1):36–42.
61. Porter JB, Rafique R, Srichairatanakool S, et al. Recent insights into interactions of deferoxamine with cellular and plasma iron pools: implications for clinical use. Ann N Y Acad Sci 2005;1054:155–68.
62. Lee P, Mohammed N, Abeysinghe RD, et al. Intravenous infusion pharmacokinetics of desferrioxamine in thalassaemia patients. Drug Metab Dispos 1993; 21:640–4.
63. Porter JB, Faherty A, Stallibrass L, et al. A trial to investigate the relationship between DFO pharmacokinetics and metabolism and DFO-related toxicity. Ann N Y Acad Sci 1998;850:483–7.

64. Evans P, Kayyali R, Hider RC, et al. Mechanisms for the shuttling of plasma non-transferrin bound iron (NTBI) onto deferoxamine by deferiprone Transl Res 2010;156(2):55–67.

65. Zanninelli G, Breuer W, Cabantchik ZI. Daily labile plasma iron as an indicator of chelator activity in Thalassaemia major patients. Br J Haematol 2009;147: 744–51.

66. Pippard M, Johnson D, Callender S, et al. Ferrioxamine excretion in iron loaded man. Blood 1982;60:288–94.

67. Cappellini MD, Cohen A, Piga A, et al. A phase 3 study of deferasirox (ICL670), a once-daily oral iron chelator, in patients with beta-thalassemia. Blood 2006; 107:3455–62.

68. Marcus RE, Davies SC, Bantock HM, et al. Desferrioxamine to improve cardiac function in iron overloaded patients with thalassaemia major. Lancet 1984;1:392–3.

69. Davies SC, Marcus RE, Hungerford JL, et al. Ocular toxicity of high-dose intra-venous desferrioxamine. Lancet 1983;2:181–4.

70. Porter JB, Davis BA. Monitoring chelation therapy to achieve optimal outcome in the treatment of thalassaemia. Best Pract Res Clin Haematol 2002;15:329–68.

71. Pennell DJ, Berdoukas V, Karagiorga M, et al. Randomized controlled trial of deferiprone or deferoxamine in beta-thalassemia major patients with asymptomatic myocardial siderosis. Blood 2006;107:3738–44.

72. Pennell DJ, Porter JB, Cappellini MD, et al. Efficacy and safety of deferasirox (exjade®) in reducing cardiac iron in patients with β-thalassemia major: results from the cardiac substudy of the EPIC trial [abstract]. Blood 2008;112:abstract 3873.

73. Tanner MA, Galanello R, Dessi C, et al. A randomized, placebo-controlled, double-blind trial of the effect of combined therapy with deferoxamine and deferiprone on myocardial iron in thalassemia major using cardiovascular magnetic resonance. Circulation 2007;115:1876–84.

74. Porter JB, Huehns ER. The toxic effects of desferrioxamine. Baillieres Clin Haematol 1989;2:459–74.

75. Cunningham MJ, Macklin EA, Neufeld EJ, et al. Complications of beta-thalassemia major in North America. Blood 2004;104:34–9.

76. Olivieri NF, Buncic JR, Chew E, et al. Visual and auditory neurotoxicity in patients receiving subcutaneous deferoxamine infusions. N Engl J Med 1986;314: 869–73.

77. Blake DR, Winyard P, Lunec J, et al. Cerebral and ocular toxicity induced by desferrioxamine. Q J Med 1985;56:345–55.

78. Porter JB, Jaswon MS, Huehns ER, et al. Desferrioxamine ototoxicity: evaluation of risk factors in thalassaemic patients and guidelines for safe dosage. Br J Haematol 1989;73:403–9.

79. De Virgilis S, Congia M, Frau F, et al. Desferrioxamine-induced growth retardation in patients with thalassaemia major. J Pediatr 1988;113:661–9.

80. Piga A, Luzzatto L, Capalbo P, et al. High dose desferrioxamine as a cause of growth failure in thalassaemic patients. Eur J Haematol 1988;40:380–1.

81. Olivieri NF, Koren G, Harris J, et al. Growth failure and bony changes induced by deferoxamine. Am J Pediatr Hematol Oncol 1992;14:48–56.

82. Hider RC, Choudhury R, Rai BL, et al. Design of orally active iron chelators. Acta Haematol 1996;95:6–12.

83. Olivieri NF, Koren G, Hermann C, et al. Comparison of oral iron chelator L1 and desferrioxamine in iron-loaded patients. Lancet 1990;336:1275–9.

84. Kontoghiorghes GJ, Goddard JG, Bartlett AN, et al. Pharmacokinetic studies in humans with the oral iron chelator 1,2-dimethyl-3-hydroxypyrid-4-one. Clin Pharmacol Ther 1990;48:255–61.

85. Fischer R, Longo F, Nielsen P, et al. Monitoring long-term efficacy of iron chelation therapy by deferiprone and desferrioxamine in patients with beta-thalassaemia major: application of SQUID biomagnetic liver susceptometry. Br J Haematol 2003;121:938–48.

86. Collins AF, Fassos FF, Stobie S, et al. Iron-balance and dose-response studies of the oral iron chelator 1,2- dimethyl-3-hydroxypyrid-4-one (L1) in iron-loaded patients with sickle cell disease. Blood 1994;83:2329–33.

87. Roberts D, Brunskill S, Doree C, et al. Oral deferiprone for iron chelation in people with thalassaemia. Cochrane Database Syst Rev 2007;3:CD004839.

88. Olivieri NF, Brittenham GM, Matsui D, et al. Iron-chelation therapy with oral deferiprone in patients with thalassemia major. N Engl J Med 1995;332:918–22.

89. Olivieri NF, Brittenham GM, McLaren CE, et al. Long-term safety and effectiveness of iron-chelation therapy with deferiprone for thalassemia major. N Engl J Med 1998;339:417–23.

90. Maggio A, D'Amico G, Morabito A, et al. Deferiprone versus deferoxamine in patients with thalassemia major: a randomized clinical trial. Blood Cells Mol Dis 2002;28:196–208.

91. Gomber S, Saxena R, Madan N. Comparative efficacy of desferrioxamine, deferiprone and in combination on iron chelation in thalassemic children. Indian Pediatr 2004;41:21–7.

92. Ha SY, Chik KW, Ling SC, et al. A randomized controlled study evaluating the safety and efficacy of deferiprone treatment in thalassemia major patients from Hong Kong. Hemoglobin 2006;30:263–74.

93. Mazza P, Amurri B, Lazzari G, et al. Oral iron chelating therapy. A single center interim report on deferiprone (L1) in thalassemia. Haematologica 1998;83:496–501.

94. Ceci A, Baiardi P, Felisi M, et al. The safety and effectiveness of deferiprone in a large-scale, 3-year study in Italian patients. Br J Haematol 2002;118:330–6.

95. Goel H, Girisha KM, Phadke SR. Long-term efficacy of oral deferiprone in management of iron overload in beta thalassemia major. Hematology 2008;13:77–82.

96. Hoffbrand AV, AL-Refaie F, Davis B, et al. Long-term trial of deferiprone in 51 transfusion-dependent iron overloaded patients. Blood 1998;91:295–300.

97. Borgna-Pignatti C, Cappellini MD, De Stefano P, et al. Cardiac morbidity and mortality in deferoxamine- or deferiprone-treated patients with thalassemia major. Blood 2006;107:3733–7.

98. Piga A, Gaglioti C, Fogliacco E, et al. Comparative effects of deferiprone and deferoxamine on survival and cardiac disease in patients with thalassemia major: a retrospective analysis. Haematologica 2003;88:489–96.

99. Porter J, Cohen A, Kwiatkowski J. Transfusion and iron chelation. In: Steinberg M, Forget B, Higgs D, et al, editors. Disorders of hemoglobin. New York: Cambridge University Press; 2009. p. 689–744.

100. Al-Refaie FN, Hershko C, Hoffbrand AV, et al. Results of long-term deferiprone (L1) therapy: a report by the international study group on oral iron chelators. Br J Haematol 1995;91:224–9.

101. Hoyes KP, Jones HM, Abeysinghe RD, et al. In vivo and in vitro effects of 3-hydroxypyridin-4-one chelators on murine hemopoiesis. Exp Hematol 1993;21:86–92.

102. Naithani R, Chandra J, Sharma S. Safety of oral iron chelator deferiprone in young thalassaemics. Eur J Haematol 2005;74:217–20.

103. Agarwal MB, Gupte SS, Viswanathan C, et al. Long-term assessment of efficacy and safety of L1, an oral iron chelator, in transfusion dependent thalassaemia: Indian trial. Br J Haematol 1992;82:460–6.

104. Choudhry VP, Pati HP, Saxena A, et al. Deferiprone, efficacy and safety. Indian J Pediatr 2004;71:213–6.

105. Cohen AR, Galanello R, Piga A, et al. Safety and effectiveness of long-term therapy with the oral iron chelator deferiprone. Blood 2003;102:1583–7.

106. Link G, Konijn AM, Breuer W, et al. Exploring the "iron shuttle" hypothesis in chelation therapy: effects of combined deferoxamine and deferiprone treatment in hypertransfused rats with labeled iron stores and in iron-loaded rat heart cells in culture. J Lab Clin Med 2001;138:130–8.

107. Galanello R, Kattamis A, Piga A, et al. A prospective randomized controlled trial on the safety and efficacy of alternating deferoxamine and deferiprone in the treatment of iron overload in patients with thalassemia. Haematologica 2006;91:1241–3.

108. Aydinok Y, Ulger Z, Nart D, et al. A randomized controlled 1-year study of daily deferiprone plus twice weekly desferrioxamine compared with daily deferiprone monotherapy in patients with thalassemia major. Haematologica 2007;92:1599–606.

109. Daar S, Pathare AV. Combined therapy with desferrioxamine and deferiprone in beta thalassemia major patients with transfusional iron overload. Ann Hematol 2006;85:315–9.

110. El-Beshlawy A, Manz C, Naja M, et al. Iron chelation in thalassemia: combined or monotherapy? the Egyptian experience. Ann Hematol 2008;87:545–50.

111. Kattamis A, Ladis V, Berdousi H, et al. Iron chelation treatment with combined therapy with deferiprone and deferioxamine: a 12-month trial. Blood Cells Mol Dis 2006;36:21–5.

112. Telfer P, Coen PG, Christou S, et al. Survival of medically treated thalassemia patients in Cyprus. Trends and risk factors over the period 1980–2004. Haematologica 2006;91:1187–92.

113. Origa R, Bina P, Agus A, et al. Combined therapy with deferiprone and desferrioxamine in thalassemia major. Haematologica 2005;90:1309–14.

114. Porter JB. Deferasirox: an effective once-daily orally active iron chelator. Drugs Today (Barc) 2006;42:623–37.

115. Nick H, Acklin P, Lattmann R, et al. Development of tridentate iron chelators: from desferrithiocin to ICL670. Curr Med Chem 2003;10:1065–76.

116. Wood JC, Aguilar M, Otto-Duessel M, et al. Influence of iron chelation on R1 and R2 calibration curves in gerbil liver and heart. Magn Reson Med 2008;60:82–9.

117. Galanello R, Piga A, Alberti D, et al. Safety, tolerability, and pharmacokinetics of ICL670, a new orally active iron-chelating agent in patients with transfusion-dependent iron overload due to beta-thalassemia. J Clin Pharmacol 2003;43:565–72.

118. Nisbet-Brown E, Olivieri NF, Giardina PJ, et al. Effectiveness and safety of ICL670 in iron-loaded patients with thalassaemia: a randomised, double-blind, placebo-controlled, dose-escalation trial. Lancet 2003;361:1597–602.

119. Waldmeier F, Bruin GJ, Glaenzel U, et al. Pharmacokinetics, metabolism, and disposition of deferasirox in beta-thalassemic patients with transfusion-dependent iron overload who are at pharmacokinetic steady state. Drug Metab Dispos 2010;38:808–16.

120. Piga A, Galanello R, Forni GL, et al. Randomized phase II trial of deferasirox (Exjade, ICL670), a once-daily, orally-administered iron chelator, in comparison

to deferoxamine in thalassemia patients with transfusional iron overload. Haematologica 2006;91:873–80.

121. Galanello R, Piga A, Cappellini MD, et al. Effect of food, type of food, and time of food intake on deferasirox bioavailability: recommendations for an optimal deferasirox administration regimen. J Clin Pharmacol 2008;48:428–35.

122. Vichinsky E, Onyekwere O, Porter J, et al. A randomised comparison of deferasirox versus deferoxamine for the treatment of transfusional iron overload in sickle cell disease. Br J Haematol 2007;136:501–8.

123. Deugnier Y, Turlin B, Ropert M, et al. Semi-quantitative assessment of hemosiderin distribution accurately reflects reductions in liver iron concentration following therapy with deferasirox (exjade®, icl670) or deferoxamine in patients with transfusion-dependent anemia [abstract]. Blood 2005;106(Suppl 11): abstract 2708.

124. Cappellini MD, Porter J, El-Beshlawy A, et al. Tailoring iron chelation by iron intake and serum ferritin: the prospective EPIC study of deferasirox in 1744 patients with transfusion-dependent anemias. Haematologica 2010;95:557–66.

125. Porter JB, Tanner MA, Pennell DJ, et al. Improved myocardial t2* in transfusion dependent anemias receiving ICL670 (deferasirox) [abstract]. Blood 2005;106: abstract 3600.

126. Pennell D, Porter J, Cappellini M, et al. Efficacy and safety of deferasirox (exjade®) in β-thalassemia patients with myocardial siderosis: 2-year results from the epic cardiac sub-study [abstract]. Blood 2009;114:abstract 4062.

127. Alpendurada F, Carpenter JP, Deac M, et al. Relation of myocardial T2* to right ventricular function in thalassaemia major. Eur Heart J 2010;31(3):1648–54.

128. Pennell D, Porter J, Cappellini M, et al. Continued improvement in cardiac t2* with deferasirox treatment over 2 years: results from the extension of epic cardiac substudy in beta-thalassaemia patients with myocardial siderosis [abstract]. Haematologica 2010;95(Suppl 2):abstract 0498.

129. Piga A, Forni G, Kattamis A, et al. Deferasirox (exjade®) in pediatric patients with β-thalassemia: update of 4.7-year efficacy and safety from extension studies [abstract]. Blood 2008;112:abstract 3883.

130. Cappellini M, R G, A P. Efficacy and safety of deferasirox (exjade®) with up to 4.5 years of treatment in patients with thalassemia major: a pooled analysis [abstract]. Blood 2008;112:abstract 5411.

131. Taher A, Cappellini MD, Vichinsky E, et al. Efficacy and safety of deferasirox doses of >30 mg/kg per d in patients with transfusion-dependent anaemia and iron overload. Br J Haematol 2009;147:752–9.

Pharmacologic Induction of Fetal Hemoglobin Production

George Atweh, MD[a], Hassana Fathallah, PhD[b],*

KEYWORDS

- Fetal hemoglobin expression • Gene regulation • Globin
- Sickle cell • Thalassemia

Human hemoglobin is a tetrameric molecule comprised of two pairs of identical polypeptide subunits, each pair encoded by a different family of genes. The human α-like globin genes (ζ, $\alpha1$, and $\alpha2$) are located on chromosome 16 and the β-like globin genes (ε, $^G\gamma$, $^A\gamma$, δ, and β) are located on chromosome 11. During development, sequential switches take place in both the α- and β-like globin clusters that result in the production of six different types of hemoglobins. Synthesis of hemoglobin begins during the first weeks of embryonic development in the yolk sac where three different hemoglobins are made: (1) Hb Gower 1 ($\zeta2\varepsilon2$); (2) Hb Portland ($\zeta2\gamma2$); and (3) Hb Gower 2 ($\alpha2\varepsilon2$). By the 13th week of gestation, the site of erythropoiesis shifts from the embryonic yolk sac to the fetal liver where fetal hemoglobin (HbF; $\alpha2\gamma2$) starts to accumulate as the embryonic ε-globin gene is turned off. Shortly before birth, a second switch occurs as the site of erythropoiesis shifts from the fetal liver to the bone marrow. As a result of this second switch, the two adult hemoglobins (HbA, $\alpha2\beta2$; and HbA$_2$, $\alpha2\delta2$) gradually replace HbF. By the end of the first year of life, the hemoglobin composition is approximately 97.5% HbA, 2% HbA$_2$, and 0.5% HbF.

In adult life, the residual amounts of HbF are distributed unevenly among red cells. HbF is concentrated in a subpopulation of erythrocytes known as "F cells." The amount of HbF and the number of F cells are genetically determined and vary within a relatively narrow range in normal individuals. Such factors as acute blood loss, pregnancy, and bone marrow transplantation that lead to erythropoietic stress can result in an increase in baseline levels of HbF. In addition, inheritance of a variety of genetic

[a] Division of Hematology and Oncology, Department of Internal Medicine, University of Cincinnati, 231 Albert Sabin Way, PO Box 670562, Cincinnati, OH 45267–0562, USA
[b] Division of Hematology and Oncology, Department of Internal Medicine, The Vontz Center for Molecular Studies, University of Cincinnati, 3125 Eden Avenue, Cincinnati, OH 45267–0508, USA
* Corresponding author.
E-mail address: Hassana.fathallah@uc.edu

Hematol Oncol Clin N Am 24 (2010) 1131–1144
doi:10.1016/j.hoc.2010.08.001
0889-8588/10/$ – see front matter © 2010 Elsevier Inc. All rights reserved.

hemonc.theclinics.com

determinants, such as sickle cell disease (SCD), thalassemia, and hereditary persistence of HbF, can also lead to higher levels of HbF and F cells in adult life.[1]

The levels of HbF in erythrocytes account for a large part of the clinical heterogeneity observed in patients with SCD[2,3] and β-thalassemia.[4,5] Patients with SCD from certain regions of Saudi Arabia[6] and India[7] have an unusually mild clinical sickling disorder associated with high levels of HbF. Moreover, the large multicenter study of the natural history of SCD (Cooperative Study of SCD) identified HbF as a major predictor of several complications, including painful events,[2,8] acute chest syndrome,[9] and mortality.[10] In addition, patients with SCD or β-thalassemia who co-inherit a genetic determinant for hereditary persistence of HbF usually have a mild clinical disorder.[4,5] These clinical and epidemiologic observations provided important clues about the beneficial role of HbF in modulating the pathophysiology of these disorders. In SCD, a high level of HbF interferes with the polymerization of HbS and prevents sickling of red blood cells. On the other hand, in β-thalassemia, a high level of γ-globin chain synthesis decreases non-α:α chain imbalance and ameliorates the anemia. Based on all these observations, it was proposed that pharmacologic induction of HbF production might be an effective therapeutic strategy for ameliorating the severity of SCD and β-thalassemia.

REGULATION OF γ-GLOBIN GENE EXPRESSION

Gene transcription of the γ-globin genes, and of other globin genes present in the β-globin cluster, is controlled by complex molecular mechanisms involving *cis*-acting elements, represented by specific nucleotide sequences, such as the cluster control region (LCR) and the promoters of the different globin genes and *trans*-acting elements, such as transcription factors and chromatin remodeling proteins.

The LCR consists of at least five DNase I hypersensitive sites (HS1–HS5). Each HS contains one or more binding motifs for three erythroid-specific transcription factors (GATA-1, NF-E2,[11–13] and EKLF[14,15]) in addition to binding sites for ubiquitous DNA binding proteins. HS1 to HS4 are formed only in erythroid cells.[16–18] The transcriptional-enhancer activity of the LCR resides mostly in HS2 and HS3. HS3 is believed to be involved in γ-globin activation during fetal-stage development[19] and in β-globin activation during adult life.[20] It is postulated that EKLF bound to HS3 may provide a competitive advantage for the interaction of the LCR with the β-globin promoter over its interactions with the γ-globin promoter, facilitating hemoglobin switching after birth.[21] The role of the LCR in switching has been conceptualized by the competition model based on the presence of developmental stage-specific transcription factors that mediate its interactions with the individual globin gene promoters.[22–24] However, significant uncertainty exists regarding the potential effects of the LCR on chromatin conformation in the β-globin gene cluster. In patients with Hispanic δβ-thalassemia in which the LCR is deleted, the β-globin cluster chromatin domain is in a closed, DNase I-resistant, transcriptionally inactive conformation, suggesting that the LCR functions to open chromatin in addition to its direct role in globin gene activation.[25] However, when the β-globin LCR was deleted from the endogenous mouse β-globin cluster in embryonic stem cells and somatic cell lines, β-like globin transcript levels were reduced, whereas the switching pattern during development remained normal and the chromatin of the β-globin gene cluster existed in an open DNase I–sensitive conformation.[26] These studies suggest that the LCR is not necessary for the establishment of an open chromatin cluster and that its primary function is that of an enhancer for transcriptional activation of the globin genes. Furthermore, these studies also suggested that the sequences conferring developmental stage-specific expression reside in the regions immediately flanking the globin genes.[26] These findings are consistent with previous studies by Arcasoy and coworkers,[27] who found autonomous silencing of the γ-globin genes in adult transgenic mice despite the absence of the LCR.

GATA-1, EKLF, and NF-E2 are the best-characterized tissue-specific transcription factors involved in the regulated expression of the β-like globin genes. All these factors bind to DNA elements in the β-like globin genes. GATA-1 and EKLF are essential for active chromatin hub formation. Contacts between the LCR and the β-like globin genes do not form in their absence.[28] In contrast, NF-E2 seems to be dispensable for β-globin active chromatin hub formation.[29] The essential role of GATA-1 in inducing β-globin LCR chromatin structure remodeling is also supported by recent studies of enforced GATA-1 expression in nonerythroid cells.[30] Transcription factors that activate the γ-globin gene promoter include the FKLF2,[31] NF-E4, and SSP.[32,33] Other studies have provided evidence that long-range interactions between the LCR and the active β-globin genes requires the binding to the LCR of a multimeric transcriptional complex formed by the nuclear protein Nuclear LIM interactor and its erythroid binding partners GATA-1, TAL-1, and LMO2.[34]

Pharmacologic Reactivation of HbF Synthesis

During the last two decades, a great deal of effort has been focused on the pharmacologic induction of HbF in patients with hemoglobin disorders. Multiple drugs including 5-azacytidine,[35,36] hydroxyurea,[37,38] erythropoietin,[39,40] and butyrate[41,42] were found to have in vivo activity in patients with these disorders. Histone deacetalyse (HDAC) inhibitors, such as butyrate, and related compounds and DNA methylation inhibitors, such as 5-azacytidine and decitabine, are believed to exert their effects through epigenetic modifications in the β-globin gene cluster (**Fig. 1**). Despite

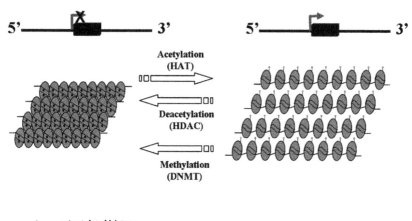

Fig. 1. Methylation of CpG dinucleotides (by DNA methyltransferases [DNMT]) and hypoacetylation of histones (by histone deacetylases [HDAC]) result in a closed chromatin configuration that represses gene expression. Hypomethylated DNA and hyperacetylated histones (by histone acetyltransferases [HAT]) result in an open chromatin structure that allows gene expression.

the controversy over the exact mechanism of induction of HbF by 5-azacytidine and hydroxyurea, considerable progress has been made in the development of these agents as drugs that can induce HbF in patients with hemoglobin disorder.

DNA Methyltransferase Inhibitors

DNA methylation is a mechanism of gene silencing in which methyl groups become covalently attached to the 5-carbon position of a cytosine residue at a "CpG" site. This epigenetic process occurs during S phase and is catalyzed by the DNA methyltransferase family of enzymes. Genes with heavily methylated promoter regions cannot be transcribed and are effectively silenced (see **Fig. 1**).

Several studies that were published in the early 1980s showed a strong inverse correlation between γ-globin gene expression and DNA methylation at the γ-globin gene promoters. During the embryonic and adult stages of development, methylation of the γ-globin promoters was shown to correlate with silencing of the γ-globin genes. In contrast, hypomethylation of the γ-globin gene promoters during the fetal stage was shown to correlate with expression of the γ-globin genes. Similarly, the inactive β-globin gene was shown to be methylated in fetal life, whereas the active β-globin gene was shown to be hypomethylated in adult life.[43,44] These observations support a model in which differences in the methylation pattern of the γ-globin gene in differentiating erythroblasts at different stages of development may be the result of fetal stage-specific demethylation associated with transcription activation. Therefore, considerable efforts have been focused on the use of DNA hypomethylating agents for the pharmacologic stimulation of HbF production in adult life.

5-Azacytidine was the first prototype of an agent that induces HbF by targeting epigenetic gene silencing. This drug was first used in the United States during the 1970s as an antileukemic agent and later in the 1980s as an HbF inducer in patients with hemoglobin disorders. 5-Azacytidine was recently approved by the Food and Drug Administration for the treatment of patients with myelodysplastic syndrome, although the mechanisms responsible for its beneficial effects in this disorder remain unknown.[45,46] The ability of 5-azacytidine to stimulate HbF production was first demonstrated in the anemic baboon where HbF levels increased up to 70% to 80% of total hemoglobin after treatment with this drug.[47,48] These observations provided strong support for the hypothesis that γ-globin gene expression could be pharmacologically induced in vivo by DNA hypomethylation at the promoters of the γ-globin genes, resulting in increased levels of HbF. These encouraging data led to clinical trials of 5-azacytidine in a small number of patients with SCD and β-thalassemia. This treatment resulted in significant increases in HbF levels (7%–23%); F cells (11%–50%); and total hemoglobin (1–4 g/dL). The therapeutic effects of this drug were associated with a decrease in the percentage of dense cells in patients with SCD and of the non-α:α chain imbalance and transfusion requirements in patients with β-thalassemia.[35,36,49,50] Despite these promising results, clinical trials with this agent were not continued because of concerns over potential carcinogenic effects of 5-azacytidine, which was previously shown to increase the incidence of tumors in an animal model.[51]

The more recent introduction of decitabine as a DNA hypomethylating agent resulted in renewed interest in the use of DNA hypomethylation for the induction of HbF (**Fig. 2**). Three clinical trials have been reported by the same group in which decitabine was administered to patients with SCD. In the first two studies, the drug was administered to a total of 15 patients by intravenous injections at doses of 0.15 to 0.3 mg/kg/day.[52,53] In the third study, decitabine was administered to eight patients by subcutaneous injections at doses similar to those used in the previous studies.[54] This therapy resulted in significant increases in mean γ-globin synthesis, HbF levels,

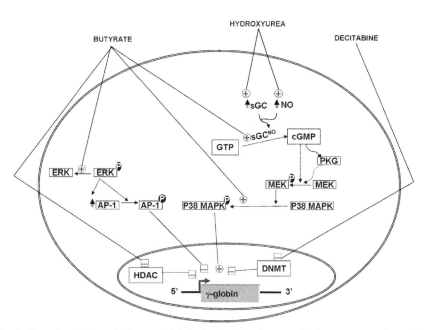

Fig. 2. Experimental model for γ-globin induction by pharmacologic agents. A schematic is shown of the molecular mechanisms for γ-globin activation in erythroid progenitor–derived cells. Butyrate mediates histone hyperacetylation by inhibition of HDAC, stimulates p38 MAPK phosphorylation and ERK MAPK dephosphorylation, and activates the sGC/cGMP pathway resulting in the activation of γ-globin expression. Hydroxyurea activates the sGC/cGMP pathway leading to the activation of γ-globin expression. Decitabine mediates DNA hypomethylation by inhibition of DNMT, inducing γ-globin expression. sGC, soluble guanlyl cyclase; cGMP, cyclic guanosine monophosphate; GTP, guanosine triphosphate; NO, nitric oxide; PKG, protein kinase G; P, phosphorylation; HDAC, histone deacetylase; DNMT, DNA methyltransferase; +, activation; −, inhibition; ↑, increase.

and F cells by 10%, 13%, and 33%, respectively. Interestingly, 100% of patients with SCD showed an increase in HbF production in response to decitabine, including several patients who had previously failed to respond to hydroxyurea. With decitabine treatment, total hemoglobin levels increased by 2 g/dL, whereas the reticulocyte count decreased, suggesting a decrease in hemolysis. The increase in the levels of HbF was associated with significant improvement in several parameters that are important in the pathophysiology of vasoocclusion, such as red blood cell adhesion, endothelial damage, and activation of the coagulation pathway. The authors also demonstrated a decrease in DNA methylation at the promoters of the γ-globin genes. The only toxicity that was observed in these studies was transient neutropenia. Interestingly, the platelet count and the proportion of megakaryocytes and erythroid cells in the marrow increased, without a corresponding decrease in marrow cellularity. The significance of these observations is not yet clear.

Despite these encouraging short-term studies, the clinical effectiveness and the potential long-term toxicities of decitabine treatment are not known at this stage. An early study reported that this agent was not carcinogenic in the rat model.[51] Other relatively short-term studies by Yang and colleagues[55] in patients with leukemia treated with decitabine did not show an increase in incidence of secondary tumors at 2 to 5 years after initiation of therapy. More recent studies have suggested that treatment of mice with a genetic disposition for colon or lung cancer with decitabine results in a marked reduction in tumor formation.[56,57] It is speculated that this reduction in tumorogenesis may be a reflection of the prevention of methylation of tumor-suppressor genes, a process that is believed to be important in the pathogenesis of some cancers. These studies suggested that decitabine may have some potential in the chemoprevention of cancer. Larger and longer-term studies are needed to confirm the safety and efficacy of decitabine in patients with hemoglobin disorders.

The molecular mechanisms of induction of HbF by 5-azacytidine and decitabine are not fully understood. These agents were first introduced based on their ability to inhibit methylation of newly synthesized DNA within the promoters of the γ-globin genes.[35,36,49,54,58] One of the five CpGs within the promoters of the fetal γ-globin genes that could be hypomethylated on exposure to these agents coincides with a DNA sequence that is occupied by proteins that participate in the switch from fetal to adult globin expression.[59,60] Methylation of this CpG favors the binding of a repressor, which might be responsible in part for γ-globin repression in adult erythroid cells. In contrast, hypomethylation of this same CpG can enhance the binding of an activator of γ-globin gene expression. In addition, recent experiments in baboons showed that DNA hypomethylation induced by treatment with decitabine is associated with histone hyperacetylation at the γ-globin promoters.[61] Taken together, these data suggest that DNA methylation may result in changes in chromatin structure that enhance the binding of transcription factors, leading to derepression and transcriptional activation of γ-globin gene expression in adult life (see **Fig. 2**).

Despite these data, the causal role of DNA hypomethylation in the induction of HbF expression by these analogs remains controversial. It is well known that a partial switch from adult to fetal hemoglobin production takes place during accelerated erythropoiesis, as seen following acute blood loss. This results in augmented F-reticulocytosis and a corresponding increase in HbF levels. Thus, some investigators proposed that 5-azacytidine treatment may result in injury to bone marrow progenitors, leading to accelerated erythropoiesis and an increase in HbF levels. In support of this hypothesis, hydroxyurea, another S-phase–specific chemotherapeutic agent, was shown to increase HbF levels in anemic baboons.[62] Because hydroxyurea does not have a direct effect on DNA methylation, it was proposed that the induction of HbF by 5-azacytidine is unlikely to be a result of its DNA hypomethylating activity.[63] Moreover, molecular examination of DNA methylation in bone marrow cells from a patient who failed to respond to 5-azacytidine with increased γ-globin synthesis revealed hypomethylation of the γ-globin promoters.[58] Thus, the exact mechanism of induction of HbF by hypomethylating agents remains shrouded in controversy.[64]

Histone Deacetylase Inhibitors

The acetylation of histones and nonhistone proteins at the ε-amino group of lysine residues is a reversible posttranslational process. Acetylation of histones is commonly associated with transcriptional activation of genes and is thought to be responsible both for a local "open chromatin" structure required for promoter activation and for impacting the binding of multiple transcription factors directly. Histone acetylation can be achieved either by acetyltransferases alone or by adenosine triphosphate-dependent nucleosome remodeling complexes, such as SWI-SNF complexes. In contrast, removal of acetyl groups by HDACs frequently accompanies suppression of gene activity, and HDACs are often found as components of transcriptional repressor complexes. Different signaling events may switch the association patterns from acetyltransferases to deacetylases, or vice versa, providing a potential mechanism for dynamic control of acetylation in vivo. The comparative analysis of the histone acetylation patterns in the human β-globin cluster between the fetal and adult stages of development showed that the LCR was acetylated at the same level in both fetal and adult erythroblasts, whereas the acetylation in the globin promoter regions correlated with the state of transcription.[65,66]

Several lines of experimental evidence have suggested that HDAC inhibition results in increased HbF synthesis. In vitro studies performed in erythroleukemia cell lines and in primary erythroid cultures have shown that several HDAC inhibitors, such as TSA,[67,68] MS-275, scriptaid,[69] and apicidin,[70] simulate HbF synthesis. In vivo, butyrate, a natural short-chain fatty acid and a well-known HDAC inhibitor, was shown to increase embryonic globin gene expression in chicken adult erythroid cells pretreated with 5-azacytidine.[71] Furthermore, infants of diabetic mothers were shown to have a delay in γ- to β-globin switch after birth. This was attributed to the elevated plasma α-amino butyric acid levels that result from ketosis during pregancy.[72,73] Moreover, exposure to butyrate was shown to result in increase HbF synthesis in adult baboons[74] and the fetal to adult globin gene switch was significantly delayed in butyrate-treated lamb fetuses.[75]

In 1993, arginine butyrate was administered to six patients, three with SCD and three with β-thalassemia.[42] This initial study provided evidence that arginine butyrate infusion can increase HbF production in vivo in patients with hemoglobin disorders. However, a subsequent study showed that the continuous infusion of arginine butyrate did not result in a sustained HbF production and did not improve the hematologic parameters in patients with SCD or β-thalassemia.[76] However, when arginine butyrate was administered intermittently at lower doses in a subsequent study in patients with SCD, this resulted in a sustained induction of HbF production in most patients.[41] The success of this regimen was attributed to its ability to avoid toxicity to erythroid precursors that might result from continuous exposure to high levels of butyrate. However, not all patients with SCD responded to butyrate treatment: interestingly, all patients whose baseline HbF levels were greater than 2% responded to treatment, whereas all patients with HbF levels less than 2% were resistant to this treatment.[41] Although pulse administration of butyrate can result in a significant improvement in the anemia in patients with β-thalassemia, most treated patients continue to suffer from profound anemia.[77]

Given the difficulty of administration of large volumes of arginine butyrate through central venous catheters, orally administered butyrate compounds have been tested to treat patients with SCD and β-thalassemia. Both sodium phenylbutyrate[78] and isobutyramide[79] resulted in some stimulation of HbF synthesis. However, the induction of HbF with these agents was modest and patient compliance was a significant challenge. As a result, clinical development of these agents did not go forward.

It is widely believed that butyrate increases γ-globin gene expression by increasing histone acetylation at their promoters. Recently, using primary erythroid cultures derived from peripheral blood of normal donors and patients with SCD, the authors analyzed the epigenetic changes induced by butyrate at the promoters of different genes of the β-globin cluster.[65] This analysis showed that butyrate exposure results in a true reversal of the normal developmental switch from γ- to β-globin expression. This is associated with increased histone acetylation and decreased DNA methylation of the γ-globin genes, with opposite changes at the promoter of the β-globin gene.[65] In vivo foot-printing studies performed in erythroblasts of patients who responded to butyrate by increasing HbF production revealed alterations in DNA binding at the proximal region of the γ-globin gene promoter.[80] Butyrate was also shown to activate signaling through the activation of soluble guanylate cyclase (sGC)[81] and p38 MAP kinase[68] pathways and inhibition of ERK MAP kinase pathway (see **Fig. 2**).[82] However, it is not yet clear how these signaling activities lead to the transcriptional activation of the γ-globin genes. More recently, butyrate was also shown to increase HbF production in patients with SCD by increasing the efficiency of translation of γ-globin mRNA.[83]

HYDROXYUREA

Hydroxyurea is a potent inhibitor of ribonucleotide reductase that interferes with cellular DNA synthesis and promotes cell death. It is orally bioavailable and had been used for many years as a chemotherapeutic agent for the treatment of patients with myeloproliferative disorders. Controversy over the mechanism of action of 5-azacytidine and concerns about its potential toxicity led investigators to explore the potential of hydroxyurea as an inducer of HbF in baboons, and later in patients with SCD and β-thalassemia. It was also widely believed, although never proved, that hydroxyurea has less carcinogenic effects than 5-azacytidine. Hydroxyurea is now the only drug approved by the Food and Drug Administration for the treatment of adult patients with moderate or severe SCD.

The ability of hydroxyurea to induce HbF synthesis both in anemic monkeys[62] and in small-scale studies in patients with SCD[38,84,85] led to a randomized placebo-controlled multicenter study of this agent in SCD. This study showed a marked decrease in the frequency of painful crises and acute chest syndrome in patients with moderate to severe disease.[86,87] More recently, Steinberg and colleagues[86] reported improved survival in patients with SCD treated with hydroxyurea. Hydroxyurea seems to have much more modest activity in patients with HbE/β-thalassemia,[37] Hb Lepore/β-thalassemia,[88] and thalassemia intermedia.[89–91] The major short-term toxicities of hydroxyurea were a reversible bone marrow suppression manifested as a decrease of white blood cell counts and platelet counts. The use of recombinant erythropoietin as a single agent in SCD is without any proved benefit, although it may increase the induction of HbF when used with hydroxyurea at extremely high doses.[84] Interestingly, higher baseline HbF levels predicted a better chance of response to hydroxyurea in children[92] but not in adults with SCD. Overall, the response to hydroxyurea is variable and around 30% of patients with β-hemoglobin disorders do not respond at all.

The mechanism by which hydroxyurea stimulates HbF synthesis has been explored in several studies. It was first proposed that the induction of HbF by hydroxyurea may be a result of perturbations in the kinetics of eryhtoid differentiation. Several studies suggested that hydroxyurea may exert its stimulatory effect on HbF synthesis through the guanosine 3′,5′-cyclic monophosphate (cGMP) signaling pathway (see **Fig. 2**). Previous studies had shown that exposure to hydroxyurea results in the induction of the sGC- and cGMP-dependent protein kinase signaling pathways.[93] Hydroxyurea was also shown to induce nitric oxide–dependent activation of sGC in cultured CD34+ human progenitors.[93] However, hydroxyurea was shown to increase nitric oxide and cGMP levels in the blood of patients with sickle cell anemia.[94,95] A more recent study has provided evidence that hydroxyurea was able to nitrosylate and activate sGC in human erythroid cells. More specifically, this study showed that hydroxyurea can directly interact with the deoxyheme of sGC by a free-radical nitroxide pathway.[96] Other studies have shown that in addition to its effect on cGMP, hydroxyurea also increases cyclic adenosine monophosphate (cAMP) levels.[97] Agents that increase either cGMP or cAMP levels in primary erythroid cells induce HbF production.[97,98] It was suggested that cGMP and cAMP may stimulate γ-gene expression by different molecular mechanisms: the former at the posttranscriptional level and the latter at the transcriptional level. A recent study suggested a pivotal role for the hydroxyurea-induced small GTP-binding protein, secretion-associated, and RAS-related (SAR) protein, in γ-globin induction by hydroxyurea.[99] This protein exerts its effect by inducing apoptosis and G1/S phase arrest by inhibition of PI3K and ERK phosphorylation and increased p21 and GATA-2 expression.[99]

FUTURE DIRECTIONS

Although a number of pharmacologic agents have been shown to induce HbF in patients with SCD, the impact of these new therapies on the natural history of hemoglobin disorders globally, especially in developing countries where these disorders are much more common, has been rather modest. There is ample epidemiologic and clinical evidence that suggests that higher HbF levels are associated with better amelioration of the clinical disorders.[2,4–7,100] Thus, more effective agents that can induce higher HbF levels are needed. Moreover, the complexity of the mechanisms of regulation of globin gene expression suggests that combination therapy consisting of two or more drugs, each with a different mechanism of action, may be more effective for the induction of very high levels of HbF. Methylation induces recruitment of HDACs, which results in more profound inhibition of transcription. The combination of a DNMT inhibitor, such as decitabine, with an HDAC inhibitor, such as butyrate, might result in more potent activation of γ-globin expression. Because these agents induce HbF production by modifying the epigenetic composition of the globin genes, it might be possible one day to personalize the therapy by custom-designing a drug combination based on the patient's own epigenetic configuration. Alternatively, a combination of DNMT inhibitors with agents, such as erythropoietin or hydroxyurea, which increase HbF by different mechanisms may also be more effective than treatment with a single agent. Finally, combination of agents that increase HbF levels with agents that target other aspects of the pathophysiology of hemoglobin disorders, such as cell adhesion or cell dehydration, may prove to be highly effective therapeutic approaches. After several decades of research to develop new therapies for hemoglobin disorders, clinicians may be at the dawn of a new era in which it might be possible to customize therapies to address the unique aspects of the pathophysiology in individual patients.

REFERENCES

1. Rochette J, Craig JE, Thein SL. Fetal hemoglobin levels in adults. Blood Rev 1994;8:213–24.
2. Bailey K, Morris JS, Thomas P, et al. Fetal haemoglobin and early manifestations of homozygous sickle cell disease. Arch Dis Child 1992;67:517–20.
3. Stevens MC, Hayes RJ, Vaidya S, et al. Fetal hemoglobin and clinical severity of homozygous sickle cell disease in early childhood. J Pediatr 1981;98:37–41.
4. Bollekens JA, Forget BG. Delta beta thalassemia and hereditary persistence of fetal hemoglobin. Hematol Oncol Clin North Am 1991;5:399–422.
5. Serjeant GR. Natural history and determinants of clinical severity of sickle cell disease. Curr Opin Hematol 1995;2:103–8.
6. Perrine RP, Pembrey ME, John P, et al. Natural history of sickle cell anemia in Saudi Arabs. A study of 270 subjects. Ann Intern Med 1978;88:1–6.
7. Kar BC, Satapathy RK, Kulozik AE, et al. Sickle cell disease in Orissa State, India. Lancet 1986;2:1198–201.
8. Platt OS, Thorington BD, Brambilla DJ, et al. Pain in sickle cell disease. Rates and risk factors. N Engl J Med 1991;325:11–6.

9. Castro O, Brambilla DJ, Thorington B, et al. The acute chest syndrome in sickle cell disease: incidence and risk factors. The cooperative study of sickle cell disease. Blood 1994;84:643–9.

10. Platt OS, Brambilla DJ, Rosse WF, et al. Mortality in sickle cell disease. Life expectancy and risk factors for early death. N Engl J Med 1994;330:1639–44.

11. Goodwin AJ, McInerney JM, Glander MA, et al. In vivo formation of a human beta-globin locus control region core element requires binding sites for multiple factors including GATA-1, NF-E2, erythroid Kruppel-like factor, and Sp1. J Biol Chem 2001;276:26883–92.

12. Martin DI, Orkin SH. Transcriptional activation and DNA binding by the erythroid factor GF-1/NF-E1/Eryf 1. Genes Dev 1990;4:1886–98.

13. Ney PA, Sorrentino BP, Lowrey CH, et al. Inducibility of the HS II enhancer depends on binding of an erythroid specific nuclear protein. Nucleic Acids Res 1990;18:6011–7.

14. Im H, Grass JA, Johnson KD, et al. Chromatin domain activation via GATA-1 utilization of a small subset of dispersed GATA motifs within a broad chromosomal region. Proc Natl Acad Sci U S A 2005;102:17065–70.

15. Zhou D, Pawlik KM, Ren J, et al. Differential binding of erythroid Krupple-like factor to embryonic/fetal globin gene promoters during development. J Biol Chem 2006;281:16052–7.

16. Forrester WC, Takegawa S, Papayannopoulou T, et al. Evidence for a locus activation region: the formation of developmentally stable hypersensitive sites in globin-expressing hybrids. Nucleic Acids Res 1987;15:10159–77.

17. Grosveld F, van Assendelft GB, Greaves DR, et al. Position-independent, high-level expression of the human beta-globin gene in transgenic mice. Cell 1987;51:975–85.

18. Kollias G, Wrighton N, Hurst J, et al. Regulated expression of human A gamma-, beta-, and hybrid gamma beta-globin genes in transgenic mice: manipulation of the developmental expression patterns. Cell 1986;46:89–94.

19. Navas PA, Peterson KR, Li Q, et al. Developmental specificity of the interaction between the locus control region and embryonic or fetal globin genes in transgenic mice with an HS3 core deletion. Mol Cell Biol 1998;18:4188–96.

20. Miller IJ, Bieker JJ. A novel, erythroid cell-specific murine transcription factor that binds to the CACCC element and is related to the Kruppel family of nuclear proteins. Mol Cell Biol 1993;13:2776–86.

21. Jackson DA, McDowell JC, Dean A. Beta-globin locus control region HS2 and HS3 interact structurally and functionally. Nucleic Acids Res 2003;31:1180–90.

22. Enver T, Raich N, Ebens AJ, et al. Developmental regulation of human fetal-to-adult globin gene switching in transgenic mice. Nature 1990;344:309–13.

23. Strouboulis J, Dillon N, Grosveld F. Developmental regulation of a complete 70-kb human beta-globin locus in transgenic mice. Genes Dev 1992;6:1857–64.

24. Townes TM, Behringer RR. Human globin locus activation region (LAR): role in temporal control. Trends Genet 1990;6:219–23.

25. Forrester WC, Epner E, Driscoll MC, et al. A deletion of the human beta-globin locus activation region causes a major alteration in chromatin structure and replication across the entire beta-globin locus. Genes Dev 1990;4:1637–49.

26. Bender MA, Bulger M, Close J, et al. Beta-globin gene switching and DNase I sensitivity of the endogenous beta-globin locus in mice do not require the locus control region. Mol Cell 2000;5:387–93.

27. Arcasoy MO, Romana M, Fabry ME, et al. High levels of human gamma-globin gene expression in adult mice carrying a transgene of deletion-type hereditary persistence of fetal hemoglobin. Mol Cell Biol 1997;17:2076–89.

28. Drissen R, Palstra RJ, Gillemans N, et al. The active spatial organization of the beta-globin locus requires the transcription factor EKLF. Genes Dev 2004;18:2485–90.

29. Kooren J, Palstra RJ, Klous P, et al. Beta-globin active chromatin Hub formation in differentiating erythroid cells and in p45 NF-E2 knock-out mice. J Biol Chem 2007;282:16544–52.

30. Layon ME, Ackley CJ, West RJ, et al. Expression of GATA-1 in a non-hematopoietic cell line induces beta-globin locus control region chromatin structure remodeling and an erythroid pattern of gene expression. J Mol Biol 2007; 366(3):737–44.

31. Asano H, Li XS, Stamatoyannopoulos G. FKLF-2: a novel Kruppel-like transcriptional factor that activates globin and other erythroid lineage genes. Blood 2000; 95:3578–84.

32. Zhou W, Clouston DR, Wang X, et al. Induction of human fetal globin gene expression by a novel erythroid factor, NF-E4. Mol Cell Biol 2000;20:7662–72.

33. Zhou W, Zhao Q, Sutton R, et al. The role of p22 NF-E4 in human globin gene switching. J Biol Chem 2004;279:26227–32.

34. Song SH, Hou C, Dean A. A positive role for NLI/Ldb1 in long-range beta-globin locus control region function. Mol Cell 2007;28:810–22.

35. Ley TJ, DeSimone J, Anagnou NP, et al. 5-azacytidine selectively increases gamma-globin synthesis in a patient with beta+ thalassemia. N Engl J Med 1982;307:1469–75.

36. Ley TJ, DeSimone J, Noguchi CT, et al. 5-Azacytidine increases gamma-globin synthesis and reduces the proportion of dense cells in patients with sickle cell anemia. Blood 1983;62:370–80.

37. Fucharoen S, Siritanaratkul N, Winichagoon P, et al. Hydroxyurea increases hemoglobin F levels and improves the effectiveness of erythropoiesis in beta-thalassemia/hemoglobin E disease. Blood 1996;87:887–92.

38. Charache S, Dover GJ, Moore RD, et al. Hydroxyurea: effects on hemoglobin F production in patients with sickle cell anemia. Blood 1992;79:2555–65.

39. Olivieri NF, Freedman MH, Perrine SP, et al. Trial of recombinant human erythropoietin: three patients with thalassemia intermedia. Blood 1992;80:3258–60.

40. Nagel RL, Vichinsky E, Shah M, et al. F reticulocyte response in sickle cell anemia treated with recombinant human erythropoietin: a double-blind study. Blood 1993;81:9–14.

41. Atweh GF, Sutton M, Nassif I, et al. Sustained induction of fetal hemoglobin by pulse butyrate therapy in sickle cell disease. Blood 1999;93:1790–7.

42. Perrine SP, Ginder GD, Faller DV, et al. A short-term trial of butyrate to stimulate fetal-globin-gene expression in the beta-globin disorders. N Engl J Med 1993; 328:81–6.

43. Mavilio F, Giampaolo A, Care A, et al. Molecular mechanisms of human hemoglobin switching: selective undermethylation and expression of globin genes in embryonic, fetal, and adult erythroblasts. Proc Natl Acad Sci U S A 1983; 80:6907–11.

44. van der Ploeg LH, Flavell RA. DNA methylation in the human gamma delta beta-globin locus in erythroid and nonerythroid tissues. Cell 1980;19:947–58.

45. Kaminskas E, Farrell AT, Wang YC, et al. FDA drug approval summary: azacitidine (5-azacytidine, Vidaza) for injectable suspension. Oncologist 2005;10: 176–82.

46. Silverman LR, Demakos EP, Peterson BL, et al. Randomized controlled trial of azacitidine in patients with the myelodysplastic syndrome: a study of the cancer and leukemia group B. J Clin Oncol 2002;20:2429–40.

47. DeSimone J, Heller P, Hall L, et al. 5-Azacytidine stimulates fetal hemoglobin synthesis in anemic baboons. Proc Natl Acad Sci U S A 1982;79:4428–31.

48. DeSimone J, Heller P, Schimenti JC, et al. Fetal hemoglobin production in adult baboons by 5-azacytidine or by phenylhydrazine-induced hemolysis is associated with hypomethylation of globin gene DNA. Prog Clin Biol Res 1983;134:489–500.

49. Charache S, Dover G, Smith K, et al. Treatment of sickle cell anemia with 5-aza-cytidine results in increased fetal hemoglobin production and is associated with nonrandom hypomethylation of DNA around the gamma-delta-beta-globin gene complex. Proc Natl Acad Sci U S A 1983;80:4842–6.

50. Lowrey CH, Nienhuis AW. Brief report: treatment with azacitidine of patients with end-stage beta-thalassemia. N Engl J Med 1993;329:845–8.

51. Carr BI, Rahbar S, Asmeron Y, et al. Carcinogenicity and haemoglobin synthesis induction by cytidine analogues. Br J Cancer 1988;57:395–402.

52. DeSimone J, Koshy M, Dorn L, et al. Maintenance of elevated fetal hemoglobin levels by decitabine during dose interval treatment of sickle cell anemia. Blood 2002;99:3905–8.

53. Koshy M, Dorn L, Bressler L, et al. 2-deoxy 5-azacytidine and fetal hemoglobin induction in sickle cell anemia. Blood 2000;96:2379–84.

54. Saunthararajah Y, Hillery CA, Lavelle D, et al. Effects of 5-aza-2'-deoxycytidine on fetal hemoglobin levels, red cell adhesion, and hematopoietic differentiation in patients with sickle cell disease. Blood 2003;102:3865–70.

55. Yang AS, Estecio MR, Garcia-Manero G, et al. Comment on "Chromosomal instability and tumors promoted by DNA hypomethylation" and "Induction of tumors in nice by genomic hypomethylation". Science 2003;302:1153 [author reply 1153].

56. Belinsky SA, Klinge DM, Stidley CA, et al. Inhibition of DNA methylation and histone deacetylation prevents murine lung cancer. Cancer Res 2003;63: 7089–93.

57. Laird PW, Jackson-Grusby L, Fazeli A, et al. Suppression of intestinal neoplasia by DNA hypomethylation. Cell 1995;81:197–205.

58. Humphries RK, Dover G, Young NS, et al. 5-Azacytidine acts directly on both erythroid precursors and progenitors to increase production of fetal hemo-globin. J Clin Invest 1985;75:547–57.

59. Jane SM, Gumucio DL, Ney PA, et al. Methylation-enhanced binding of Sp1 to the stage selector element of the human gamma-globin gene promoter may regulate development specificity of expression. Mol Cell Biol 1993;13:3272–81.

60. Sengupta PK, Lavelle D, DeSimone J. Increased binding of Sp1 to the gamma-globin gene promoter upon site-specific cytosine methylation. Am J Hematol 1994;46:169–72.

61. Lavelle DE. The molecular mechanism of fetal hemoglobin reactivation. Semin Hematol 2004;41:3–10.

62. Letvin NL, Linch DC, Beardsley GP, et al. Augmentation of fetal-hemoglobin production in anemic monkeys by hydroxyurea. N Engl J Med 1984;310:869–73.

63. Stamatoyannopoulos G. Control of globin gene expression during development and erythroid differentiation. Exp Hematol 2005;33:259–71.

64. Mabaera R, Greene MR, Richardson CA, et al. Neither DNA hypomethylation nor changes in the kinetics of erythroid differentiation explain 5-azacytidine's ability to induce human fetal hemoglobin. Blood 2008;111:411–20.

65. Fathallah H, Weinberg RS, Galperin Y, et al. Role of epigenetic modifications in normal globin gene regulation and butyrate-mediated induction of fetal hemo-globin. Blood 2007;110:3391–7.

66. Yin W, Barkess G, Fang X, et al. Histone acetylation at the human {beta}-globin locus changes with developmental age. Blood 2007;110(12):4101–7.
67. Cao H, Stamatoyannopoulos G, Jung M. Induction of human gamma globin gene expression by histone deacetylase inhibitors. Blood 2004;103:701–9.
68. Pace BS, Qian XH, Sangerman J, et al. p38 MAP kinase activation mediates gamma-globin gene induction in erythroid progenitors. Exp Hematol 2003;31: 1089–96.
69. Cao H. Pharmacological induction of fetal hemoglobin synthesis using histone deacetylase inhibitors. Hematology 2004;9:223–33.
70. Witt O, Monkemeyer S, Ronndahl G, et al. Induction of fetal hemoglobin expression by the histone deacetylase inhibitor apicidin. Blood 2003;101:2001–7.
71. Ginder GD, Whitters MJ, Pohlman JK. Activation of a chicken embryonic globin gene in adult erythroid cells by 5-azacytidine and sodium butyrate. Proc Natl Acad Sci U S A 1984;81:3954–8.
72. Bard H, Prosmanne J. Relative rates of fetal hemoglobin and adult hemoglobin synthesis in cord blood of infants of insulin-dependent diabetic mothers. Pediatrics 1985;75:1143–7.
73. Perrine SP, Greene MF, Faller DV. Delay in the fetal globin switch in infants of diabetic mothers. N Engl J Med 1985;312:334–8.
74. Constantoulakis P, Knitter G, Stamatoyannopoulos G. On the induction of fetal hemoglobin by butyrates: in vivo and in vitro studies with sodium butyrate and comparison of combination treatments with 5-AzaC and AraC. Blood 1989;74:1963–71.
75. Perrine SP, Rudolph A, Faller DV, et al. Butyrate infusions in the ovine fetus delay the biologic clock for globin gene switching. Proc Natl Acad Sci U S A 1988;85:8540–2.
76. Sher GD, Ginder GD, Little J, et al. Extended therapy with intravenous arginine butyrate in patients with beta-hemoglobinopathies. N Engl J Med 1995;332: 1606–10.
77. Perrine SP, Yang YM, Piga A, et al. Butyrate + EPO in beta thalassemia intermedia: interim findings of a phase II trial. Blood 2002;100:47a.
78. Collins AF, Pearson HA, Giardina P, et al. Oral sodium phenylbutyrate therapy in homozygous beta thalassemia: a clinical trial. Blood 1995;85:43–9.
79. Reich S, Buhrer C, Henze G, et al. Oral isobutyramide reduces transfusion requirements in some patients with homozygous beta-thalassemia. Blood 2000;96:3357–63.
80. Ikuta T, Kan YW, Swerdlow PS, et al. Alterations in protein-DNA interactions in the gamma-globin gene promoter in response to butyrate therapy. Blood 1998;92:2924–33.
81. Ikuta T, Ausenda S, Cappellini MD. Mechanism for fetal globin gene expression: role of the soluble guanylate cyclase-cGMP-dependent protein kinase pathway. Proc Natl Acad Sci U S A 2001;98:1847–52.
82. McElveen RL, Lou TF, Reese K, et al. Erk pathway inhibitor U0126 induces gamma-globin expression in erythroid cells. Cell Mol Biol (Noisy-le-grand) 2005;51:215–27.
83. Weinberg RS, Ji X, Sutton M, et al. Butyrate increases the efficiency of translation of gamma-globin mRNA. Blood 2005;105:1807–9.
84. Rodgers GP, Dover GJ, Noguchi CT, et al. Hematologic responses of patients with sickle cell disease to treatment with hydroxyurea. N Engl J Med 1990; 322:1037–45.
85. Platt OS, Orkin SH, Dover G, et al. Hydroxyurea enhances fetal hemoglobin production in sickle cell anemia. J Clin Invest 1984;74:652–6.

86. Steinberg MH, Lu ZH, Barton FB, et al. Fetal hemoglobin in sickle cell anemia: determinants of response to hydroxyurea. Multicenter Study of Hydroxyurea. Blood 1997;89:1078–88.

87. Charache S, Terrin ML, Moore RD, et al. Effect of hydroxyurea on the frequency of painful crises in sickle cell anemia. Investigators of the Multicenter Study of Hydroxyurea in Sickle Cell Anemia. N Engl J Med 1995;332:1317–22.

88. Rigano P, Manfre L, La Galla R, et al. Clinical and hematological response to hydroxyurea in a patient with Hb Lepore/beta-thalassemia. Hemoglobin 1997; 21:219–26.

89. Cario H, Wegener M, Debatin KM, et al. Treatment with hydroxyurea in thalassemia intermedia with paravertebral pseudotumors of extramedullary hematopoiesis. Ann Hematol 2002;81:478–82.

90. de Paula EV, Lima CS, Arruda VR, et al. Long-term hydroxyurea therapy in beta-thalassaemia patients. Eur J Haematol 2003;70:151–5.

91. Hajjar FM, Pearson HA. Pharmacologic treatment of thalassemia intermedia with hydroxyurea. J Pediatr 1994;125:490–2.

92. Zimmerman SA, Schultz WH, Davis JS, et al. Sustained long-term hematologic efficacy of hydroxyurea at maximum tolerated dose in children with sickle cell disease. Blood 2004;103:2039–45.

93. Cokic VP, Smith RD, Beleslin-Cokic BB, et al. Hydroxyurea induces fetal hemoglobin by the nitric oxide-dependent activation of soluble guanylyl cyclase. J Clin Invest 2003;111:231–9.

94. Conran N, Oresco-Santos C, Acosta HC, et al. Increased soluble guanylate cyclase activity in the red blood cells of sickle cell patients. Br J Haematol 2004;124:547–54.

95. Nahavandi M, Tavakkoli F, Wyche MQ, et al. Nitric oxide and cyclic GMP levels in sickle cell patients receiving hydroxyurea. Br J Haematol 2002;119:855–7.

96. Cokic VP, Andric SA, Stojilkovic SS, et al. Hydroxyurea nitrosylates and activates soluble guanylyl cyclase in human erythroid cells. Blood 2008;111:1117–23.

97. Keefer JR, Schneidereith TA, Mays A, et al. Role of cyclic nucleotides in fetal hemoglobin induction in cultured CD34+ cells. Exp Hematol 2006;34:1151–61.

98. Bailey L, Kuroyanagi Y, Franco-Penteado CF, et al. Expression of the gamma-globin gene is sustained by the cAMP-dependent pathway in beta-thalassaemia. Br J Haematol 2007;138:382–95.

99. Tang DC, Zhu J, Liu W, et al. The hydroxyurea-induced small GTP-binding protein SAR modulates gamma-globin gene expression in human erythroid cells. Blood 2005;106:3256–63.

100. Powars DR, Weiss JN, Chan LS, et al. Is there a threshold level of fetal hemoglobin that ameliorates morbidity in sickle cell anemia? Blood 1984;63:921–6.

Allogeneic Cellular Gene Therapy for Hemoglobinopathies

Javid Gaziev, MD*, Guido Lucarelli, MD

KEYWORDS

• Thalassemia • Sickle cell anemia • Stem cell transplantation
• Cellular gene therapy

β-Thalassemia and sickle cell anemia (SCA) are among the most widespread single gene disorders worldwide. Globally it is estimated that approximately 7% of the world's population are carriers of inherited hemoglobin disorders and that 300,000 to 400,000 babies with severe forms of these diseases are born each year. The β-thalassemias are caused by more than 200 different β-globin gene mutations that either reduce or abolish production of the β-globin chain, which lead to the development of ineffective erythropoiesis and hemolytic anemia.[1] The most severe form of disease is characterized by the complete absence of β-globin production and results from the inheritance of 2 β^0 thalassemia alleles, in the homozygous or compound heterozygous states. These combinations usually result in β-thalassemia major; the patients present within 6 months of life with severe anemia and if not treated with regular blood transfusions, die within the first 2 years. The current conventional treatment of β-thalassemia major consists of lifelong regular blood transfusions combined with iron chelation therapy. In developed countries, the optimization of transfusion support and iron chelation therapy have improved the survival of patients with thalassemia converting a previously fatal disease with early death into a chronic, although progressive disease compatible with prolonged survival, eventually for a few decades. Conversely, in less well developed countries where most of these patients reside, most children die before the age of 20 years because of the unavailability of safe blood products and/or expensive iron-chelating drugs. Despite the prolonged life expectancy, a recent study from the United Kingdom Thalassemia Registry showed a steady decline in survival starting from the second decade, with fewer than 50% of patients remaining alive beyond 35 years mainly because of poor compliance

The authors have nothing to disclose.
International Center for Transplantation in Thalassemia and Sickle Cell Anemia, Mediterranean Institute of Hematology, Policlinico Tor Vergata, Viale Oxford 81, Rome- 00133, Italy
* Corresponding author.
E-mail address: j.gaziev@fondazioneime.org

Hematol Oncol Clin N Am 24 (2010) 1145–1163
doi:10.1016/j.hoc.2010.08.004
0889-8588/10/$ – see front matter © 2010 Elsevier Inc. All rights reserved.

with chelation therapy.[2] Allogeneic hematopoietic stem cell transplantation (HSCT) is the only definitively curative therapeutic modality for the treatment of β-thalassemia major.[3,4] HSCT is a form of gene therapy that uses allogeneic stem cells as vectors for genes essential for normal hematopoiesis. Eventually the vector may well be autologous stem cells transformed by the insertion of normal genes, but there is no indication that this approach will be a widely available clinical option in the foreseeable future. It should be acknowledged that the risk of serious acute and chronic complications of transplantation can present a therapeutic dilemma in light of the observation that, in developed countries where patients with thalassemia receive up-to-date medical treatment, the use of regular blood transfusion and optimal chelation therapy results in a very good survival rate.[5,6] However, many such patients with increasing age currently experience poor outcomes with conventional treatment, even in countries with universal access to optimal medical treatment.[2,7]

Patients with SCA have an abnormal hemoglobin (hemoglobin S) that polymerizes under hypoxic conditions, causing increased viscosity, deformation, and membrane damage of the erythrocyte that results in vascular occlusion due to adhesion of sickle cells to each other and to vascular endothelium.[8] The natural history of SCA is characterized by severe chronic hemolytic anemia, acute painful crises, and shortened life-span.[9,10] Acute stroke, silent cerebral infarcts, acute chest syndrome, and avascular bone necrosis are among the most disabling complications occurring in SCA patients.[9,11] Several advances such as early penicillin prophylaxis, antipneumococcal vaccine, better blood transfusion practice, and treatment with hydroxyurea in the last 2 decades have contributed both to improved quality of life and to an increase in the life expectancy at least for those patients with access to treatment.[12,13] Although medical treatments are life-extending, end-organ damage cannot be avoided in most of these patients over time. In fact, a recent prospective longitudinal study over more than 4 decades of observation showed that by the fifth decade of age, nearly 50% of patients had documented irreversible damage of at least one organ.[14] The most common cause of death in children is pneumococcal sepsis, whereas adult patients usually succumb to stroke, multiorgan failure, or acute chest syndrome. At present, HSCT is the only recognized curative therapy for patients with SCA. However, there has been slow progress in the use of HSCT for SCA. Indeed, so far only approximately 250 SCA patients have received HSCT worldwide. The higher individual variability of disease severity, some advances of medical treatment, the lack of universally accepted criteria for transplantation, and the lack of a suitable HLA-identical donor are obstacles for expanding HSCT to many potential candidates.[15,16] Consequently, HSCT has been mainly offered to pediatric patients with a significant clinical complication such as stroke, recurrent vaso-occlusive events, or anemia requiring chronic blood transfusions. A recent survey among 30 adult patients with sickle cell disease (SCD) about their feelings toward receiving a reduced-intensity bone marrow transplant (BMT)[17] showed that 62% were willing to accept a 10% transplant-related mortality (TRM), one-third of patients were willing to accept a 30% TRM, and 62% accepted a 10% risk of graft failure. Fifty percent accepted infertility, but only 20% considered chronic graft-versus-host disease (GVHD) as an acceptable alternative. Overall, 60% of patients were willing to accept a clinical trial of reduced-intensity BMT. This survey reflects a high morbidity rate among patients with SCD and shows inadequacy of current conservative management strategies to control long-term disease complications. The survey further indicates that many patients with SCD are willing to accept even high toxicities for a potentially curative therapy.

HEMATOPOIETIC STEM CELL TRANSPLANTATION FOR THALASSEMIA
HSCT Transplantation Tailored to the Patient's Clinical Condition: Risk Class Approach

In 1988, the authors analyzed the influence of pretransplant characteristics on the outcome of transplantation in 116 consecutive patients aged 16 years or younger who were all treated with exactly the same conditioning regimen and GVHD prophylaxis, starting in June 1985.[18] In a multivariate analysis hepatomegaly and portal fibrosis were associated with a significantly reduced probability of survival, whereas a history of poor compliance with the chelation regimen could not be distinguished from hepatomegaly as a predictor of survival and event-free survival. The influence of pretransplant characteristics on the outcome of transplantation was reexamined in late 1989,[19] by which time 167 patients aged less than 17 years had been treated with the same regimen which, in addition to the previous revealed 2 risk factors, showed a strong statistically significant correlation between a history of iron chelation and survival. The quality of chelation was characterized as regular when desferoxamine therapy was initiated no later than 18 months after the first transfusion and administered subcutaneously for 8 to 10 hours continuously for at least 5 days each week, and any deviation from this regimen was considered as irregular. The degree of hepatomegaly (greater than or not greater than 3 cm), the presence or absence of portal fibrosis in the pretransplant liver biopsy, and the quality of chelation (regular or irregular) given through the years before transplant were identified as variables permitting the categorization of patients into 3 risk classes. Class 1 patients had none of these adverse risk factors, class 3 patients had all 3, and class 2 patients had 1 or 2 adverse risk factors. The results of these studies have allowed the authors to apply treatment protocols tailored to the patient's clinical condition related to the quality of previous conventional treatment.

The first 2 BMT from HLA-matched sibling donors were performed in Seattle, USA on December 3, 1981 and in Pesaro, Italy on December 17, 1981. The 14-month-old child transplanted in Seattle had received only 250 mL of packed red blood cells (RBCs) at the time of transplantation. The patient had successful engraftment and was cured of thalassemia.[3] The Pesaro approach was based on an assessment that restricting transplants to untransfused patients was impractical, and a 16-year-old thalassemic patient who had received 150 RBC transfusions was given a marrow graft from his HLA-matched brother. This patient rejected the graft and was the first of an extensive series of transplants for thalassemia performed to date.

EXPERIENCE OF THE FIRST 20 YEARS (1982–2002)
HSCT in Class 1 and Class 2 Patients

Between 1985 and 1992, 412 class 1 (n = 124) and class 2 (n = 297) patients were treated with busulfan (BU), 3.5 mg/kg/d for 4 consecutive days and cyclophosphamide (CY), 50 mg/kg/d for the subsequent 4 days. As GVHD prophylaxis they received cyclosporine (CSA) and low-dose methylprednisolone. The thalassemia-free survival rates in class 1 and class 2 patients treated during this time frame were 91% and 84%, respectively.[20] The results of transplantation in class 1 and class 2 patients have remained unchanged in subsequent years.

HSCT in Class 3 Patients

Before the risk class approach was adopted, class 3 younger patients (age <17 years) treated with the same preparatory regimen as class 1 and class 2 patients

(BU14/CY200) experienced a decreased rate of thalassemia-free survival (53%) and a higher probability of TRM (39%), mainly due to drug-related toxicity.[21] Therefore, the authors reduced the total dose of CY to 120 to 160 mg/kg in the conditioning regimen for class 3 patients to overcome the increased TRM. In fact, this modification improved the probability of overall survival in class 3 younger patients from 53% to 79%, but was associated with an increase in the probability of graft rejection from 7% to 30%, probably due to inadequate immunosuppression and failure to eradicate the massive erythroid hyperplasia characteristic of these patients.[20,21] The results obtained were not satisfactory and subsequent efforts were made to optimize the treatment protocol for class 3 patients. In April 1997 a new preparatory regimen (Protocol 26) was adopted for class 3 younger patients in an attempt to decrease the higher rejection rate through reducing erythroid expansion and increasing immunosuppression over time to avoid unacceptable peritransplant drug toxicity.[22] This novel treatment regimen involved an intensified preparation with 3 mg/kg of azathioprine and 30 mg/kg hydroxyurea daily from day -45 from the transplant, fludarabine (FLU) 20 mg/m^2 from day -17 through day -13, followed by the administration of BU 14 mg/kg total dose and CY 160 mg/kg total dose. GVHD prophylaxis consisted of CSA, low-dose methylprednisolone, and a modified "short course" of methotrexate (MTX). In addition, patients received hypertransfusion and intravenous chelation and growth factors (granulocyte colony-stimulating factor and erythropoietin) twice weekly to maintain stem cell proliferation in the face of hypertransfusion, thereby facilitating the effect of the hydroxyurea. Importantly this new treatment regimen improved thalassemia-free survival for class 3 patients younger than 17 years from 58% to 85% together with a reduction in the probability of rejection from 30% to 8% as compared with previous preparative regimens.

HSCT in Adult Patients

The authors consider as adult patients those who are 17 years or older. These patients have more advanced disease and treatment-related organ damage, mainly due to prolonged exposure to iron overload and/or hepatitis C. Consequently, most adult patients belong to the class 3 risk group. Since September 1996, 107 adult patients, with a median age of 20 years (range, 17–35 years), received transplants from HLA-identical siblings.[23,24] There were 18 class 2 patients treated with BU 14 mg/kg and CY 200 mg/kg, and 89 class 3 patients treated with BU 14 to 16 mg/kg and CY 120 to 160 mg/kg as preparatory regimen. An analysis of this cohort of patients showed the probability of survival, thalassemia-free survival, rejection, and nonrejection mortality to be 66%, 62%, 4%, and 37%, respectively. Of note, unlike class 3 younger patients, adult patients treated with the same conditioning regimens had a low graft rejection rate (4%), suggesting that donor-host tolerance might be induced even among extensively transfused patients. This was an unexpected observation indicating that adult patients could benefit from less intensive conditioning regimens with reduced transplant-related toxicity. Therefore, the authors subsequently reduced the total dose of cyclophosphamide to 90 mg/kg in the conditioning regimen for adults and decided to administer to them the preconditioning phase of the Protocol 26 preparatory regimen. A recent analysis of 15 high-risk adult patients treated with this regimen showed a probability of survival, thalassemia-free survival, rejection, and nonrejection mortality of 65%, 65%, 7%, and 28%, respectively.[25]

At present, BMT programs for thalassemia have been established in several countries worldwide, with results similar to those obtained in Pesaro.[26–35]

CURRENT EXPERIENCE OF HSCT FOR THALASSEMIA

In 2004, the authors of this article and 2 other transplant physicians moved from Pesaro to Rome where they started a new Transplant Program in the International Center for Transplantation in Thalassemia and Sickle Cell Anemia at the Mediterranean Institute of Hematology. Whereas the Pesaro experience was predominantly done on an Italian patient population, the Rome experience was characterized by 2 features: the patients were ethnically very heterogeneous, and the vast majority of these patients was not regularly transfused/chelated, or highly sensitized due to receiving RBC transfusions without the use of leukodepletion filters. Therefore, these patients were likely to have a higher risk of graft rejection as a result of sensitization to HLA antigens. Taking these characteristics into consideration, the authors modified the treatment protocols for transplantation of such patients (**Table 1**). As of September 2009, 20 class 1, 38 class 2 and 42 class 3 patients, younger than 17 years, received a first HSCT from an HLA-matched family donor at the authors' institution. **Figs. 1–3** show the probability of survival, thalassemia-free survival, rejection, and TRM for class 1, class 2, and class 3 patients, with a median follow-up of 35 months (range, 6–63 months) for surviving patients. The results of this new experience confirmed those obtained in Pesaro, and most importantly, showed the reproducibility of the Pesaro experience in other centers.

HSCT FROM ALTERNATIVE DONORS FOR THALASSEMIA
HSCT from Alternative Related Donors

One of the major obstacles to successful transplantation is the limited number of HLA-matched related donors within families. Approximately 70% of patients lack a suitable family donor. Some of these patients could benefit from HSCT from matched unrelated donors. However, the chance of finding of a matched unrelated donor is strongly dependent on the ethnic background of the patient. The curative potential of HSCT for thalassemia and the limited number of HLA-matched related donors have led to the use of stem cell transplantation from alternative donors in

Table 1
Current treatment protocols

	Preconditioning	Conditioning (mg/kg)	GVHD Prophylaxis
Thalassemia			
Class 1 & class 2 age >4 years	None	ivBu Cy 200	CSA/MP/short MTX
Class 1 & class 2 age ≤4 years	None	ivBu TT 10 Cy 200	CSA/MP/short MTX
Class 3 age <17 years	d −35 to −11 Az, Hu; d −16 to −11 Flu 150	ivBu TT 10 Cy 160	CSA/MP/short MTX
Adults (age ≥17 years) class 2–3	d −35 to −12 Az, Hu; d −16 to −12 Flu 150	ivBu TT 10 Cy 90	CSA/MP/short MTX
Sickle Cell Disease			
	None	ivBu Cy 200 ATG 10	CSA/MP/short MTX

Abbreviations: ATG, thymoglobulin; Az, azathioprine; Bu, busulfan; CSA, cyclosporine; Cy, cyclophosphamide; Flu, fludarabine; GVHD, graft-versus-host disease; Hu, hydroxyurea; iv, intravenous; MP, methylprednisolone; MTX, methotrexate; TT, thiotepa.

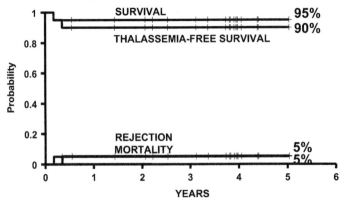

Fig. 1. Estimates of survival, thalassemia-free survival, transplant-related mortality, and rejection for 20 class 1 patients younger than 17 years.

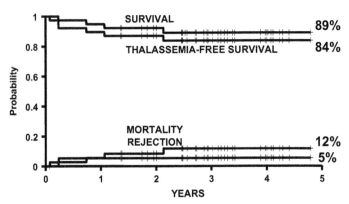

Fig. 2. Estimates of survival, thalassemia-free survival, transplant-related mortality, and rejection for 38 class 2 patients younger than 17 years.

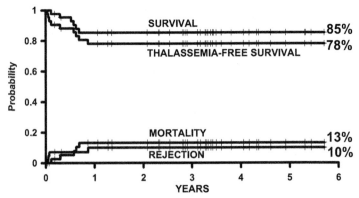

Fig. 3. Estimates of survival, thalassemia-free survival, transplant-related mortality, and rejection for 42 class 3 patients younger than 17 years.

thalassemia. The authors analyzed the results of HSCT in 29 patients with β-thalassemia major who received a marrow graft from HLA phenotypically matched relatives (n = 6), HLA-mismatched siblings (n = 13), parents (n = 8), or relatives (n = 2).[36] Fifteen out of 29 patients received one antigen-mismatched graft. The conditioning regimen consisted of BU/CY in combination with total body irradiation (TBI) or total lymphoid irradiation (TLI). Nine patients also received antilymphocyte globulin. There were high rates of graft failure and TRM (55% and 34%, respectively) and a low thalassemia-free survival rate (21%), showing that these preparative regimens were not adequately myeloablative and immunosuppressive to ensure a high sustained engraftment rate and consequently an adequate probability of disease-free survival.

HSCT from Haploidentical Family Donors

In 2002, the authors' group started a Haploidentical Transplant program for thalassemia. Patients who lacked an HLA-matched family or unrelated donor were eligible for this study. Between 2002 and 2008, 22 patients with transfusion-dependent thalassemia and median age of 7 years (range, 3–14 years) were given stem cell grafts from haploidentical mothers (n = 20) or brothers (n = 2). All of the patients received an intensified preparative regimen consisting of 3 mg/kg azathioprine and 60 mg/kg hydroxyurea daily from day −59 from the transplant, and fludarabine (FLU) 30 mg/m^2 from day −17 through day −13, aimed at reducing hyperplastic bone marrow and gradually increasing immunosuppression to avoid unacceptable peritransplant drug toxicity. During this time frame, the patients also received hypertransfusion to suppress endogenous erythropoiesis, and granulocyte colony-stimulating factor and erythropoietin to maintain stem cell proliferation, thus facilitating the effect of hydroxyurea. As conditioning regimen, they received BU14/thiotepa (TT)10/CY200 and antithymocyte globulin (ATG). All patients received cyclosporine for GVHD prophylaxis for the first 2 months after transplantation. As stem cell source, 8 patients received T-cell–depleted peripheral blood stem cells (PBSC) (CD34+ immunoselected) and CD3+/CD19+ immunodepleted bone marrow stem cells. The last 14 patients received CD34+ selected peripheral and bone marrow stem cells, using the CliniMACS procedure. Median infused cell doses were: CD34+ 15.2 × 10^6/kg, CD3+ 1.8 × 10^5/kg, and CD19+ 0.27 × 10^6/kg in the first 8 patients, and CD34+14.2 × 10^6/kg, CD3+ 2 × 10^5/kg, and CD19+ 0.19 × 10^6/kg in the last 14 patients. Overall, 6 patients rejected their grafts, 2 patients died of Epstein-Barr virus–related cerebral lymphoma or cytomegalovirus pneumonia, and 14 patients are alive and cured of thalassemia. The rates of survival, thalassemia-free survival, rejection, and nonrejection mortality were 90%, 61%, 29%, and 14% respectively.[37] In this pediatric patient population, immune reconstitution, especially CD4+ cell recovery, was delayed. These data showed the feasibility of haploidentical stem cell transplantation for patients with thalassemia and, therefore, this procedure should be considered for those younger patients who lack a suitable HLA-matched related or unrelated donor.

Cord Blood Transplantation from Related Donors

Cord blood as an alternative source of hematopoietic stem cells has successfully been used to treat hematological malignant and nonmalignant diseases.[38,39] The use of umbilical cord blood for transplantation in thalassemia is discussed in greater detail elsewhere in this issue, in the article by Kanathezhath and Walters. A recent study from the Eurocord cooperative group analyzed the outcome of 33 patients with class 1 or class 2 thalassemia, and 11 with SCD who received cord blood cells from a sibling.[40] The majority of patients received BU and CY and ATG, and the remaining patients had BU and FLU as conditioning regimen. In 17 patients TT was added to

BU/CY or BU/FLU. Seven (21%) out of 33 patients with thalassemia experienced graft failure. No patient died of transplant-related complications. A low percentage of patients experienced either acute (11%) or chronic (6%) GVHD, which is encouraging. The 2-year estimate of event-free survival was 79%. Although transplanted patients were in the low to intermediate risk classes, the incidence of graft rejection was high. An increased risk of graft failure after cord blood transplantation, compared with that in patients given BMTs, has previously been reported. The one log lower cell dose in cord blood grafts, which is a well known disadvantage, probably has a negative influence on sustained engraftment in recipients with nonmalignant diseases.

HSCT from HLA-Matched Unrelated Donors

At present, many patients who need an allogeneic HSCT and do not have a suitable family donor could benefit from HLA-matched unrelated donor transplantation. Results of HSCT from unrelated donors for the treatment of malignant diseases have improved steadily, mainly due to the introduction of high-resolution molecular techniques for histocompatibility testing and improvements in the management of posttransplant complications. In a recent study, the outcome of BMT from matched unrelated donors prospectively selected using high-resolution molecular typing for HLA class I and class II loci for 68 patients with thalassemia major who received BU/CY or BU/FLU and/or TT as conditioning regimen has been reported.[41] There were 14 class 1, 16 class 2, and 38 class 3 patients. Overall rates of survival, thalassemia-free survival, rejection, and TRM for entire cohort of patients were 79.3%, 65.8%, 14.4%, and 20.7%, respectively. The incidence of acute grade II to IV or grade III to IV GVHD was 40% and 17%, respectively. Ten of 56 evaluable patients (18%) developed chronic GVHD. Class 1 and class 2 patients had much better overall and disease-free survival (96.7% and 80%, respectively) than class 3 patients (65.5% and 54.5%, respectively). These investigators have also recently reported encouraging results in adult patients with thalassemia who received bone marrow from matched unrelated donors, with rates of survival, thalassemia-free survival, TRM, and rejection of 70%, 70%, 30%, and 4%, respectively.[42] Similar results were reported in another study from Asia that included 21 children who received transplants from a matched unrelated donor, as well as 28 patients who received transplants from matched related donors.[35] The 2-year thalassemia-free survival for patients who received transplants from matched unrelated donors was 71%, compared with 82% for patients who received transplants from matched related donors. Although a limited number of patients have been transplanted thus far, these data show that HSCT using HLA-matched unrelated donors, not only in younger but also in adult patients with well-selected donors, may offer success rates similar to those obtained with HLA-identical sibling donors. The main limitation of the experience with matched unrelated donors for HSCT in thalassemia is that, using stringent criteria of HLA matching, only about one-third of thalassemia patients who started the search found a suitable donor in a median time of 3 to 4 months. Using less stringent HLA matching criteria for donor selection, such as allowing 1 or 2 allele mismatches, could increase the donor pool, but the results of such transplants remain to be determined.

Cord Blood Transplantation from Unrelated Donors

Encouraging preliminary results of sibling cord blood transplantation for children with nonmalignant diseases including thalassemia and accumulating experience of successful application of unrelated mismatched cord blood in hematological malignancies and nonmalignant diseases[38,39] have led to the use of unrelated cord blood transplantation in patients with thalassemia. Recently, the outcome of unrelated cord blood transplantation for 45 patients with nonmalignant diseases, with a median age of 4.5 years (range, 0.1–16.2 years), has been reported.[43] Cord blood units were matched at 4 (or more) out of 6 HLA-A, HLA-B, and HLA-DRB1 loci. There were 32 transfusion-dependent thalassemia patients, 21 with class 1 characteristics and 9 with class 2 characteristics (2 patients were unclassified). The conditioning regimen for these patients consisted of intravenous busulfan, 14 mg/kg total dose and cyclophosphamide, 200 mg/kg total dose. Five patients (16%) had primary (n = 3) or secondary (n = 2) graft failure and all 5 had sustained engraftment following a second transplantation. The incidence of grade II to IV and grade III to IV acute GVHD was 76% and 42%, respectively. The overall incidence of chronic GVHD was 35%, with only 1 patient experiencing extensive disease. TRM at 2 years was 12%. The results of this study are encouraging, and the high rates of graft rejection and of grade III to IV acute GVHD observed in these patients could probably be reduced by using better matched (5/6 or 6/6) unrelated cord blood units.

Mixed Chimerism Following HSCT for Thalassemia

Mixed hematopoietic chimerism (MC) is an interesting phenomenon after HSCT for thalassemia. The authors' group has evaluated MC in 335 patients who received BMT from HLA-matched family donors for thalassemia. The incidence of MC at 2 months after transplant was 32.2%.[20] Of the 227 patients with complete donor chimerism, none rejected their grafts while 35 of 108 patients (32.4%) with MC lost the graft, indicating that MC is a risk factor for graft rejection in patients with thalassemia. The percentage of residual host hematopoietic cells (RHCs) determined at 2 months after transplant was predictive for graft rejection, with nearly all patients experiencing graft rejection when RHCs exceeded 25%, and only 13% of patients having graft rejection when RHCs were less than 10%.[44,45] The risk of rejection for patients who had RHCs between 10% and 25% was 41%.

Unlike hematological malignancies in which residual host cells are predictive of relapse, patients with thalassemia can have lifelong stable mixed chimerism without rejection following transplantation. Ten percent of patients receiving BMT for thalassemia following myeloablative conditioning became persistent mixed chimeras and became transfusion-independent, suggesting that a limited number of engrafted donor cells might be sufficient to provide significant improvement of disease phenotype in patients with thalassemia major once donor-host tolerance has been established.

TRANSPLANT-RELATED COMPLICATIONS
Graft Failure or Rejection

Patients with thalassemia have a substantial incidence of graft rejection after most myeloablative preparatory regimens, and this seems to be related to the stage of their disease at the time of transplantation. In fact, whereas the probability of graft rejection is low in class 1 patients (3%), it occurred in 8% to 38.5% of class 3 younger patients.[22,46] Patients with engraftment failure and without functioning marrow have a bleak prognosis because an early second transplant with a second course of conditioning is usually not a reasonable option. Patients who reject their grafts and have a return of host hematopoiesis do not have an urgent need for second transplants, and such interventions can be delayed until the toxic effects of the conditioning regimen for the first transplant have subsided. At least 1 year should be allowed to pass between the first and second transplant. The historical experience of the authors with second transplants showed a low thalassemia-free survival rate and high rate of graft rejection.[47,48] In 2003, they devised a new treatment protocol for second transplants in patients with thalassemia aimed at reducing the high graft rejection rate and increasing disease-free survival. Sixteen patients with thalassemia recurrence following rejection of the first graft, with a median age of 9 years (range, 4–20 years), were given second transplants using bone marrow or PBSC.[49] All but 2 patients received stem cells from the same donor. The sustained engraftment rate was high (94%), with only 1 patient having graft failure. The rates of survival, thalassemia-free survival, graft failure, and TRM were 79%, 79%, 6%, and 16%, respectively. This treatment protocol for second transplants from the same donor in patients with recurrence of thalassemia major following a first transplant is highly effective in terms of sustained engraftment and event-free survival.

Graft-Versus-Host Disease

GVHD is the principal cause of morbidity and mortality after allogeneic HSCT. The incidence of grade II to IV acute GVHD was significantly lower (17%) in patients given cyclosporine (CSA) and a short course of MTX as compared with patients receiving CSA and methylprednisolone (32%) as GVHD prophylaxis.[50] Cumulative incidence of moderate or severe chronic GVHD was 8% and 2%, respectively. A recent study[51] showed that class 1 and class 2 thalassemia patients given PBSC had significantly higher incidence of grade II to IV (75%) and grade III to IV (36%) acute GVHD than patients receiving BMT (57% and 22%, respectively). All patients received CSA/MTX as GVHD prophylaxis. The incidence of chronic GVHD was also significantly higher in the PBSC group (49%) than in the BMT group (17%). Taken together, these data indicate that the use of PBSC as stem cell source may not be the preferred choice in patients with thalassemia.

Management of the Ex-Thalassemics

Patients with thalassemia treated successfully with HSCT have been called "ex-thalassemic." Ex-thalassemics still carry the clinical complications acquired during years of transfusion and chelation therapy. Iron overload, chronic hepatitis, liver fibrosis, and endocrine dysfunction are among the issues requiring long-term management in ex-thalassemics. The authors have shown that iron stores in class 2 and class 3 patients remain elevated even 7 years after transplantation.[52] Natural history of liver fibrosis following BMT for thalassemia showed that ion overload and hepatitis C virus (HCV) infection are independent risk factors for progression of liver fibrosis, and their concomitant presence results in a striking increase in risk for this complication.[53] Therefore, the toxic effect of iron overload contributing to progression of already present organ damage should be avoided as soon as possible using posttransplant iron depletion. Either regular phlebotomy or chelation therapy can successfully remove excess iron from the body by normalizing the iron pool.[54,55]

Growth failure and endocrine dysfunction are common and well-known complications occurring in thalassemia patients treated by conventional treatment. Children receiving HSCT before 8 years of age showed a normal growth rate, whereas older children, class 3 patients, and patients who developed chronic GVHD had impaired growth.[56] Gonadal damage is a common side effect of BU/CY conditioning. Indeed, approximately one-third of boys and two-thirds of girls failed to spontaneously enter puberty following HSCT.[57] Nevertheless, some patients can achieve fertility after transplant, as evidenced by the authors' observations of 5 successful pregnancies and 4 paternities in ex-thalassemics, a finding that indicates patients exposed to BU/CY conditioning regimens are not inevitably infertile.

Infection with HCV is common in thalassemic patients, particularly in those transfused before second-generation enzyme-linked immunosorbent assay tests became available for detecting HCV in donated blood. Liver damage due to HCV infection is exacerbated by iron overload, and liver disease is a recognized cause of mortality and morbidity. Thus, avoidance of progression of liver damage to cirrhosis must be a primary goal. Therefore ex-thalassemics should be offered current treatment with peginterferon α-2b/ribavirin after they have completed their iron depletion program.

Another important issue in ex-thalassemics is lifelong monitoring for posttransplant malignancies, although their incidence in this patient population is low (0.8%). In their ex-thalassemics, the authors have observed 4 cases of non-Hodgkin's lymphomas (3 early and 1 late occurring), and 5 cases of solid tumors.

HEMATOPOIETIC STEM CELL TRANSPLANTATION FOR SICKLE CELL ANEMIA

The first successful HSCT for SCA was performed in 1984 in an 8-year-old girl who suffered from both acute myeloid leukemia and SCA, and resulted in the cure of the SCD.[58] Since then, there has been slow progress in stem cell transplantation for SCA, with only approximately 250 transplants performed to date worldwide. One of the major reasons of this very conservative approach to transplantation for SCA is the absence of universally accepted indications for transplantation. In addition, high individual variability of disease severity and a limited number of HLA-identical donors have had a negative impact on decision making by both patients and treating physicians. Consequently, transplantation has been offered primarily to younger patients with overt symptomatology from the disease. Current selection criteria for transplantation in patients with SCD include that patients should be younger than 16 years, have an HLA-identical related donor, and have at least one of the following signs or symptoms: stroke or a central nervous system event lasting longer than 24 hours, acute chest syndrome, recurrent severe painful episodes, impaired neuropsychological function and abnormal cerebral magnetic resonance imaging scan (without severe residual functional neurologic impairment), stage I or II sickle lung disease, sickle nephropathy, bilateral proliferative retinopathy, osteonecrosis of multiple joints, or red blood cell alloimmunization during the course of long-term transfusion therapy.[59] Despite the characteristics of this patient population with preexisting organ damage, the results of HSCT after myeloablative conditioning in children have been very encouraging, with disease-free survival in most studies of approximately 85% and TRM rate of less than 10% (**Table 2**). The results of transplantation might be even better if HSCT were performed in children prior to the development of irreversible sickle vasculopathy-related complications. In fact, the overall survival (OS) and disease-free survival (DFS) rates in 14 asymptomatic children transplanted at a young age were 100% and 93%, respectively.[61] These data and recent advances in transplantation strategies require revision of inclusion criteria to offer transplantation to potential candidates.

Mixed Chimerism Following Myeloablative HSCT for SCA

The development of stable mixed donor-host chimerism in patients with nonmalignant diseases has curative potential. The principal risk of mixed chimerism in these patients is graft rejection usually occurring within the first year after transplantation, as has been well documented in patients with thalassemia.[20] However, a subgroup of patients developed lifelong stable mixed chimerism once donor-host tolerance was

Table 2
Worldwide experience of myeloablative HSCT for sickle cell disease

Reference	No. of Patients (Hb genotypes)	Median Age, Years	Donor Source	Conditioning	OS, n (%)	DFS, n (%)	Rejection, n (%)	Deaths, n (%)	aGVHD, n (%)	cGVHD, n (%)
Giardini et al[60]	18 (5 HbSS, 4 HbSβ0, 9 HbS β+)	7 (4–38)	Sib/BM	BuCy (17) BuCyALG (1)	4 (78)	13 (72)	1 (6)	4 (22)	3 (17.6)	1 (5.8)
Vermylen et al[61]	50 (HbSS)	7.5 (0.9–23)	Sib/BM (48) Sib/cord (2)	Bu/Cy ± TLI or ATG	46 (93)	42 (85)	5 (10)	2 (4)	20 (40)	10 (20)
Walters et al[59,62]	50 (48 HbSS, 1 HbS β+; 1 HbS/O)	9.9 (3.3–15.9)	Sib/BM	BuCy ± ATG (horst or rabbit) or CAMPATH	47 (94)	42 (84)	5 (10)	3 (6)	NA	NA
Bernaudin[63]	87 (85 HbSS, 2 HbSβ0)	8.8 (2.2–22)	Sib/BM (74) Sib/cord (12) Sib/PBSC (1)	BuCy (12) BuCy/rabbit ATG (75)	80 (92)	74 (86)	7 (5)	6 (7)	17 (20)	11 (12.6)
Majumdar et al[64]	10 (8 HbSS; 2 HbSβ0)	9 (2.8–16.3)	Sib/BM	BuCyATG	9 (90)	7 (77)	1 (10)	1 (10)	4 (40)	5 (5)
Panepinto et al[65] CIBMTR study	67 (59 HbSS; 1 HbSβ+; 7 other)	10 (2–27)	Sib/BM (54) Sib/PBSC (9) Cord blood (4)	BuCy (63) Others (4)	64 (97)	55 (85)	9 (13)	3 (4.4)	10 (4–19)	22 (13–34)
McPherson et al[66]	25 (HbSS)	8.6 (3.3–17.4)	Sib/BM	BuCyATG	96	96	0	1 (4)	4 (16)	NA

Abbreviations: aGVHD, acute graft-versus-host disease; ALG, antilymphocyte disease; ATG, antithymocyte globulin; BM, bone marrow; Bu, busulfan; CAMPATH, anti-CD52 antibodies; cGVHD, chronic graft-versus-host disease; Cy, cyclophosphamide; DFS, disease-free survival; NA, not available; OS, overall survival; PBSC, peripheral blood stem cells; Sib, sibling; TLI, total lymphoid irradiation.

established.[44,45] Walters and colleagues[67] have observed stable mixed chimerism in 13 of 50 patients (26%) who survived free of SCD, for a median duration of 6.9 years (range, 4.2–13 years). Of note, among these patients 5 had mixed donor chimerism of less than 75% (range, 11%–74%) and none of them developed sickle cell–related complications during a follow-up period that ranged from 22 to 70.2 months (median, 36.3 months). There was no apparent association between the development of mixed chimerism and graft rejection in this series. Wu and colleagues[68] reported on 9 patients with mixed chimerism after BMT for SCD who showed improvement, following transplantation, in markers of intravascular hemolysis, as well as markers of vascular function (eg, plasma nitric oxide and soluble vascular adhesion molecule-1 levels). These data demonstrate that mixed chimerism, if maintained, can result in clinical improvement in patients with SCD.

Reduced-Intensity HSCT for SCD

Reduced-intensity conditioning regimens were initially developed for patients not eligible for allogeneic stem cell transplantation following high-dose myeloablative therapy. In a recent study, 7 patients (18 years or younger) with high-risk SCD were given a bone marrow graft from an HLA-matched sibling donor.[69] Conditioning regimen consisted of BU 6.4 mg/kg (intravenous) or 8 mg/kg (orally) total dose, FLU 175 mg/m^2 total dose, equine ATG 130 mg/kg total dose, and TLI 500 cGy. Regimen-related toxicity was minimal. All but one patient had sustained engraftment. None of the patients developed greater than grade 2 acute GVHD or extensive chronic GVHD. Five out of 7 patients developed mixed chimerism. At a follow-up of 2 to 8.5 years after HSCT, all patients were alive and 6 of the 7 patients had no laboratory or clinical evidence of disease. These data are encouraging in terms of sustained engraftment with minimal toxicity. However, it should be acknowledged that unlike adult patients, children with thalassemia and SCD tolerate myeloablative regimens without significant toxicities. Furthermore, unfavorable outcomes of adults with SCD given a reduced-intensity conditioning regimen have been reported.[70]

Nonmyeloablative Stem Cell Transplantation for SCD

In 2 recent studies, the feasibility of nonmyeloablative conditioning regimen including low-dose TBI (ie, 200 cGy), FLU, and/or ATG for patients with SCD (n = 9), or β-thalassemia has been investigated.[71,72] The patients' ages varied between 3 and 30 years. Nine patients received bone marrow and 2 patients PBSC from HLA-matched donors. Ten of 11 patients showed donor chimerism from 25% to 100%. However, all but 1 patient lost their grafts after discontinuation of immunosuppression. There was one death following a second transplant. These results indicated that, using nonmyeloablative regimens, sustained donor engraftment is more difficult to achieve in patients with hemoglobinopathies, at least with these conditioning regimens. More recently, however, a successful novel nonmyeloablative conditioning regimen in adults with SCD has been reported.[73] Ten adults with a median age of 26 years (range, 16–45 years) and severe SCD underwent nonmyeloablative transplantation with PBSC from HLA-matched siblings. The conditioning regimen included alemtuzumab, 1 mg/kg total dose on day −7 to −3 and TBI of 300 cGy on day −2. As GVHD prophylaxis, recipients received sirolimus initiated on day −1 at a dose of 5 mg every 4 h for 3 doses then 5 mg daily. Patients received 5.51–23.8 × 10^6 CD34+ cells/kg. Nine of 10 patients had sustained engraftment and 1 had rejection. No patient died. None of the patients had full donor chimerism in both lymphoid and myeloid lines. Acute or chronic GVHD did not develop in any patient. Severe arthralgia and pneumonia attributed to the administration of sirolimus were important adverse events observed in these patients. Of note, patients with a history of cerebrovascular events before transplantation did not experience such events after transplantation. One patient became pregnant 30 months after transplantation and delivered a healthy baby. The investigators proposed that the success of transplantation was due to the conditioning regimen using TBI of 300 cGy creating enough marrow space for engraftment of donor cells, alemtuzumab helping to prevent graft rejection, and sirolimus promoting the differentiation of regulatory T cells and T-helper cells that play key roles in minimizing the risk of GVHD. The results of this study are very encouraging, and enable physicians to offer HSCT to adult SCD patients who until recently were excluded from allogeneic stem cell transplantation.

Related or Unrelated Cord Blood Transplantation for SCD

In a Eurocord study, 11 patients with SCD underwent related donor cord blood transplantation following a BU/CY/ATG conditioning regimen.[40] Nine of the donor cord blood units were fully HLA-matched but 2 were mismatched at high resolution for the HLA-A locus. All but one patient had sustained engraftment, with a 2-year OS and DFS of 100% and 90%, respectively.

A recent publication reviewed the experience from 4 United States centers on unrelated cord blood transplantation for 7 children (aged 3.4–16.8 years) with SCD, who received 1 or 2 antigen-mismatched cord blood.[74] Four patients received a myeloablative conditioning with BU/CY ± FLU and ATG, and the remaining 3 patients received a reduced-intensity regimen with FLU, ATG, TLI, and either BU (8 mg/kg) or CY. Four children experienced graft failure with autologous reconstitution. Three patients had donor engraftment, 1 died of multiorgan failure, and 2 are alive free of disease. One patient with a primary graft failure after reduced-intensity regimen received a second unrelated cord blood transplant, and is alive and cured from SCD. These results indicate that although the outcome of cord blood transplantation for SCD from related HLA-matched donors is similar to that obtained with BMT, unrelated mismatched cord blood transplantation for SCD resulted in a substantial risk of morbidity and mortality.

Long-Term Results of Myeloablative BMT for SCD

A recent study evaluated pulmonary, gonadal, and central nervous system (CNS) status following an HLA-matched sibling bone marrow transplantation in 55 long-term survivors.[75] This study showed that patients with a prior stroke who had stable engraftment of donor cells experienced no subsequent strokes after BMT, and brain magnetic resonance imaging demonstrated stable or improved appearance. Pulmonary function in most patients remained unchanged or improved. Evaluation of gonadal function showed hypogonadotrophic hypogonadism in most males and primary ovarian failure in most females after BMT. However, one female had a successful pregnancy 13 years after BMT, and another female who rejected her graft gave birth to a healthy baby following preimplantation genetic diagnosis 14 years after BMT. The study concluded that patients who had stable donor engraftment did not experience sickle-related complications after BMT, and were protected from progressive CNS and pulmonary disease. Bernaudin and colleagues[76] reported that only 5 of 17 girls had spontaneous puberty, while 12 needed hormonal treatment for puberty induction after BMT for SCD. Of importance is that the girls who had spontaneous puberty were younger at the time of transplantation than the girls who required hormonal treatment, indicating that ovarian function could be preserved in most patients if HSCT is performed at a much younger age before pubertal development.

SUMMARY

Allogeneic HSCT still remains the only definitively curative option for patients with thalassemia and SCD. A transplant approach in thalassemia based on risk classes resulted in defining the best treatment protocol for class 1 and class 2 patients, with a high DFS rate. This approach also allowed determination of the best treatment protocol for class 3 patients, leading to success rates in these patients similar to those obtained in class 1 and class 2 patients. Results of HSCT in thalassemia using matched unrelated donors, especially in class 1 and class 2 patients, are similar to those obtained with sibling donors. Advances in transplantation biology have made it possible to perform haploidentical stem cell transplantation in patients with thalassemia who lack a related or unrelated HLA-matched donor, with very encouraging results. Children with SCD receiving HSCT following current myeloablative conditioning protocols achieve a high cure rate. The recently developed novel nonmyeloablative transplantation protocol for SCD patients could serve as a platform for its wide application not only in adults but also in high-risk pediatric patients with SCD.

REFERENCES

1. Weatheral DJ, Clegg JB. The thalassemia syndromes. 4th edition. Oxford (UK): Blackwell Science; 2001.
2. Modell B, Khan M, Darlison M. Survival in beta-thalassemia major in the UK: data from the UK Thalassemia Register. Lancet 2000;355:2051–2.
3. Thomas ED, Buckner CD, Sanders JE, et al. Marrow transplantation for thalassaemia. Lancet 1982;ii:227–9.
4. Lucarelli G, Galimberti M, Polchi P, et al. Marrow transplantation in patients with advanced thalassemia. N Engl J Med 1987;316:1050–5.
5. Borgna- Pignatti C, Rugolotto S, DeStefano P, et al. Survival and complications in patients with thalassemia major treated with transfusions and desferrioxamine. Haematologica 2004;89:1187–93.
6. Pennell DJ, Berdoukas V, Karagiorga M, et al. Randomized controlled trial of deferiprone or desferoxamine in beta-thalassemia major patients with asymptomatic myocardial siderosis. Blood 2006;107:3738–44.
7. Cunningham MJ, Macklin EA, Neueld EJ, et al. Thalassemia Clinical Research Network. Complications of beta-thalassemia major in North America. Blood 2002;99:36–43.
8. Gavins F, Yilmaz G, Granger DN. The evolving paradigm for blood cell-endothelial cell interactions in the cerebral microcirculation. Microcirculation 2007;14:667–81.
9. Platt OS, Brambilla DJ, Rosse WF, et al. Mortality in sickle cell disease. Life expectancy and risk factors for early death. N Engl J Med 1994;330:1639–44.
10. Wierenga KJJ, Hambleton IR, Lewis NA. Survival estimates for patients with homozygous sickle-cell disease in Jamaica: a clinic-based population study. Lancet 2001;357:680–3.
11. Verduzco LA, Nathan DG. Sickle cell disease and stroke. Review article. Blood 2010;114:5117–25.
12. Vichinsky E. New therapies in sickle cell disease. Lancet 2002;360:629–31.
13. Zimmerman SA, Schultz WH, Davis JS, et al. Sustained long-term hematological efficacy of hydroxyurea at maximum tolerated dose in children with sickle cell disease. Blood 2004;103:2039–45.
14. Powars DR, Chan LS, Hiti A, et al. Outcome of sickle cell anemia. A 4-decade observational study of 1056 patients. Medicine 2005;84:363–76.

15. Walters MC, Patience M, Leisenring W, et al. Barriers to bone marrow transplantation for sickle cell anemia. Biol Blood Marrow Transplant 1996;2:100–4.
16. Sullivan KM, Parkman R, Walters MC. Bone marrow transplantation for non-malignant disease. Hematology Am Soc Hematol Educ Program 2000;319–38.
17. Chakrabarti S, Bareford D. A survey on patient perception of reduced-intensity transplantation in adults with sickle cell disease. Bone Marrow Transplant 2007; 39:447–51.
18. Lucarelli G, Galimberti M, Polchi P, et al. Bone marrow transplantation in patients with thalassemia. N Engl J Med 1990;322:417–21.
19. Lucarelli G, Galimberti M, Polchi P, et al. Bone marrow transplantation in thalassemia. Hematol Oncol Clin North Am 1991;5(3):549–56.
20. Lucarelli G, Andreani M, Angelucci E. The cure of thalassemia by bone marrow transplantation. Blood Rev 2002;16:81–5.
21. Lucarelli G, Clift R, Galimberti M, et al. Marrow transplantation for patients with thalassemia: results in Class 3 patients. Blood 1996;87:2082–8.
22. Sodani P, Gaziev J, Polchi P, et al. New approach for bone marrow transplantation in patients with class 3 thalassemia aged younger than 17 years. Blood 2004;104: 1201–3.
23. Lucarelli G, Galimberti M, Polchi P, et al. Bone marrow transplantation in adult thalassemia. Blood 1992;80:1603–7.
24. Lucarelli G, Clift RA, Galimberti M, et al. Bone marrow transplantation in adult thalassemic patients. Blood 1999;93:1164–7.
25. Gaziev J, Sodani P, Polchi P, et al. Bone marrow transplantation in adults with thalassemia. Treatment and long-term follow-up. Ann N Y Acad Sci 2005;1054: 196–205.
26. Di Bartolomeo P, Santarone S, Di Bartolomeo P, et al. Long-term of survival in patients with Thalassemia major treated with bone marrow transplantation. Am J Hematol 2008;83(7):528–30.
27. Argiolu F, Sanna MA, Cossu F, et al. Bone marrow transplant in thalassemia. The experience of Cagliari. Bone Marrow Transplant 1997;19(Suppl 2):65–7.
28. Clift RA, Johnson FL. Marrow transplants for thalassemia. The USA experience. Bone Marrow Transplant 1997;19(Suppl 2):57–9.
29. Lawson SE, Roberts IAG, Amrolia P, et al. Bone marrow transplantation for β-thalassemia major: the UK experience in two paediatric centers. Br J Haematol 2003; 120:289–95.
30. Ghavamzadeh A, Bahar B, Djahani M, et al. Bone marrow transplantation of thalassemia, the experience in Tehran (Iran). Bone Marrow Transplant 1997;19(Suppl 2): 71–3.
31. Dennison D, Srivastava A, Chandy M. Bone marrow transplantation for thalassaemia in India. Bone Marrow Transplant 1997;19(Suppl 2):70.
32. Lin HP, Chan LL, Lam SK, et al. Bone marrow transplantation for thalassemia. The experience from Malaysia. Bone Marrow Transplant 1997;19(Suppl 2):74–7.
33. Li CK, Shing MK, Chik KW, et al. Haematopoietic stem cell transplantation for thalassaemia major in Hong Kong: prognostic factors and outcome. Bone Marrow Transplant 2002;29:101–5.
34. Issaragrisil S, Suvatte V, Visuthisakchai S, et al. Bone marrow and cord blood stem cell transplantation for thalassemia in Thailand. Bone Marrow Transplant 1997;19(Suppl 2):54–6.
35. Hongeng S, Pakakasama S, Chuansumrit A, et al. Outcomes of transplantation with related and unrelated-donor stem cells in children with severe thalassemia. Biol Blood Marrow Transplant 2006;12:683–7.

36. Gaziev D, Galimberti M, Lucarelli G, et al. Bone marrow transplantation from alternative donors for thalassemia: HLA-phenotypically identical relative and HLA nonidentical sibling or parent transplants. Bone Marrow Transplant 2000;25(8):815–21.
37. Sodani P, Isgro A, Gaziev J, et al. Purified T-depleted, CD34+ peripheral blood and bone marrow cell transplantation from haploidentical mother to child with Thalassemia. Blood 2010;115:1296–302.
38. Glukman E, Rocha E, Boyer-Chammard A, et al. Outcome of cord-blood transplantation from related and unrelated donors. Eurocord Transplant Group and the European Blood and Marrow Transplantation Group. N Engl J Med 1997; 337:373–81.
39. Rocha V, Cornish J, Sievers EL, et al. Comparison of outcomes of unrelated bone marrow and umbilical cord blood transplants in children with acute leukemia. Blood 2001;97:2962–71.
40. Locatelli F, Rocha V, Reed W, et al. Related umbilical cord blood transplantation in patients with thalassemia and sickle cell disease. Blood 2003;101:2137–43.
41. La Nasa G, Argiolu F, Giardini C, et al. Unrelated bone marrow transplantation for beta-thalassemia patients: the experience of the Italian Bone Marrow Transplant Group. Ann N Y Acad Sci 2005;1054:186–95.
42. La Nasa G, Caocci G, Argiolu F, et al. Unrelated donor stem cell transplantation in adult patients with thalassemia. Bone Marrow Transplant 2005;36:971–5.
43. Jaing T-H, Chen SH-H, Tsai MH, et al. Transplantation of unrelated donor umbilical cord blood for nonmalignant diseases: a single institution's experience with 45 patients. Biol Blood Marrow Transplant 2010;16:102–7.
44. Andreani M, Manna M, Lucarelli G, et al. Persistence of mixed chimerism in patients transplanted for the treatment of thalassemia. Blood 1996;87:3494–9.
45. Andreani M, Nesci S, Lucarelli G, et al. Long-term survival of ex-thalassemic patients with persistent mixed chimerism after marrow transplantation. Bone Marrow Transplant 2000;25:401–4.
46. Chandy M, Mathews V, George B, et al. Reduced intensity conditioning with fludarabine, busulfan and cyclophosphamide for high risk patients with thalassemia major undergoing allogeneic bone marrow transplantation results in high rejection rates. Blood 2007;110:594a.
47. Gaziev D, Polchi P, Lucarelli G, et al. Second marrow transplants for graft failure in patients with thalassemia. Bone Marrow Transplant 1999;24:1299–306.
48. Gaziev J, Giardini C, Polchi P, et al. New approaches to the second transplant for thalassemia. Bone Marrow Transplant 2004;33(Suppl 1):S153.
49. Gaziev J, Sodani P, Lucarelli G, et al. Second stem cell transplantation for Thalassemia recurrence following graft rejection of the first graft. Bone Marrow Transplant 2008;42:397–404.
50. Gaziev D, Polchi P, Galimberti M, et al. Graft-versus-host disease after bone marrow transplantation for thalassemia: an analysis of incidence and risk factors. Transplantation 1997;63:854–60.
51. Ghavamzadeh A, Iravani M, Ashouri A, et al. Peripheral blood versus bone marrow as a source of hematopoietic stem cells for allogeneic transplantation in children with class I and II beta thalassemia. Biol Blood Marrow Transplant 2008;14:301–8.
52. Lucarelli G, Angelucci E, Giardini C, et al. Fate of iron stores in thalassemia after bone marrow transplantation. Lancet 1993;342:1388–91.
53. Angelucci E, Muretto P, Nicolucci A, et al. Effects of iron overload and hepatitis C virus positivity in determining progression of liver fibrosis in thalassemia following bone marrow transplantation. Blood 2002;100:17–21.

54. Angelucci E, Muretto P, Lucarelli G, et al. Phlebotomy to reduce iron overload in patients cured of thalassemia by bone marrow transplantation. Italian Cooperative Group for Phlebotomy Treatment of Transplanted Thalassemia Patients. Blood 2002;90(3):994–8.

55. Giardini C, Galimberti M, Lucarelli G, et al. Desferrioxamine therapy accelerates clearance of iron deposits after bone marrow transplantation for thalassemia. Br J Haematol 1995;89:868–73.

56. Gaziev D, Galimberti M, Giardini C, et al. Growth in children after bone marrow transplantation for thalassemia. Bone Marrow Transplant 1993;12(Suppl 1): 100–1.

57. De Sanctis V, Galimberti M, Lucarelli G, et al. Growth and development in ex-thalassemic patients. Bone Marrow Transplant 1997;19(Suppl 2):126–7.

58. Johnson FL, Look AT, Gockerman J, et al. Bone marrow transplantation in a patient with sickle-cell anemia. N Engl J Med 1984;311(12):780–3.

59. Walters MC, Patience M, Leisenring W, et al. Bone marrow transplantation for sickle cell disease. N Engl J Med 1996;335(6):369–76.

60. Giardini C, Galimberti M, Lucarelli G, et al. Bone marrow transplantation in sickle cell disorders in Pesaro. Bone Marrow Transplant 1997;19(Suppl 2):106–9.

61. Vermylen C, Cornu G, Frester A, et al. Haematopoietic stem cell transplantation for sickle cell anaemia: the first 50 patients transplanted in Belgium. Bone Marrow Transplant 1998;22:1–6.

62. Walters MC, Storb R, Patience M, et al. Impact of bone marrow transplantation for symptomatic sickle cell disease: an interim report. Blood 1999;95(6):1918–24.

63. Bernaudin F, Socie G, Kuentz M, et al. Long-term results of related myeloablative stem-cell transplantation to cure sickle cell disease. Blood 2007;110(7):2749–56.

64. Majumdar S, Robertson Z, Robinson A, et al. Outcome of hematopoietic cell transplantation in children with sickle cell disease, a single center's experience. Bone Marrow Transplant 2009;45:1–6.

65. Panepinto JA, Walters MC, Carreras J, et al. Matched-related donor transplantation for sickle cell disease: report from the Center for International blood and transplant research. Br J Haematol 2007;137:479–85.

66. McPherson ME, Hutcherson D, Olson E, et al. Safety and efficacy of targeted busulfan therapy in children undergoing myeloablative matched sibling donor BMT for sickle cell disease. Bone Marrow Transplant 2010. DOI:10.1038/bmt 2010.60.

67. Walters MC, Patience M, Leisenring W, et al. Stable mixed hematopoietic chimerism after bone marrow transplantation for sickle cell anemia. Biol Blood Marrow Transplant 2001;7:665–73.

68. Wu CJ, Gladwin M, Tisdale J, et al. Mixed hematopoietic chimerism for sickle cell disease prevents intravascular haemolysis. Br J Haematol 2007;139:504–7.

69. Krishnamurti L, Kharbanda S, Biernacki M, et al. Stable long-term donor engraftment following reduced-intensity hematopoietic cell transplantation for sickle cell disease. Biol Blood Marrow Transplant 2008;14:1270–8.

70. van Beisen K, Bartholomew A, Stock W, et al. Fludarabine-based conditioning regimen for allogeneic transplantation in adults with sickle cell disease. Bone Marrow Transplant 2000;26:445–9.

71. Iannone R, Casella JF, Fuchs EJ, et al. Results of minimally toxic nonmyeloablative transplantation in patients with sickle cell anemia and beta-thalassemia. Biol Blood Marrow Transplant 2003;9:519–28.

72. Horan JT, Liesveld JL, Fenton P, et al. Hematopoietic stem cell transplantation for multiply transfused patients with sickle cell disease and thalassemia after

low-dose total body irradiation, fludarabine, and rabbit anti-thymocyte globulin. Bone Marrow Transplant 2005;35:171–7.

73. Hsieh MM, Kang EM, Fitzhugh CD, et al. Allogeneic hematopoietic stem-cell transplantation for sickle cell disease. N Engl J Med 2009;361(24):2309–17.

74. Adamkiewicz TV, Szabolcs P, Haight A, et al. Unrelated cord blood transplantation in children with sickle cell disease: review of four-center experience. Pediatr Transplant 2007;11:641–4.

75. Walters MC, Hardy K, Edwards S, et al. Pulmonary, gonadal, and central nervous system status after bone marrow transplantation for sickle cell disease. Biol Blood Marrow Transplant 2010;16:263–72.

76. Bernaudin F, Kuentz M, Socie G. Late effects of myeloablative stem cell transplantation or late effects of sickle cell disease itself? Blood 2008;111(3):1744.

Umbilical Cord Blood Transplantation for Thalassemia Major

Bindu Kanathezhath, MD[a], Mark C. Walters, MD[b],*

KEYWORDS

- Hematopoietic cell transplantation • Thalassemia major
- Graft-versus-host disease • Umbilical cord blood

After the initial demonstration nearly 30 years ago[1] that bone marrow transplantation has curative potential for thalassemia major (discussed in the article by Gaziev and Lucarelli elsewhere in this issue), subsequent efforts have focused on methods to improve the safety of hematopoietic cell transplantation and to broaden its availability. These activities have included the investigation of alternative sources of hematopoietic stem cells that might be used in lieu of bone marrow. This effort was driven in part by the recognition that graft-versus-host disease (GVHD) is a leading cause of morbidity and mortality after conventional marrow transplantation and that most individuals with thalassemia major lack an HLA-identical sibling donor. The possibility that umbilical cord blood (UCB) might help investigators achieve both objectives was first suggested by the report of successful UCB transplantation for another hereditary hematologic disorder, Fanconi anemia, in 1989.[2] Since then, more than 20,000 transplantation procedures have been performed from unrelated donor UCB units, and more than 450,000 UCB units have been collected and banked by approximately 50 cord blood banks worldwide (reviewed by Rocha and Gluckman[3]). Although the bulk of the clinical application of UCB transplantation has been in the treatment of recurrent or refractory malignant hematologic disorders, UCB also has the potential to emerge as an important alternative source of donor hematopoietic cells in the treatment of thalassemia major. This possibility hinges on exploiting the favorable characteristics of UCB, which include a lowered incidence of GVHD and a rapid tempo of immune reconstitution after transplantation,[4] and on establishing novel approaches to reduce the problem of graft rejection after UCB transplantation.

[a] Hematology/Oncology, Children's Hospital & Research Center, Oakland, 747 52nd Street, Oakland, CA 94609, USA
[b] Children's Hospital & Research Center, Oakland, 747 52nd Street, Oakland, CA 94609, USA
* Corresponding author.
E-mail address: mwalters@mail.cho.org

Hematol Oncol Clin N Am 24 (2010) 1165–1177
doi:10.1016/j.hoc.2010.08.006
0889-8588/10/$ – see front matter © 2010 Elsevier Inc. All rights reserved.

CHARACTERISTICS OF THE UCB GRAFT

UCB has several properties that make it an attractive alternative to marrow as a source of allogeneic cells for transplantation, particularly for nonmalignant disorders, such as thalassemia major, where GVHD offers no benefit. These advantages, as articulated in the review by Rocha and Locatelli,[5] include a lower incidence and severity of acute and chronic GVHD; the possibility of extending the number of HLA-antigen mismatches to 1 to 2 of the 6 HLA loci currently considered in UCB transplantation; a lower risk of transmitting latent virus infections, such as cytomegalovirus and Epstein-Barr virus, in the harvested hematopoietic cell collection; the elimination of clinical risk to the donor during hematopoietic stem cell procurement procedures; and a higher frequency of rare HLA haplotype representation in the donor pool compared with bone marrow registries as a result of targeting UCB collections from under-represented ethnic minorities. These advantages are balanced by a disadvantage, however, which is a higher risk of graft rejection and delayed hematopoietic recovery after transplantation that can contribute to serious infections. This risk follows from the reduced number of hematopoietic progenitor cells contained in a typical UCB collection compared with marrow harvesting and from the possibility that the naive immune system in UCB translates into a blunted allogeneic effect elicited by donor T lymphocytes and that is required for overcoming host immunologic barriers to engraftment. This limitation is significant in thalassemia major because pretransplantation exposures to minor histocompatibility antigens by chronic red blood cell transfusions seem to contribute to a high rate of graft rejection after conventional bone marrow transplantation for thalassemia major. Thus, graft rejection is predicted to pose a significant barrier to the wider application of UCB transplantation for thalassemia major.

GRAFT REJECTION AND UCB TRANSPLANTATION

Several strategies have been used to mitigate the risk of graft rejection after UCB transplantation (discussed later). Almost all the published clinical series of unrelated donor UCB transplantation in children and adults with hematologic malignancies showed that the total nucleated cell (TNC) dose contained in a UCB unit has a profound impact on engraftment, as measured by preprocessing or the post-thaw TNC dose infused.[6–8] Similarly, other direct measurements of the cellular content of the UCB unit, such as colony-forming unit activity and CD34+ cell content (a surrogate cell surface marker for the hematopoietic stem cell), were positively correlated with donor engraftment.[9] An effect of TNC on other transplant-related complications, such as infection risk and survival, was also observed.[10,11] In addition, the degree of HLA matching seemed to have an independent impact on outcome, with those recipients who had greater than 2 HLA mismatches experiencing the worst outcomes (the degree of matching in UCB transplantation is assessed by low-resolution HLA typing methods at HLA-A and HLA-B loci and by high-resolution at HLA-DRB1). The indication for UCB transplantation also had an impact on outcome, and those recipients with advanced-stage malignant diseases experienced the worst outcomes. As the factors that affect outcome became more widely appreciated, decision making about the selection of UCB donor units and suitable transplantation recipients was adjusted and these changes have improved outcomes over the past 2 decades, as assessed by the year the transplantation was conducted (**Fig. 1**).[3] In addition, improved supportive care and wider experience at individual centers also seem to have contributed to the improved outcomes.

Children who had nonmalignant disorders experienced a higher rate of graft rejection after UCB transplantation compared with those with a malignant disorder.[12,13] In

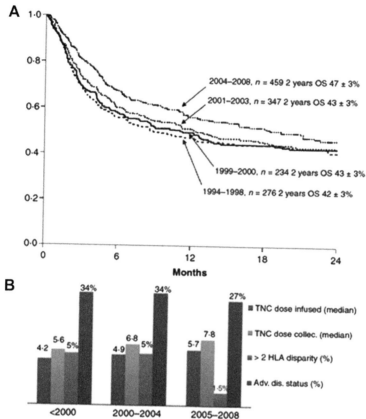

Fig. 1. (*A*) Survival after unrelated UCB transplantation for children with hematologic malignancies by year of treatment. (*B*) Median of collected and infused total nucleated cells per kg recipient weight (10^7/kg), number of HLA disparities, and status of the disease in children with hematologic malignancies. Adv. dis., advanced disease; OS, overall survival. (*Reproduced from* Rocha V, Gluckman E. Improving outcomes of cord blood transplantation: HLA matching, cell dose and other graft- and transplantation-related factors. Br J Haematol 2009;147(2):262–74; with permission.)

the setting of a nonmalignant disorder, the degree of HLA matching also influenced the probability of engraftment.[5] This effect was more important in children with nonmalignant disorders compared with those malignant disorders, because a higher of incidence of GVHD associated with HLA mismatching translated into a graft-versus-malignancy effect that lowered the risk of relapse after UCB transplantation. For this reason, the degree of HLA matching (that is, 0, 1, or 2 HLA antigen mismatches) does not seem to influence the outcome in children with acute leukemia. In the nonmalignant disorders, however, HLA mismatching had a major impact on the incidence and severity of GVHD, engraftment, and survival, which was only partially overcome by increasing the cell dose.[3,5] Based on Eurocord data that included 1204 UCB transplant recipients with malignant (N = 925) and nonmalignant (N = 279) conditions, the outcome after UCB transplantation was unacceptably poor in nonmalignant disease recipients who received a TNC dose less than 3.5×10^7/kg and if HLA matching occurred at 4 of 6 HLA antigens. For this reason, optimizing the TNC dose in the

UCB unit is generally agreed on as a key component in the decision-making process that precedes transplantation.

The cell dose limitation is particularly difficult to overcome in adult recipients and was a principal reason why UCB transplantation initially was restricted to children during its early development. In an effort to expand UCB transplantation, the transplantation team in Minneapolis reasoned that using 2 UCB units might facilitate engraftment and mitigate the difficulties associated with delayed engraftment or non-engraftment when also preceded by the application of a reduced intensity preparative regimen.[14,15] A target cell dose of 3×10^7 TNC/kg recipient weight was achieved in 85% of the study participants by identifying 2 UCB units that were matched at 4 of 6 HLA antigens with the recipient and 3 of 6 HLA antigens between the 2 UCB units. Of 110 patients with hematologic diseases who were treated, 92% experienced neutrophil engraftment a median of 12 days after transplantation. More recently, outcomes after consecutive UCB transplantation in 155 adult recipients with hematologic malignancies were analyzed.[5,16] In this cohort that also received a reduced intensity conditioning regimen, 38% received transplantation with 2 UCB units to fulfill minimum cell dose targets. Eighty percent of the patients had a neutrophil recovery greater than $500/mm^3$ by 60 days after transplantation and 14% experienced graft rejection and autologous recovery of hematopoiesis. The factors associated with a better rate of neutrophil recovery included an elevated CD34+ cell dose, HLA compatibility, and having received a previous autologous stem cell transplantation. Together, these series show that it is possible to use 2 UCB units when the UCB cell content is otherwise limiting and that the cell dose and HLA compatibility are key factors that influence the engraftment of donor cells, particularly in recipients with nonmalignant hematologic disorders.

CORD BLOOD TRANSPLANTATION FOR THALASSEMIA MAJOR—SIBLING DONORS

As in other nonmalignant indications for transplantation, the potential for delayed or failed engraftment after cord blood transplantation (CBT) for thalassemia major is balanced by the benefit of a lowered risk of GVHD, a complication that offers no apparent benefit in thalassemia.[7,8,17] Thus, the initial reports of CBT for thalassemia focused on the tempo and durability of engraftment and on rates of acute and chronic GVHD. In one retrospective survey of sibling donor cord blood transplantation, 7 of 33 children with thalassemia developed graft rejection after transplantation with an event-free survival of 79%.[18] The rates of acute and chronic GVHD were low, however, and only 4 of 38 evaluable children with sickle cell disease or thalassemia developed acute GVHD after CBT, and 2 of these 4 had an HLA-disparate donor. The Kaplan-Meier probability of chronic GVHD was 6%. Thus, as predicted, the higher incidence of graft rejection after CBT was balanced by a lower incidence of GVHD when compared with rates historically observed after bone marrow transplantation from an HLA-identical sibling donor. Moreover, the low rate of GVHD was associated with excellent survival probability, and none of the 33 patients with thalassemia died after CBT.

The graft rejection risk after sibling CBT for thalassemia was analyzed with respect to the chemotherapeutic agents of the conditioning regimen and postgrafting immunosuppression regimens. When the conditioning regimen included busulfan (BU) and cyclophosphamide (CY) with or without antithymocyte globulin (ATG), there was a significant association with graft rejection after UCB transplantation for thalassemia. The event-free survival was improved if a combination of BU, CY and thiotepa (TT) or BU, fludarabine (Flu), and TT was administered (94% vs 62%, $P = .03$) (**Fig. 2**).[18] In addition, recipients with sickle cell disease and thalassemia who received

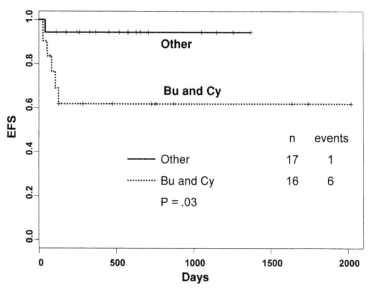

Fig. 2. Kaplan-Meier estimates of the probability of event-free survival after UCB transplantation for thalassemia. Patients who were prepared for transplantation with a standard combination of BU/CY with or without ATG were compared with patients who received an alternative combination of BU/CY/TT or BU/Flu/TT. The time in days after transplantation is depicted in the X axis. (*Reproduced from* Locatelli F, Rocha V, Reed W, et al. Related umbilical cord blood transplantation in patients with thalassemia and sickle cell disease. Blood 2003;101(6):2137–43; with permission.)

methotrexate (MTX) as part of GVHD prophylaxis had a poorer event-free survival compared with those who did not receive MTX (55% vs 90%, P = .005) (**Fig. 3**). Thus, good outcomes were observed among those who did not receive MTX for GVHD prophylaxis and in those who received a modulated conditioning regimen. In a contemporary cohort recently treated from Pavia, Italy, children with thalassemia were prepared for CBT with a combination of BU, Flu, and TT and received cyclosporine alone for postgrafting immunosuppression.[18] All 27 survived free of thalassemia, and none experienced acute or chronic GVHD. The majority of these individuals had stable mixed donor-host chimerism that persisted after UCB transplantation; thus, mixed chimerism early after UCB transplantation was not a predictor of graft rejection (**Fig. 4**).

These initial impressions about excellent outcomes after sibling CBT for thalassemia was confirmed in a recent retrospective analysis comparing outcomes after sibling donor marrow and cord blood transplantation.[19] This cohort included recipients with sickle cell disease and thalassemia major and compared outcomes in 389 marrow (259 with thalassemia) and 70 cord blood (44 with thalassemia) recipients who were treated between 1994 and 2005 in 13 different centers. There was no difference in overall survival between the 2 groups, but individuals who received cord blood were less likely to develop GVHD (10 ± 4% vs 20 ± 2%) and had a slower tempo of blood count recovery, although the overall probability of neutrophil recovery was little different (90 ± 4% vs 93 ± 1%). For this reason, families affected by thalassemia major should be offered the option of pursuing sibling donor UCB collection and cyropreservation, and there are resources in the United States to support this activity through the Stem Cell Therapeutic and Research Act of 2005 administered by the Health Resources

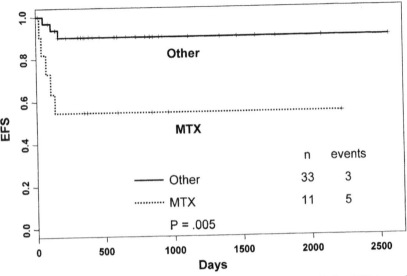

Fig. 3. Kaplan-Meier estimates of the probability of event-free survival after UCB transplantation for hemoglobinopathies in patients who received or did not receive MTX for GVHD prophylaxis. The time in days after transplantation is depicted in the X axis. (*Reproduced from* Locatelli F, Rocha V, Reed W, et al. Related umbilical cord blood transplantation in patients with thalassemia and sickle cell disease. Blood 2003;101(6):2137–43; with permission.)

and Services Administration and by selected family cord blood banking companies. Families with thalassemia seem motivated to pursue this option, and a transplantation use rate of 44% was observed when the thalassemia donor-recipient pairs were HLA identical, compared with 1.4% in children with acute lymphoblastic leukemia.[13]

Another method to improve cell dose in sibling UCB transplantation is to combine the cord blood unit with marrow from the same sibling donor, thereby enhancing the stem cell content of the combined graft.[20] This approach was selected in a series of 13 patients with nonmalignant disorders, 7 of whom had thalassemia major.[21] None of the recipients had graft rejection after UCB transplantation and there was no GVHD. Thus, the modification of pretransplantation and postgrafting immunosuppressive regimens seems to have optimized outcomes after UCB transplantation for thalassemia. In addition, in cases where it is feasible to augment the cord blood unit with marrow from the same donor, this too seems a safe and effective means to promote engraftment. Finally, it has been shown recently that the human placenta is a rich source of hematopoietic stem cells, and the development of methods to harvest placental cells that lack maternal cell contamination as a strategy to expand the cellular content of UCB collections would have considerable usefulness.[22]

CORD BLOOD TRANSPLANTATION FOR THALASSEMIA MAJOR—UNRELATED DONORS

Investigations to expand UCB transplantation for thalassemia by using unrelated donors are ongoing but, as in the sibling UCB transplantation setting, modification of the transplantation strategy may be necessary to improve on the initial experience. The first reports demonstrated the feasibility of unrelated donor UCB transplantation, documented by case reports or small series of patients (**Table 1**).[23,24] Thalassemia

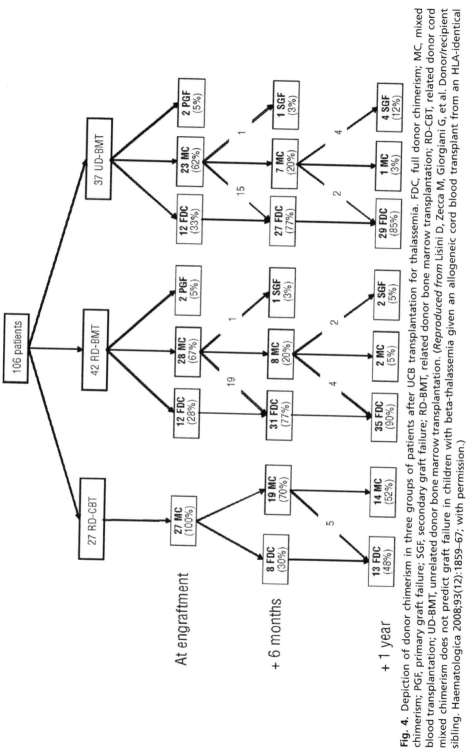

Fig. 4. Depiction of donor chimerism in three groups of patients after UCB transplantation for thalassemia. FDC, full donor chimerism; MC, mixed chimerism; PGF, primary graft failure; SGF, secondary graft failure; RD-BMT, related donor bone marrow transplantation; RD-CBT, related donor cord blood transplantation; UD-BMT, unrelated donor bone marrow transplantation. (*Reproduced from* Lisini D, Zecca M, Giorgiani G, et al. Donor/recipient mixed chimerism does not predict graft failure in children with beta-thalassemia given an allogeneic cord blood transplant from an HLA-identical sibling. Haematologica 2008;93(12):1859–67; with permission.)

Table 1
Outcomes after unrelated CBT for thalassemia major

	Jaing et al, 2010	Jaing et al, 2008	Jaing et al, 2007	Jaing et al, 2005	Vanichsetakul et al, 2004
No. patients	32	51	5	5	6
Risk group	Class 1—21 Class 2—9 Unk—2	Class 1—20 Class 2—11 Class 3—1 Unk—19	Unk—5	Class 1—5	Class 1—1 Class 2—2 Class 3—3
Median age (range)	4.5 (0.1-16.2)[a]	4.3 (0.3-20)	11.1 (10-13.1)	3.7 (2.3-11.4)	5.5 (2-15)
Conditioning regimen	BU/CY/ATG	BU/CY/ATG	BU/CY/ATG	BU/CY/ATG	BU/CY ± Flu
aGVHD	76% (95% CI, 0.65-0.82)[a]	N/A	100%	100%	40%
cGVHD	35% (95% CI, 0.29-0.42)[a]	N/A	100% (limited)	0%	0%
Double CBT	12[a]	12	5	0	0
Graft rejection	5/32 (16%)	21.6%	20%	0	0
Survival	88% (5-year)[a]	74.5%	80%	100%	83.3%
Event-free survival	77% (5-year)[a]	N/A	60%	100%	83.3%

Abbreviations: aGVHD, acute graft-versus-host disease; cGVHD, chronic graft-versus-host disease; N/A, not available; No, number; Unk, unknown.
[a] This report combined 32 patients with thalassemia major and 13 patients with other nonmalignant hematological disorders.
Data from Refs.[23–28,41]

recipients typically received unrelated cord blood units matched at 4 of 6 and 5 of 6 HLA antigens and were prepared with a conventional combination of BU/CY/ATG. The largest series published in 2004 and 2005 from Asian centers reported that 10 of 11 patients survived free of thalassemia after successful UCB transplantation, and none of the survivors had chronic GVHD. In 2007, another small series showed the potential for a successful outcome after double UCB transplantation, in which five children with thalassemia received cord blood units matched at 2 of 6 to 4 of 6 HLA antigens after preparation with BU/CY/ATG.[25] One of the five died of complications related to GVHD and pulmonary hemorrhage, and another had a late graft rejection. All four survivors had limited chronic GVHD after the double cord blood transplantation. More recently, dual-unit CBT was also successful in rescuing from an initial graft failure after unrelated donor UCB transplantation in three children with thalassemia major.[26] A larger series of 51 children with a median age of 4.3 years (range 0.3–20 years) from 14 Asian centers was updated in 2008.[27] The times to having an absolute neutrophil count greater than 500/mm^3 and platelet count greater than 20,000/μL independent of transfusion support were 17 and 40 days, respectively. The transplant-related mortality was 13.7% and 38 of 51 (75%) patients survived after UCB transplantation. Eleven (21.6%) patients had graft failure or autologous recovery after unrelated UCB transplantation. Together, these retrospective data showed the possibility of a successful outcome after unrelated UCB transplantation but also underscore a need to identify safer and more effective transplantation regimens and to address the problem of graft rejection after unrelated UCB transplantation.

The largest single series of unrelated UCB transplantation was reported by a team in Taiwan that treated 32 consecutive patients and was included in a larger description of a total of 45 patients with nonmalignant disorders.[28] The recipients had Pesaro class I (N = 21), class II (N = 9), or unknown risk class (N = 2) assigned before UCB transplantation and all were prepared with BU/CY/ATG (see **Table 1**). To increase the cell dose delivered, 12 of 45 patients received double cord blood units for transplantation. The cord blood units were matched at 6 of 6 HLA antigens (N = 11), 5 of 6 (N = 25), and 4 of 6 or fewer HLA antigens (N = 27). The median TNC and CD34+ cell doses before thawing the UCB unit were 7.6×10^7/kg and 4.0×10^5/kg, respectively. The probability of neutrophil and platelet engraftment after UCB transplantation was 88% and 82%, respectively. The overall and event-free survival rates at 5 years were 88% and 77%, respectively, with a median follow-up of 25 months. The transplant-related mortality was 12%; 76% had grades II-IV acute GVHD and 35% had chronic GVHD at 1 year after UCB transplantation. Five of 32 thalassemia patients (16%) had a graft rejection after transplantation and all five were successfully treated by a second hematopoietic cell transplantation. In four cases, the patients received double UCB transplantation and in one case, HLA-haploidentical mobilized peripheral blood stem cells were used in the second rescue transplantation. All 55 survived independent of RBC transfusions with stable engraftment of donor cells, although all five have chronic GVHD (limited distribution in four). This single-center experience suggests that increasing the cell dose by using double cord blood unit transplantation mitigated the risk of graft rejection, at the expense, however, of causing more frequent GVHD. Nonetheless, this experience suggests that it is possible to improve the outcome after unrelated UCB transplantation by modulating the graft content, as was observed in the sibling donor setting. Additional studies are needed, however, to identify an optimal conditioning regimen.

The authors have investigated an alternative strategy to ensure engraftment after HLA-mismatched UCB transplantation that uses photochemically modified donor

T lymphocytes to promote engraftment. The authors hypothesized that it might be possible to ensure engraftment without a significant risk of severe GVHD after donor-mismatched UCB transplantation by using add-backs of amotosalen (S-59)–treated T lymphocytes with donor cord blood. S-59 is a water soluble, nontoxic synthetic psoralen that has been used for pathogen inactivation in platelet and plasma products.[29–35] S-59 forms covalent monoadducts and cross-links between the pyrimidine bases of the DNA and RNA on illumination with long wavelength UV-A light. When treated with nanomolar concentration of S-59, photochemically treated T lymphocytes demonstrate near complete abrogation of lymphocyte proliferation, even in the presence mitogens.[36] In a preclinical murine model of thalassemia, S-59–treated donor lymphocytes facilitated engraftment without GVHD after mismatched bone marrow transplantation.[37] These preclinical studies recently were extended to a murine model of UCB transplantation across a major histocompatibility barrier that the authors think are sufficiently encouraging to develop a clinical investigation of this methodology.

Another requirement of wider access to UCB transplantation for thalassemia major is increasing the size of the UCB donor inventory. Similar efforts in the unrelated marrow donor registries might also be pursued, except that the large size of these registries has effectively diminished the return on recruiting additional volunteers. It has been estimated that with a registry size of 10 million donors, approximately 7 million additional donors would need to be recruited to increase the likelihood of identifying an HLA-matched donor by 1%.[38] The current donor inventory, according to the Bone Marrow Donors Worldwide Web site, is 13.8 million (http://www.bmdw.org). In contrast, many fewer additional UCB units are required to have a significant impact on the probability of identifying a suitable donor.[39] In addition, by collecting UCB units from large obstetric centers that match the ethnic representation of a targeted disorder, the likelihood of accumulating UCB units that might be suitable for transplantation should be increased. Based on empirical calculations derived from the 50% rate of successfully identifying suitable UCB units (HLA 4 of 6 or 5 of 6 matched donors with a minimum cell dose of 2.5×10^7 TNC/kg recipient weight) from an inventory of more than 20,000 units searched by approximately 16,000 requests, one analysis projected that an inventory of 55,000 to 60,000 units from a representative ethnic sampling should generate at least 1 suitable UCB unit in 80% of the searches.[40] Thus, the development of UCB as an alternate source of hematopoietic cells in transplantation for thalassemia major also must be linked to an effort to increase the UCB inventory with high-quality units collected from an ethnically representative population.

SUMMARY

UCB transplantation for thalassemia major is in an early stage of development. UCB has properties, however, that make it an attractive alternative to bone marrow stem cells, in particular, a decreased incidence of GVHD. This benefit, however, is balanced by a greater risk of graft rejection, due in part to a restricted number of hematopoietic stem cells. This risk can be overcome in part by selecting UCB units that contain a large number of cells and by selecting units that are closely matched at the HLA loci. Recent results show excellent outcomes after HLA-identical sibling UCB transplantation, stressing the importance of collecting cord blood in families when a child is affected by thalassemia. Even when the UCB unit collected after a sibling birth is combined with a marrow harvest from the same donor, the results are excellent, with low rates of GVHD. The use of double UCB transplantation from unrelated donors might also be useful as another approach to optimize the donor hematopoietic stem cell content. The future development of UCB transplantation is likely to focus on defining the best conditioning regimen to use and on defining optimum UCB unit characteristics.

REFERENCES

1. Thomas ED, Buckner CD, Sanders JE, et al. Marrow transplantation for thalassaemia. Lancet 1982;2(8292):227–9.
2. Gluckman E, Broxmeyer HA, Auerbach AD, et al. Hematopoietic reconstitution in a patient with Fanconi's anemia by means of umbilical-cord blood from an HLA-identical sibling. N Engl J Med 1989;321(17):1174–8.
3. Rocha V, Gluckman E. Improving outcomes of cord blood transplantation: HLA matching, cell dose and other graft- and transplantation-related factors. Br J Haematol 2009;147(2):262–74.
4. Cohen G, Carter SL, Weinberg KI, et al. Antigen-specific T-lymphocyte function after cord blood transplantation. Biol Blood Marrow Transplant 2006;12(12):1335–42.
5. Rocha V, Locatelli F. Searching for alternative hematopoietic stem cell donors for pediatric patients. Bone Marrow Transplant 2008;41(2):207–14.
6. Michel G, Rocha V, Chevret S, et al. Unrelated cord blood transplantation for childhood acute myeloid leukemia: a Eurocord Group Analysis. Blood 2003; 102(13):4290–7.
7. Gluckman E, Rocha V, Boyer-Chammard A, et al. Outcome of cord-blood transplantation from related and unrelated donors. Eurocord transplant group and the European blood and marrow transplantation group. N Engl J Med 1997; 337(6):373–81.
8. Rubinstein P, Carrier C, Scaradavou A, et al. Outcomes among 562 recipients of placental-blood transplants from unrelated donors. N Engl J Med 1998;339(22): 1565–77.
9. Wagner JE, Barker JN, DeFor TE, et al. Transplantation of unrelated donor umbilical cord blood in 102 patients with malignant and nonmalignant diseases: influence of CD34 cell dose and HLA disparity on treatment-related mortality and survival. Blood 2002;100(5):1611–8.
10. Rocha V, Sanz G, Gluckman E. Umbilical cord blood transplantation. Curr Opin Hematol 2004;11(6):375–85.
11. Gluckman E, Rocha V, Arcese W, et al. Factors associated with outcomes of unrelated cord blood transplant: guidelines for donor choice. Exp Hematol 2004; 32(4):397–407.
12. Gluckman E, Rocha V, Ionescu I, et al. Results of unrelated cord blood transplant in fanconi anemia patients: risk factor analysis for engraftment and survival. Biol Blood Marrow Transplant 2007;13(9):1073–82.
13. Walters MC, Quirolo L, Trachtenberg ET, et al. Sibling donor cord blood transplantation for thalassemia major: experience of the sibling donor cord blood program. Ann N Y Acad Sci 2005;1054:206–13.
14. Brunstein CG, Barker JN, Weisdorf DJ, et al. Umbilical cord blood transplantation after nonmyeloablative conditioning: impact on transplantation outcomes in 110 adults with hematologic disease. Blood 2007;110(8):3064–70.
15. Barker JN, Weisdorf DJ, DeFor TE, et al. Transplantation of 2 partially HLA-matched umbilical cord blood units to enhance engraftment in adults with hematologic malignancy. Blood 2005;105(3):1343–7.
16. Rocha V, Mohty M, Gluckman E, et al. Reduced-intensity conditioning regimens before unrelated cord blood transplantation in adults with acute

leukaemia and other haematological malignancies. Curr Opin Oncol 2009;21 (Suppl 1):S31–4.

17. Pinto FO, Roberts I. Cord blood stem cell transplantation for haemoglobinopathies. Br J Haematol 2008;141(3):309–24.

18. Locatelli F, Rocha V, Reed W, et al. Related umbilical cord blood transplantation in patients with thalassemia and sickle cell disease. Blood 2003;101(6):2137–43.

19. Kabbara N, Locatelli F, Rocha V, et al. A multicentric comparative analysis of outcomes of HLA-identical related cord blood and bone marrow transplantation in patients with beta-thalassemia or sickle cell disease. Biol Blood Marrow Transplant 2008;14(2):3–4.

20. Bernaudin F, Socie G, Kuentz M, et al. Long-term results of related myeloablative stem-cell transplantation to cure sickle cell disease. Blood 2007;110(7): 2749–56.

21. Soni S, Cowman MJ, Edwards S, et al. Co-Infusion of matched sibling donor cord blood and bone marrow as stem cell source for allogeneic stem cell transplantation in pediatric non-malignant disorders. Biol Blood Marrow Transplant 2008; 14(2):75–6.

22. Serikov V, Hounshell C, Larkin S, et al. Human term placenta as a source of hematopoietic cells. Exp Biol Med (Maywood) 2009;234(7):813–23.

23. Jaing TH, Hung IJ, Yang CP, et al. Rapid and complete donor chimerism after unrelated mismatched cord blood transplantation in 5 children with beta-thalassemia major. Biol Blood Marrow Transplant 2005;11(5):349–53.

24. Vanichsetakul P, Wacharaprechanont T, O-Charoen R, et al. Umbilical cord blood transplantation in children with beta-thalassemia diseases. J Med Assoc Thai 2004;87(Suppl 2):S62–7.

25. Jaing TH, Yang CP, Hung IJ, et al. Transplantation of unrelated donor umbilical cord blood utilizing double-unit grafts for five teenagers with transfusion-dependent thalassemia. Bone Marrow Transplant 2007;40(4):307–11.

26. Jaing TH, Hung IJ, Yang CP, et al. Second transplant with two unrelated cord blood units for early graft failure after cord blood transplantation for thalassemia. Pediatr Transplant 2009;13(6):766–8.

27. Jaing TH, Tan P, Rosenthal J, et al. Unrelated cord blood transplantation (UCBT) for transfusion-dependent thalassemia—a cibmtr audited retrospective analysis of 51 consecutive patients. Biol Blood Marrow Transplant 2008;14(2):6–7.

28. Jaing TH, Chen SH, Tsai MH, et al. Transplantation of unrelated donor umbilical cord blood for nonmalignant diseases: a single institution's experience with 45 patients. Biol Blood Marrow Transplant 2010;16(1):102–7.

29. Allain JP, Bianco C, Blajchman MA, et al. Protecting the blood supply from emerging pathogens: the role of pathogen inactivation. Transfus Med Rev 2005;19(2):110–26.

30. Lin L. Inactivation of cytomegalovirus in platelet concentrates using Helinx technology. Semin Hematol 2001;38(4 Suppl 11):27–33.

31. McCullough J, Vesole DH, Benjamin RJ, et al. Therapeutic efficacy and safety of platelets treated with a photochemical process for pathogen inactivation: the SPRINT trial. Blood 2004;104(5):1534–41.

32. Snyder E, McCullough J, Slichter SJ, et al. Clinical safety of platelets photochemically treated with amotosalen HCl and ultraviolet a light for pathogen inactivation: the SPRINT trial. Transfusion 2005;45(12):1864–75.

33. van Rhenen D, Gulliksson H, Cazenave JP, et al. Transfusion of pooled buffy coat platelet components prepared with photochemical pathogen inactivation treatment: the euroSPRITE trial. Blood 2003;101(6):2426–33.

34. Van Voorhis WC, Barrett LK, Eastman RT, et al. Trypanosoma cruzi inactivation in human platelet concentrates and plasma by a psoralen (amotosalen HCl) and long-wavelength UV. Antimicrob Agents Chemother 2003;47(2):475–9.
35. Wollowitz S. Fundamentals of the psoralen-based Helinx technology for inactivation of infectious pathogens and leukocytes in platelets and plasma. Semin Hematol 2001;38(4 Suppl 11):4–11.
36. Jordan CT, Roback JD. Separating antiviral and GVHD activities of donor T cells prior to bone marrow transplantation. Immunol Res 2004;29(1–3):209–18.
37. Kuypers FA, Watson G, Sage E, et al. Stem cell transplantation with S-59 photochemically treated T-cell add-backs to establish allochimerism in murine thalassemia. Ann N Y Acad Sci 2005;1054:214–22.
38. Hurley CK, Fernandez Vina M, Setterholm M. Maximizing optimal hematopoietic stem cell donor selection from registries of unrelated adult volunteers. Tissue Antigens 2003;61(6):415–24.
39. Querol S, Rubinstein P, Marsh SG, et al. Cord blood banking: 'providing cord blood banking for a nation'. Br J Haematol 2009;147(2):227–35.
40. Querol S, Mufti GJ, Marsh SG, et al. Cord blood stem cells for hematopoietic stem cell transplantation in the UK: how big should the bank be? Haematologica 2009; 94(4):536–41.
41. Jaing TH, Wang B, Gjertson D, et al. Unrelated cord blood transplantation (UCBT) of 30 consecutive patients with transfusion-dependent thalassemia from a single center. Biol Blood Marrow Transplant 2009;15(2):24–5.

Noninvasive Approaches to Prenatal Diagnosis of Hemoglobinopathies Using Fetal DNA in Maternal Plasma

Y.M. Dennis Lo, DM, DPhil[a,b,*], Rossa W.K. Chiu, MBBS, PhD[a,b]

KEYWORDS

• Noninvasive prenatal diagnosis • Plasma DNA • Digital PCR
• β-Thalassemia • Circulating nucleic acids

Prenatal diagnosis is an established part of modern obstetrics practice. Conventional methods for obtaining fetal genetic materials for analysis, however, such as amniocentesis and chorionic villus sampling, are invasive and constitute a risk to the fetus. Over the past few decades, there has been much effort in developing noninvasive methods for prenatal diagnosis that do not have such a risk. Early approaches focused on the isolation of fetal nucleated cells that had entered into the maternal circulation.[1,2] However, because of the rarity of such cells in the maternal circulation, typically of the order of several cells per milliliter of maternal blood,[3] it has been a challenge to obtain a robust detection of these cells. For example, in a large study designed to investigate the use of these cells for the noninvasive prenatal detection of fetal chromosomal aneuploidies, the detection of circulating male fetal nucleated cells could only be achieved with a sensitivity of 41.4%, with a false-positive rate of 11.1%.[4] As a result

This study was supported by the University Grants Committee of the Government of the Hong Kong Special Administration Region, China, under the Areas of Excellence Scheme (AoE/M-04/06).
The authors hold patents and have filed patent applications relating to the diagnostic applications of plasma nucleic acids. Part of this patent portfolio has been licensed to Sequenom Inc. YMDL is a consultant to, holds equities in, and receives research support from Sequenom Inc.
[a] Department of Chemical Pathology, The Chinese University of Hong Kong, Prince of Wales Hospital, 30-32 Ngan Shing Street, Shatin, New Territories, Hong Kong SAR, China
[b] Li Ka Shing Institute of Health Sciences, The Chinese University of Hong Kong, Prince of Wales Hospital, 30-32 Ngan Shing Street, Shatin, New Territories, Hong Kong SAR, China
* Corresponding author.
E-mail address: loym@cuhk.edu.hk

Hematol Oncol Clin N Am 24 (2010) 1179–1186
doi:10.1016/j.hoc.2010.08.007
0889-8588/10/$ – see front matter © 2010 Elsevier Inc. All rights reserved.

of such difficulties, many investigators in the field have moved away from fetal cell isolation to other approaches.

In 1997, Lo and colleagues[5] demonstrated that cell-free fetal DNA can be detected in the plasma and serum of pregnant women. Thus, Lo and colleagues were able to detect Y chromosomal DNA sequences in the plasma and serum of women carrying male fetuses. No Y chromosomal signals were seen in women carrying female fetuses. With the use of real-time quantitative polymerase chain reaction (PCR), Lo and colleagues[6] showed that fetal DNA can be detected in maternal plasma during the first trimester and at a mean fractional concentration of approximately 3%. That figure is much higher than the fractional concentration of fetal nucleated cells in maternal blood.[3] The high fractional concentration of fetal DNA in maternal plasma suggests that fetal DNA genotyping using this approach should be more readily achievable than previous methods based on the isolation of the rare fetal nucleated cells in maternal blood.

Another advantage of using plasma DNA is that fetal DNA is cleared rapidly from maternal plasma after delivery, with a half-life of approximately 16 minutes.[7] This observation indicates that there is no risk of fetal DNA persistence from one pregnancy to the next, unlike the observation that certain fetal cell populations can persist for long periods within the mother's body.[8] In other words, fetal genotype information that could be obtained from maternal plasma DNA analysis reflects that of the current pregnancy.

It is now accepted that the placenta is the principal origin of such fetal DNA in maternal plasma. This conclusion is based on several observations. First, fetal DNA in maternal plasma can be detected at normal concentrations in anembryonic pregnancies in which only the placenta, but not other fetal tissues, is present.[9] Second, fetal DNA in maternal plasma carries the DNA methylation signature of the placenta.[10–12] Third, in cases in which the placenta carries a distinctive cytogenetic signature when compared with other fetal tissues, such a signature can also be seen in maternal plasma.[13]

PRENATAL DIAGNOSTIC APPLICATIONS

The first diagnostic applications using fetal DNA in maternal plasma have focused on the detection of sequences that a fetus has inherited from the father but which are absent in the genome of the mother. Examples of such sequences involve those that are present on the Y chromosome. Several groups have reported the detection of fetal-derived Y chromosomal sequences in maternal plasma for prenatal gender determination for sex-linked diseases, such as hemophilia.[14,15] Another application of prenatal gender determination using this approach is in congenital adrenal hyperplasia in which prenatal dexamethasone treatment for the prevention of virilization is only indicated for female fetuses.[16]

Another early diagnostic application of fetal DNA in maternal plasma is for the prenatal determination of fetal RhD status in RhD-negative pregnant women.[17,18] This application has been validated by several large-scale studies.[19,20]

Due to the robustness with which fetal gender and RhD status can be determined from maternal plasma, these applications have been used diagnostically in several centers, initially in Europe and more recently in the United States.

APPLICATION TO THE HEMOGLOBINOPATHIES

Fetal DNA in maternal plasma was first applied to the hemoglobinopathies for the prenatal diagnosis of β-thalassemia.[21] Chiu and colleagues developed a real-time

PCR assay to detect the 4–base pair (bp) deletion in codons 41/42 of the human β-globin gene (HBB), which is the most common β-thalassemia mutation in China. They studied families in which the father was a carrier of this mutation whereas the mother was a carrier of another HBB mutation. Thus, the primary use of this approach is in the exclusion of β-thalassemia in the fetus, in which case the paternal mutation is not detected in maternal plasma. Provided that the assay has been optimized to have a high sensitivity for the detection of circulating fetal DNA, a negative signal indicates that no further prenatal testing is needed for a particular case. Because the diagnostic significance of this lack of detection of the paternal mutation is great, several investigators in the field have proposed developing a positive control for the detection of fetal DNA in maternal plasma (discussed later).

Conversely, if the paternal mutation is detected in maternal plasma, the only conclusion is that the fetus has inherited the paternal mutation. It is unclear, however, if a fetus is only a carrier or also has inherited the maternal mutation. This is a more challenging issue because the maternal mutation is present in maternal plasma after the release by the mother's own cells, irrespective of fetal mutational status. Recent advances in highly quantitative digital counting technologies, such as digital PCR, have allowed the solution of this problem (discussed later).

Several investigators have studied the detection other paternally inherited HBB mutations in maternal plasma. Unlike the 4-bp deletion (described previously), many of these other mutations are caused by point mutations. Hence, the specificity of the detection method, with regard to the target sequence, needs to be high. One approach with which this can be done is using variants of allele-specific or single-allele extension reactions followed by mass spectrometry.[22,23] This has been successfully implemented for the IVS2 654 (C → T), nt -28 (A → G), and CD 17 (A → T) mutations causing β-thalassemia[22] and the (GAG → AAG) missense mutation in codon 26 of the HBB gene causing hemoglobin E disease.[23] Furthermore, it has been shown that through the detection of a paternally inherited single nucleotide polymorphism (SNP) allele that is linked to the nonmutant HBB gene of the father, β-thalassemia major can be excluded.[22] Several groups have demonstrated that arrayed primer extension assays can be used for the detection of paternally inherited fetal β-thalassemia mutations and linked SNPs in maternal plasma.[24,25] Another promising approach is the use of single-molecule techniques, such as digital PCR (discussed later).[26,27]

Another strategy that has been attempted by investigators is developing technologies that allow the selective enrichment of fetal DNA in maternal plasma. For this approach to work, physical or biochemical characteristics that could differentiate fetal from maternal DNA in maternal plasma have to be found. One characteristic is the size of the DNA molecules, because Chan and colleagues[28] first reported that fetal DNA molecules in maternal plasma are shorter than their maternally derived counterparts. Li and colleagues[29] were able to obtain a relative enrichment of the circulating fetal DNA by the use of a gel-based electrophoretic system and to selectively extract the short DNA molecules from the gel. Using this approach, Li and colleagues[30,31] performed noninvasive prenatal detection of four HBB mutations in maternal plasma. This gel-based system is complex, however, and potentially prone to contamination to be used in a routine diagnostic context. Thus, it is hoped that future developments of more rapid and efficient size separation systems will allow this strategy to be used on a routine basis.[32]

Recently, a proof-of-concept report has shown that fetal DNA in maternal plasma can be used for the noninvasive prenatal exclusion of hemoglobin Bart's disease.[33] The sensitivity reported in this preliminary report, however, which is based on microsatellite polymorphisms, is only 33.3%. Because an established ultrasound-based approach is already used for this purpose, it is currently unclear if the DNA-based approach offers any additional advantage over the more conventional ultrasound-based method.[34]

UNIVERSAL FETAL DNA CONTROLS

In many of the diagnostic applications involving fetal DNA in maternal plasma (discussed previously), the absence of detectable signal from the target sequence is taken as meaning that the fetus has not inherited this sequence from its father. Another possibility, however, is that fetal DNA concentration within the maternal plasma is below the detection limit of the assay. Several investigators have proposed including a control for the presence of fetal DNA in a particular maternal plasma sample. Conceptually, the simplest system of this type is to detect the presence of a paternally inherited fetal allele for an SNP in maternal plasma.[35] Multiple SNPs, however, would be needed because each SNP is only informative in a proportion of cases.

In an effort to develop a fetal DNA marker that is gender and polymorphism independent, Poon and colleagues[36] proposed using DNA methylation differences between fetal and maternal DNA molecules in maternal plasma for this purpose. Poon and colleagues first demonstrated this concept using a locus that exhibited genomic imprinting. In 2005, Chim and colleagues[10] demonstrated that the promoter of the *SERPINB5* gene (coding for maspin) was hypomethylated in the placenta and developed hypomethylated *SERPINB5* sequences as the first gender- and polymorphism-independent fetal DNA marker in maternal plasma. This work has been followed by others reporting many DNA methylation markers that can be used in this fashion.[11,12,37–39]

Several investigators have used methylation-specific PCR to detect fetal DNA methylation markers in maternal plasma.[10,40] Methylation-specific PCR requires, however, that the plasma DNA sample be treated with bisulfite,[41] a procedure that can be associated with significant DNA degradation.[42] In an effort to circumvent this disadvantage, several investigators have focused on the use of hypermethylated fetal DNA markers, which can be detected with the use of simple digestion based on methylation-sensitive restriction enzymes.[11] Such enzymes digest the hypomethylated maternal DNA targets in maternal plasma, leaving the hypermethylated fetal DNA targets for detection.

SINGLE-MOLECULE DETECTION METHODS

As discussed previously, the most significant difficulty with the detection of fetal DNA molecules in maternal plasma is that such molecules represent a minority population in maternal plasma, being surrounded by an excess of maternally derived DNA molecules.[6] A powerful approach to tackle this problem is the use of single-molecule detection methods, in which plasma DNA molecules are analyzed individually and not interfered with by other target molecules of similar sequence.[43] One single-molecule analytic approach is digital PCR, in which a sample for analysis is diluted to an extent such that each PCR has an equivalent of 0.5 target molecule or less.[26,44] Then, many of these digital PCRs are performed in parallel. Some of these reactions have a target molecule and give rise to a positive reaction whereas those with no target molecule have a negative reaction. The number of target molecules is given by the total number of positive reactions. This approach is a powerful method for qualitative detection and quantitative analysis. The precision of such an approach for quantitative analysis is positively correlated with the number of digital PCRs.

On a qualitative level, digital PCR can be used for the detection of paternally inherited fetal mutations or polymorphisms in maternal plasma. An example is the detection of Y chromosome–derived sequences in maternal plasma.[27,45]

On a quantitative level, digital PCR can allow mutation dosage analysis of a fetus to be performed in maternal plasma. For a prenatal diagnosis of an autosomal recessive disease, the mother is typically a carrier of the mutation, with the mutant versus wild-type alleles present in a 1:1 ratio in her genome. If a fetus is homozygous for the mutant allele, then after the release of fetal DNA into maternal plasma, there is a slight over-representation of the mutant allele in maternal plasma. Provided that a sufficient number of molecules is counted in maternal plasma, digital PCR is able to detect this small allelic imbalance.[27] Conversely, if a fetus is homozygous for the wild-type allele, then there is a slight overrepresentation of the wild-type allele in maternal plasma. Finally, if a fetus is a heterozygous carrier of the mutation, then mutant and wild-type alleles remain in a 1:1 ratio in maternal plasma. This digital counting approach has been successfully implemented for the noninvasive prenatal diagnosis of *HBB* mutations causing β-thalassemia and hemoglobin E disease.[27]

One disadvantage of the digital PCR approach is that it is tedious to perform the hundreds or thousands of reactions needed to arrive at a statistically significant result. Recently, several high throughput approaches have been developed for performing such digital PCRs, including those that are based on microfluidics.[45–47]

The recent advent of massively parallel DNA sequencing technologies has provided another powerful method for the detection and counting of individual plasma DNA molecules.[48] Thus far, this approach has been used for the noninvasive prenatal diagnosis of fetal chromosomal aneuploidies.[49–51] It is expected that this method will also be used for the noninvasive prenatal diagnosis of monogenic disease, such as the hemoglobinopathies, in the near future.

SUMMARY

Since the discovery of fetal DNA in maternal plasma in 1997, various proof-of-concept studies have shown that this approach holds promise for the noninvasive prenatal diagnosis of various hemoglobinopathies. Over the next few years, the validation of these early studies by large-scale clinical trials will be essential to bring these developments into routine clinical applications.

REFERENCES

1. Bianchi DW, Flint AF, Pizzimenti MF, et al. Isolation of fetal DNA from nucleated erythrocytes in maternal blood. Proc Natl Acad Sci U S A 1990;87:3279–83.
2. Cheung MC, Goldberg JD, Kan YW. Prenatal diagnosis of sickle cell anaemia and thalassaemia by analysis of fetal cells in maternal blood. Nat Genet 1996;14: 264–8.
3. Bianchi DW, Williams JM, Sullivan LM, et al. PCR quantitation of fetal cells in maternal blood in normal and aneuploid pregnancies. Am J Hum Genet 1997; 61:822–9.
4. Bianchi DW, Simpson JL, Jackson LG, et al. Fetal gender and aneuploidy detection using fetal cells in maternal blood: analysis of NIFTY I data. National institute of child health and development fetal cell isolation study. Prenat Diagn 2002;22: 609–15.
5. Lo YM, Corbetta N, Chamberlain PF, et al. Presence of fetal DNA in maternal plasma and serum. Lancet 1997;350:485–7.

6. Lo YM, Tein MS, Lau TK, et al. Quantitative analysis of fetal DNA in maternal plasma and serum: implications for noninvasive prenatal diagnosis. Am J Hum Genet 1998;62:768–75.

7. Lo YM, Zhang J, Leung TN, et al. Rapid clearance of fetal DNA from maternal plasma. Am J Hum Genet 1999;64:218–24.

8. Bianchi DW, Zickwolf GK, Weil GJ, et al. Male fetal progenitor cells persist in maternal blood for as long as 27 years postpartum. Proc Natl Acad Sci U S A 1996;93:705–8.

9. Alberry M, Maddocks D, Jones M, et al. Free fetal DNA in maternal plasma in anembrynoic pregnancies: confirmation that the origin is the trophoblast. Prenat Diagn 2007;27:415–8.

10. Chim SS, Tong YK, Chiu RW, et al. Detection of the placental epigenetic signature of the maspin gene in maternal plasma. Proc Natl Acad Sci U S A 2005;102:14753–8.

11. Chan KC, Ding C, Gerovassili A, et al. Hypermethylated RASSF1A in maternal plasma: a universal fetal DNA marker that improves the reliability of noninvasive prenatal diagnosis. Clin Chem 2006;52:2211–8.

12. Chiu RW, Chim SS, Wong IH, et al. Hypermethylation of RASSF1A in human and rhesus placentas. Am J Pathol 2007;170:941–50.

13. Flori E, Doray B, Gautier E, et al. Circulating cell-free fetal DNA in maternal serum appears to originate from cyto- and syncytio-trophoblastic cells. Case report. Hum Reprod 2004;19:723–4.

14. Costa JM, Benachi A, Gautier E. New strategy for prenatal diagnosis of X-linked disorders. N Engl J Med 2002;346:1502.

15. Finning KM, Chitty LS. Non-invasive fetal sex determination: impact on clinical practice. Semin Fetal Neonatal Med 2008;13:69–75.

16. Rijnders RJ, van der Schoot CE, Bossers B, et al. Fetal sex determination from maternal plasma in pregnancies at risk for congenital adrenal hyperplasia. Obstet Gynecol 2001;98:374–8.

17. Lo YM, Hjelm NM, Fidler C, et al. Prenatal diagnosis of fetal RhD status by molecular analysis of maternal plasma. N Engl J Med 1998;339:1734–8.

18. Faas BH, Beuling EA, Christiaens GC, et al. Detection of fetal RHD-specific sequences in maternal plasma. Lancet 1998;352:1196.

19. Finning K, Martin P, Summers J, et al. Effect of high throughput RHD typing of fetal DNA in maternal plasma on use of anti-RhD immunoglobulin in RhD negative pregnant women: prospective feasibility study. BMJ 2008;336:816–8.

20. Rouillac-Le Sciellour C, Serazin V, Brossard Y, et al. Noninvasive fetal RHD genotyping from maternal plasma. Use of a new developed free DNA fetal kit RhD. Transfus Clin Biol 2007;14:572–7.

21. Chiu RW, Lau TK, Leung TN, et al. Prenatal exclusion of beta-thalassaemia major by examination of maternal plasma. Lancet 2002;360:998–1000.

22. Ding C, Chiu RW, Lau TK, et al. MS analysis of single-nucleotide differences in circulating nucleic acids: application to noninvasive prenatal diagnosis. Proc Natl Acad Sci U S A 2004;101:10762–7.

23. Tsang JC, Charoenkwan P, Chow KC, et al. Mass spectrometry-based detection of hemoglobin E mutation by allele-specific base extension reaction. Clin Chem 2007;53:2205–9.

24. Chan K, Yam I, Leung KY, et al. Detection of paternal alleles in maternal plasma for non-invasive prenatal diagnosis of beta-thalassemia: a feasibility study in southern Chinese. Eur J Obstet Gynecol Reprod Biol 2010;150:28–33.

25. Papasavva T, Kalikas I, Kyrri A, et al. Arrayed primer extension for the noninvasive prenatal diagnosis of beta-thalassemia based on detection of single nucleotide polymorphisms. Ann N Y Acad Sci 2008;1137:302–8.
26. Lo YM, Lun FM, Chan KC, et al. Digital PCR for the molecular detection of fetal chromosomal aneuploidy. Proc Natl Acad Sci U S A 2007;104:13116–21.
27. Lun FM, Tsui NB, Chan KC, et al. Noninvasive prenatal diagnosis of monogenic diseases by digital size selection and relative mutation dosage on DNA in maternal plasma. Proc Natl Acad Sci U S A 2008;105:19920–5.
28. Chan KC, Zhang J, Hui AB, et al. Size distributions of maternal and fetal DNA in maternal plasma. Clin Chem 2004;50:88–92.
29. Li Y, Zimmermann B, Rusterholz C, et al. Size separation of circulatory DNA in maternal plasma permits ready detection of fetal DNA polymorphisms. Clin Chem 2004;50:1002–11.
30. Li Y, Di Naro E, Vitucci A, et al. Detection of paternally inherited fetal point mutations for beta-thalassemia using size-fractionated cell-free DNA in maternal plasma. JAMA 2005;293:843–9.
31. Li Y, Di Naro E, Vitucci A, et al. Size fractionation of cell-free DNA in maternal plasma improves the detection of a paternally inherited beta-thalassemia point mutation by MALDI-TOF mass spectrometry. Fetal Diagn Ther 2009;25:246–9.
32. Hahn T, Drese KS, O'Sullivan CK. Microsystem for isolation of fetal DNA from maternal plasma by preparative size separation. Clin Chem 2009;55:2144–52.
33. Ho SS, Chong SS, Koay ES, et al. Noninvasive prenatal exclusion of haemoglobin Bart's using foetal DNA from maternal plasma. Prenat Diagn 2010;30:65–73.
34. Li DZ. Prenatal diagnosis of hemoglobin Bart's disease: what is the noninvasive approach? Prenat Diagn 2010;30:390.
35. Chow KC, Chiu RW, Tsui NB, et al. Mass spectrometric detection of an SNP panel as an internal positive control for fetal DNA analysis in maternal plasma. Clin Chem 2007;53:141–2.
36. Poon LL, Leung TN, Lau TK, et al. Differential DNA methylation between fetus and mother as a strategy for detecting fetal DNA in maternal plasma. Clin Chem 2002;48:35–41.
37. Old RW, Crea F, Puszyk W, et al. Candidate epigenetic biomarkers for non-invasive prenatal diagnosis of Down syndrome. Reprod Biomed Online 2007;15:227–35.
38. Chim SS, Jin S, Lee TY, et al. Systematic search for placental epigenetic markers on chromosome 21: towards noninvasive prenatal diagnosis of fetal trisomy 21. Clin Chem 2008;54:500–11.
39. Papageorgiou EA, Fiegler H, Rakyan V, et al. Sites of differential DNA methylation between placenta and peripheral blood: molecular markers for noninvasive prenatal diagnosis of aneuploidies. Am J Pathol 2009;174:1609–18.
40. Tong YK, Ding C, Chiu RW, et al. Noninvasive prenatal detection of fetal trisomy 18 by epigenetic allelic ratio analysis in maternal plasma: theoretical and empirical considerations. Clin Chem 2006;52:2194–202.
41. Herman JG, Graff JR, Myohanen S, et al. Methylation-specific PCR: a novel PCR assay for methylation status of CpG islands. Proc Natl Acad Sci U S A 1996;93:9821–6.
42. Grunau C, Clark SJ, Rosenthal A. Bisulfite genomic sequencing: systematic investigation of critical experimental parameters. Nucleic Acids Res 2001;29:E65.
43. Chiu RW, Cantor CR, Lo YM. Non-invasive prenatal diagnosis by single molecule counting technologies. Trends Genet 2009;25:324–31.

44. Vogelstein B, Kinzler KW. Digital PCR. Proc Natl Acad Sci U S A 1999;96: 9236–41.

45. Lun FM, Chiu RW, Chan KC, et al. Microfluidics digital PCR reveals a higher than expected fraction of fetal DNA in maternal plasma. Clin Chem 2008;54:1664–72.

46. Warren L, Bryder D, Weissman IL, et al. Transcription factor profiling in individual hematopoietic progenitors by digital RT-PCR. Proc Natl Acad Sci U S A 2006;103: 17807–12.

47. Fan HC, Quake SR. Detection of aneuploidy with digital polymerase chain reaction. Anal Chem 2007;79:7576–9.

48. Lo YM, Chiu RW. Next-Generation sequencing of plasma/serum DNA: an emerging research and molecular diagnostic tool. Clin Chem 2009;55:607–8.

49. Chiu RW, Chan KC, Gao Y, et al. Noninvasive prenatal diagnosis of fetal chromosomal aneuploidy by massively parallel genomic sequencing of DNA in maternal plasma. Proc Natl Acad Sci U S A 2008;105:20458–63.

50. Fan HC, Blumenfeld YJ, Chitkara U, et al. Noninvasive diagnosis of fetal aneuploidy by shotgun sequencing DNA from maternal blood. Proc Natl Acad Sci U S A 2008;105:16266–71.

51. Chiu RW, Sun H, Akolekar R, et al. Maternal plasma DNA analysis with massively parallel sequencing by ligation for noninvasive prenatal diagnosis of trisomy 21. Clin Chem 2010;56:459–63.

Hemoglobin Gene Therapy for β-Thalassemia

Arthur Bank, MD*

KEYWORDS

- Thalassemia • Cooley anemia • Gene therapy • Lentiviruses
- Clinical trials

Human globin gene therapy is an exciting approach to curing homozygous β-thalassemia (β-thalassemia, Cooley anemia) as well as sickle cell anemia. These diseases are particularly suitable for this approach because the specific genetic defects that cause them are known: sickle cell disease is caused by a point mutation in the human β-globin gene; most β-thalassemia mutations are also caused by single nucleotide changes, all of which lead to either decreased or absent normal β-globin protein. Human β-globin gene therapy with autologous modified stem cells has been envisioned for many years by patients, physicians, and scientists as a logical and ideal way to cure the disease. However, it is only recently that some limited success has been achieved.

The only cure for β-thalassemia (Cooley anemia) is allogeneic stem cell transplantation (ASCT), using stem cells from adult peripheral blood, bone marrow, or umbilical cord blood sources. ASCT is discussed in detail by Gaziev and Lucarelli elsewhere in this issue , as well as by Kanathezhath and Walters. ASCT is limited by immunologic differences between patients and potential donors; less than 30% of patients have suitable donors. A curative result occurs in the most eligible patients who fit the criteria for transplantation, most of whom are children. The potential development of graft-versus-host disease, a potentially life-threatening complication caused by immune reactions, has tempered the use of ASCT, especially when a completely compatible donor is not available.

There are 2 general approaches to providing normal β-globin function by gene therapy in these disorders: correction of the DNA defect in the β-globin gene by homologous recombination, or addition of a normal β-globin gene to the genome. Gene correction has the great advantage of maintaining the β-globin gene in its native

This article is adapted from a chapter in *Turning Blood Red: The Fight for Life in Cooley's Anemia*, by Arthur Bank, published by World Scientific Publishing. The author is a founder, equity holder, and consultant to Genetix Pharmaceuticals Inc, Cambridge, MA.
Columbia University, New York, NY, USA
* 4465 Douglas Avenue, New York, NY 10471.
E-mail address: ab13@columbia.edu

Hematol Oncol Clin N Am 24 (2010) 1187–1201
doi:10.1016/j.hoc.2010.08.002
0889-8588/10/$ – see front matter © 2010 Elsevier Inc. All rights reserved.

hemonc.theclinics.com

chromosomal environment, and thus is the preferred gene therapy approach. However, homologous recombination occurs at too low a frequency at present to be useful for human globin gene therapy.

Gene addition has been used successfully in human gene therapy clinical trials, with viral vectors transferring and expressing corrective genes in human hematopoietic cells. So-called γ-retroviral vectors containing Moloney viral components have been used to cure patients with severe immune disorders such as subacute combined immunodeficiency (SCID) and adenosine deaminase deficiency.[1-3] In these conditions, the gene-corrected lymphocytes are naturally selected for survival and expansion in preference to the patient's own defective cells, and even low-level transduction (infection) and expression of the corrective gene results in immune reconstitution of the affected T lymphocyte compartment, and cure.

No such selection currently exists for gene-corrected hematopoietic stem cells (HSC) containing and expressing the human β-globin gene in sickle cell disease or β-thalassemia. Thus, high levels of normal β-globin transfer and expression are required to cure these diseases.

GLOBIN GENE THERAPY

The current approach to human gene therapy for thalassemia is theoretically simple, using autotransplantation. HSC are taken from the patient, a normal hemoglobin (Hb) gene is added to the cells outside the body, and the human β-globin gene–corrected cells are returned to the patient intravenously. They automatically home and engraft in the marrow.

Gene therapy for β-thalassemia has been believed to be feasible since 1972, when β-globin complementary DNA, (cDNA), a copy of globin messenger RNA, was described.[4,5] Then, it was believed that the globin cDNA itself could be used as the source of the normal human β-globin gene sequences that could cure the disease. However, in the 1980s, it became clear that, in addition to the coding sequences present in globin cDNA, other important regulatory elements are required for successful and high-level human β-globin gene expression. These sequences include the intervening sequences within the gene, and regulatory sequences upstream and downstream of the human β-globin gene. In the late 1980s, Grosveld and colleagues[6] described important regulatory sequences far from the β-globin gene itself, called the β locus control region (β LCR) that are necessary to provide high level of expression of the human β-globin gene. The β LCR provides position-independent high-level enhancement of globin expression, and its discovery was seminal in moving β-globin gene therapy forward.[6]

Viruses as Vectors

Naked DNA can theoretically be used as the vector (or carrier) to transfer and express genes in human gene therapy, including those for human β-globin. However, viruses are much more efficient. Viruses are pieces of RNA or DNA wrapped in specialized viral proteins: after infecting cells, viruses use the host cell's molecular machinery to encode specific viral proteins, and express and assemble the proteins into viruses. Specific viral proteins on the surface of the viruses allow them to enter cells. After infection and integration, the viral DNA directs the synthesis of more of viral proteins; more viral particles assemble and are eventually extruded to infect more cells.

After infection, certain classes of viruses, adenoviruses, and, to some extent, adeno-associated viruses, remain in the cytoplasm of cells; they do not enter the nucleus and do not integrate into chromosomal DNA. These viruses are not useful for human blood stem cell gene therapy, a process that requires the corrective genes to integrate into the patient's chromosomes; this is necessary so that, when the gene-corrected stem cells divide, the corrective genes are transferred as part of the chromosomal material and maintained in daughter stem cells.

RNA viruses, called retroviruses, are most useful for human gene therapy. These viruses contain so-called *gag*, *pol*, and *env* gene sequences that lead to the production of the proteins required by the virus: gag proteins produce the core proteins of the virus; the *pol* gene specifies the enzyme, reverse transcriptase, which the viruses use to make a DNA copy of their RNA; the *env* genes code for the proteins of the viral envelope. These retroviruses also have genes that encode a protein called integrase, which enhances the integration of viral genetic material into chromosomal DNA.

Intact replication-competent retroviruses produce more viral particles after integration, often kill the cells they infect, release their viral particles from the cells, and infect more cells. Replication-competent viruses are not desirable for human gene therapy; not only can they kill the cells they transduce, but their integration at multiple sites in host chromosomes can activate cellular oncogenes in a process known as insertional mutagenesis. Instead, in human gene therapy, we use pieces of viruses, not intact viruses, in such a way that they are incapable of generating intact viral copies of themselves, while still carrying genes, such as the human β-globin gene, into cells and integrating those genes into chromosomal DNA. We make so-called replication-incompetent defective retroviruses (pseudoviruses) that, unlike their normal counterparts, are unable to reproduce themselves after they have inserted their genetic material into our chromosomes.

These defective viruses do not contain all of the proper genes and signals for new wild-type viral production on a single piece of DNA or RNA, as in replication-competent viruses. Defective viruses are created in so-called packaging cells; these are tissue culture cells into which the genes that produce the necessary viral proteins, gag, pol, env, and integrase, usually derived from Moloney leukemia viruses, are added, The viral genes encoding these proteins are added to the packaging cells on separate pieces of DNA called plasmids. The production of viral proteins in the packaging cells leads to the formation of empty viral particles with no DNA or RNA material capable of chromosomal integration.

When a suitable piece of DNA containing the corrective gene (in our case a human β-globin gene–containing gene vector) is added to these packaging cells, so-called producer cells are made. The nucleotide sequences on this vector plasmid are the only ones that are integrated into the host chromosomes after viral integration. With the production of gag, pol, env, and integrase proteins in the producer cells, retroviral particles are formed containing the RNA encoding the corrective gene. The producer cells then release intact viral particles into the medium. The pseudoviruses containing the human β-globin gene transfer their globin gene sequences into target HSC, integrate the gene sequences into chromosomal DNA, and allow the expression of potentially curative human β-globin. To reiterate, these defective viruses, unlike their normal counterparts, cannot reproduce themselves after they have inserted their genetic material into our chromosomes; components of the material necessary to produce intact viruses in this gene therapy system are on separate plasmids and cannot generate normal infectious wild-type virus.

I believed many years ago that defective viruses containing the human β-globin gene could be used as a pill that could be taken orally to cure sickle cell disease and thalassemia. I believed that the pill would uncoat in the stomach; viral particles would be released and enter the blood stream, exit at the right tissue location (in this case, the bone marrow), and integrate into HSC DNA. Several tissue-specific viruses are known. Two examples are hepatitis virus, which contains envelope proteins that target specific receptors on liver cells; and the acquired immune deficiency syndrome (AIDS) virus, which only infects T lymphocytes. However, it has not been possible to find viruses with envelopes that specifically target human HSC.

Instead, the approach has been to collect and concentrate HSC ex vivo, and use envelope proteins that can enter many different cell types, including HSC. HSC are obtained from either bone marrow or circulating blood, and our human β-globin gene–containing retrovirus is added outside the body; this provides a great advantage compared with other gene therapy applications in which the target organ cannot be removed. Exposure of the virus is limited to the gene-targeted blood cells and there is no danger of affecting non–blood cells. In addition, the ex vivo approach permits high ratios of virus to relevant HSC, levels that might not be possible if the gene therapy virus was given in vivo.

We used Moloney leukemia virus–based γ-retroviruses, to transfer and express human genes in 2 phase 1 human clinical trials to express a potential anticancer gene, the multiple drug resistance (MDR) gene, in human HSC.[7,8] For these trials, we developed safe and efficient defective packaging cell lines to produce the defective retroviruses.[9,10] We achieved the expression of the MDR gene in the bone marrow of patients, but at levels that were too low to be of clinical significance.[7,8]

Mouse Models

During the past 20 years, several groups have shown transfer and expression of a human β-globin gene into mouse HSC, occasionally at high levels, with γ-retroviral vectors.[11–14] In 1997, we reported one mouse that made 20% as much human β-globin as mouse β-globin.[14] However, this was a rare, significant, positive result among many negative ones.

Trial and error has shown that efficient globin gene therapy is not reproducible using γ-retroviral vectors. This finding is primarily because the target cell, the HSC, is largely quiescent; it divides infrequently. γ-Retroviruses require cell division to move their contents from the cytoplasm to the nucleus of cells. They are inefficient at having the viral particles enter the nucleus of HSC and integrating into the chromosomes of these cells that only occasionally divide.

To solve the problem of targeting nondividing human HSC, a special type of retrovirus, a so-called lentivirus, a virus that does not require cell division to achieve HSC target cell integration, is being used. Lentiviruses traverse the cytoplasm of nondividing cells and, after reverse transcription, lentiviral particles can move from the cytoplasm to the nucleus of cells without cell division. Sadelain and Leboulch pioneered the use of lentiviruses in human globin gene therapy.[15–18] Working independently, they showed that the anemia in mice with diseases resembling human homozygous β-thalassemia (Cooley anemia) and sickle cell disease can be alleviated significantly using lentiviruses containing a normal human β-globin gene.[15–18] These studies are the impetus for the current human globin clinical trial in Paris and proposed trials.

Sadelain and Leboulch were responsible for an earlier critical contribution to the human β-globin gene therapy field. They had previously shown that it was necessary to remove certain specific nucleotide sequences from human β-globin IVS2 for the globin retroviral vector to be appropriately reverse transcribed and expressed in target HSC.[19,20]

HUMAN GLOBIN GENE THERAPY

Human globin gene therapy is essentially autologous stem cell transplantation with gene transfer. HSC from blood or marrow are removed from the patient, transduced with the corrective human β-globin gene–containing lentivirus, and returned to the patient by vein (**Fig. 1**). This method overcomes the limitations of allogeneic transplantation because there are no immunologic barriers to engraftment, and, thus, many more patients are potentially eligible for treatment.

It is critical that human globin gene therapy specifically targets HSC, because these are the only cells capable of both cell division and HSC maintenance, as well as of erythroid differentiation. More differentiated transduced cells in the red blood cell lineage will merely continue to differentiate for days, lose their nuclei and become reticulocytes and mature red blood cells, and die.

In the past 2 decades, the environment for gene therapy research has been more favorable in France than in the United States. The unexpected death of a patient in a gene therapy trial at the University of Pennsylvania in 1999, using another type of virus, an adenovirus, had made this area of research less appealing to the scientific and medical community.[21] The first largely successful human clinical gene therapy trial was performed using γ-retroviruses in Paris in the late 1990s by Cavazzana-Calvo and colleagues.[1,2] Nine of the 10 children with X-linked SCID (X-SCID) in this trial were cured of the immunologic deficiency.[1,2]

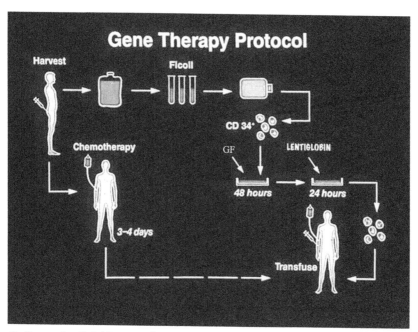

Fig. 1. Human Lentiglobin gene therapy. Bone marrow cells are harvested and purified by Ficoll gradients and exposure to anti-CD34 antibodies. The CD34+ cells are incubated with growth factors (GF) including interleukin 3, thrombopoietin, Flt3 ligand and stem cell factor for 24 to 48 hours, and then exposed to Lentiglobin, the human β-globin gene–containing virus, for 24 hours. While the cells are being processed, the patient's own bone marrow is ablated using chemotherapy. Then the gene-altered cells are transfused into the patient intravenously. (*Adapted from* Bank, A. Turning blood red: the fight for life in Cooley's anemia. Hackensack (NJ): World Scientific Publications; 2008. p. 216; with permission.)

Current Human Thalassemia Clinical Trial

The first and only ongoing human β-globin gene therapy clinical trial, is being performed in Paris.[22–24] A corrective human β-globin gene is being delivered using a proprietary lentiviral product called Lentiglobin (Genetics Pharmaceuticals Inc., Cambridge, MA). (I am a cofounder of Genetix, the primary medical consultant to it in the United States, and an equity shareholder). Lentiglobin contains the structural human β-globin gene as well as its promoter and critical elements of the human βLCR. Only these human β-globin gene–specific promoter-enhancer elements are actively transcribed after Lentiglobin sequences are integrated in the genome of gene-transduced target human HSC.[22,24]

The Lentiglobin gene–containing plasmid also contains the human immunodeficiency virus (HIV) Rev response element and other DNA elements that enhance nuclear migration of the viral DNA.[23,24] The Lentiglobin plasmid is a so-called self-inactivating (SIN) vector. It contains the 5′ HIV long terminal repeat (LTR) with its promoter and enhancer elements necessary for the transcription of Lentiglobin RNA and for the reverse transcription of this RNA as a DNA copy. However, the 3′ HIV LTR promoter–enhancer sequences in the SIN vector are rendered inactive by deletions.[22–24] As in all retroviruses, when reverse transcription occurs, the 3′ HIV LTR becomes the 5′ LTR sequences; in our case, the resulting Lentiglobin DNA 5′ LTR sequences are, thus, rendered inactive. This Lentiglobin SIN vector structure ensures that no HIV promoter or enhancer sequences are active in transcription after integration of Lentiglobin DNA into the host cell genome.

In addition, the Lentiglobin vector expresses so-called insulator sequences, short DNA sequences placed on either side of the β-globin sequences in the Lentiglobin plasmid, which prevent the activation of genes upstream or downstream of the insertion sites of the Lentiglobin vector. The cells that produce Lentiglobin virus also contain separate plasmids that encode and express lentiviral HIV gag and pol genes, and the envelope protein, vesicular stomatitis viral protein (VSV-G). The Lentiglobin virus used in the trial has been shown to express human β-globin at high levels in target human HSC in mice.[16,17]

One disadvantage of currently used lentiviral production, including Lentiglobin in the Paris trial, is that the expression of the viral HIV gag and pol proteins required are toxic to the producer cells. This toxicity requires that the Lentiglobin vector plasmid is transfected into a so-called transient packaging cell line system. In this system, the HIV gag-pol, VSV-G env, and Lentiglobin plasmids are added to the packaging cells, 293T monkey kidney cells, on separate plasmids, in small tissue culture dishes for 24 to 48 hours to transiently produce the Lentiglobin virus. Supernatants from several different tissue culture dishes are harvested and constitute the infectious Lentiglobin virus used in the trial. Pooled supernatants from the Lentiglobin virus–producing 293T cells are further purified by chromatography before being used to transduce the HSC target cells.

The use of transient lentiviral systems is not as convenient as more desirable stable producer lines developed with Moloney γ-retroviral components, in which all of the components of the virus are stably integrated into the packaging and producer cell lines; these stable lines were used in the human MDR gene therapy trials.[7,8] The lack of toxicity of Moloney gag-pol expression permits single clones of γ-retroviral stable producer lines to be isolated and grown to large volumes without cell death and used repeatedly. Several potentially useful stable lentiviral packaging lines have been described recently in which the HIV gag and pol genes are stably integrated into chromosomal DNA.[25–29] In these lines, the toxicity of the HIV gag-pol genes is circumvented by the transient and reversible expression of these genes using tetracycline control elements.[25–29] However, none of these lines is currently used in human clinical trials.

In the Paris gene therapy trial, CD34+ cells are isolated from the bone marrow or mobilized peripheral blood samples of patients; this CD34+ cell purification eliminates many differentiated cells, and concentrates the HSC. As previously noted, human HSC are the only relevant population for human globin gene therapy because only HSC can both self-renew and differentiate into erythroid cells, presumably for the life of the patient. More differentiated nucleated erythroid cells differentiate and die in days to weeks.

A Unique Human β-Globin Gene–containing Vector

In the ongoing phase 1 clinical trial in Paris, the human β-globin gene sequence in Lentiglobin has been modified by mutating a single amino acid at position 87 of the β-globin sequence.[22,24] Hb containing β87 globin (Hbβ87) has been shown to function normally in its expression and oxygen-carrying capacity.[16,17,30,31] It has also been shown that Hbβ87 acts like fetal Hb (HbF) in preferentially interfering with sickling in studies of human sickled cells, and may be particularly useful in gene therapy trials in patients with sickle cell disease.[30,31]

The major reason for using the β87 globin gene in Lentiglobin in patients with β-thalassemia is that Hbβ87 expression can easily be distinguished from that of normal Hb (HbA). Because all patients with thalassemia continue to have significant amounts of HbA in their blood as a result of transfusions after their transplantation, this distinction is extremely useful.

The amount of new β87 globin gene in the patients' cells can be measured by polymerase chain reaction (PCR). New β87 globin protein is quantitated by high-pressure liquid chromatography (HPLC). Thus, positive tests for the presence of the β87 gene by PCR, and for β87 globin by HPLC, are clear measures of the success of human β87 globin gene transfer and expression in the trial.

In the Paris trial, bone marrow is harvested from patients, CD34+ cells isolated, and Lentiglobin is transduced into these cells (see **Fig. 1**).[22,24] If adequate Lentiglobin transduction is documented in burst-forming unit, erythrocytes (BFU-E), and colony-forming units-granulocyte macrophage (CFU-GM) cultures from the patient's transduced marrow samples, the patient then undergoes full myeloablation, and the transduced cells are returned to the patient intravenously (see **Fig. 1**). The current principal investigators (PIs) in the trial are Drs Leboulch and Marina Cavazzana-Calvo. Dr Eliane Gluckman was an earlier co-PI.

Clinical trial protocols are a compromise between potential benefit and perceived or known risk: the so-called benefit/risk ratio. In the Paris trial, we accepted the increased risk of full marrow ablation to increase our chances for meaningful therapeutic benefit. This risk was accepted because previous experience in human allogeneic bone marrow transplantation (ABMT) has shown that less-than-complete ablation of a recipient's bone marrow is often insufficient to allow successful transplantation of donor cells.[32,33] It has been shown in mice that HSC transduced with retroviruses compete unfavorably with wild-type HSC for marrow engraftment.[34] This result suggests that, in human gene therapy protocols using reduced-intensity marrow ablation, the patient's residual unmodified HSC will outcompete transduced gene–corrected cells for marrow engraftment.

However, the risks of complete marrow ablation are also potentially greater than using nonmyeloablative regimens, with longer periods of leukopenia and thrombocytopenia after transplantation.

Results to Date

Two patients with thalassemia have been treated to date on the current Paris protocol.[24] The first patient, TK, is a woman with severe thalassemia. After the gene therapy procedure, she initially had evidence of a small amount of β87 globin gene transfer by PCR that was transient and too low to be clinically significant. However, her gene therapy treatment was not ideal because she received only one-third as many gene-corrected cells as planned. She survived several weeks of very low white blood cell and platelet counts, and was given antibiotics, white cell growth factors, and platelet transfusions to ameliorate these complications. She also continued to receive red blood cell transfusions to combat her anemia. She was eventually given an untransduced backup bone marrow sample (collected and stored as part of the protocol in case of the failure of the gene-corrected cells to engraft sufficiently). She has now fully recovered her white cell and platelet function.

The second patient, PLB, is a 19-year-old man, doubly heterozygous for β-thalassemia and HbE ($\alpha_2\beta^E_2$).[24] The β^E gene acts like a β^+ thalassemia allele and only provides limited output of β^E globin. The patient's HbE gene output has always been low (HbE<20% of normal HbA levels), and his limited HbE and HbF production have not prevented him from severe lifelong anemia and its complications. He required monthly transfusions since early childhood before the gene therapy procedure. He also continued to need transfusions for several months after transplantation with the β87-containing Lentiglobin vector.[24] In contrast to patient TK, he had only a short time after the gene therapy procedure of marrow hypoplasia during which his white blood cell (WBC) count and platelet count were low.

Several months after transplantation, PLB began to significantly increase his production of Hb β87.[24] This increased production has continued in the last 19 months (to June 2010), and he has not needed any blood transfusions during this time. He is the first patient with a human Hb disorder to obtain clinical benefit and become transfusion independent with human β-globin gene therapy.[24] He currently has approximately 9 to 10 g percent of Hb in his circulating blood, approximately one-third being Hb β87, one-third human HbF, and one-third HbE.[24] He has no residual transfused HbA.

Safety Issues

During the past year, analysis of the clonal composition of patient PLBs reconstituting β87-containing cells by linear amplification-mediated PCR has revealed that, although reconstitution is polyclonal, a single clone is dominant. This clone has arisen from the insertion of the Lentiglobin vector DNA into a specific gene, *Hmga2*; expression of Hb β87 by this clone in erythroid cells is largely responsible for the Hb β87 production in the patient.[23,24] Approximately 10% of the patient's CFU-GM and WBCs as well as BFU-E contain the same insertion of Lentiglobin into *Hmga2*, indicating that the clone is a multilineage clone, resembling a myeloid-biased HSC clone.[24]

Insertion of Lentiglobin into one of the introns of *Hmga2* with a loss of intronic function has occurred in this clone. This loss is similar to that occurring with other *Hmga2* mutations, some of which are associated with clonal proliferation.[24] Recent studies have shown that clonality, with loss of *Hmga2* introns, is more common than was previously believed in patients in other human gene therapy trials[35]; in most of these trials, these clones, presumably selected for their increased proliferative capacity, do not continue to expand over time.[35] The proliferation of the Lentiglobin-containing HMGA2 clone in PLB has continued at a low level in the past year. It is unknown whether the clone will expand, regress, or remain stable in the future.

The goals of human globin gene therapy are safety as well as efficacy. Experience from X-SCID trials is disconcerting in this regard. In these studies, although 9 of 10 patients in the Paris trial, and others in a similar trial in London, were cured of their disease, several patients have subsequently developed leukemia as a result of insertional mutagenesis.[2] The unacceptable events in these trials are probably related, at least in part, to the insertion of the curative gene in an HSC in the vicinity of an oncogene, a gene whose expression can cause the uncontrolled growth of cells and cancer.

In X-SCID, normal T lymphocytes lack a normal γC receptor gene, whose protein product is necessary to fight certain types of infections.[2] The curative γC receptor gene used in these gene therapy trials is expressed from a γ-retroviral promoter-enhancer LTR. In patients who developed leukemia, a rare cell inserted the γC receptor gene and its powerful nonspecific promoter-enhancer near a known oncogene, Lmo2, and activation of Lmo2 likely caused the emergence of the proliferative leukemic clone.[1]

The design of the Lentiglobin vector used in the Paris study theoretically avoids the potential problems of the γC vector in the X-SCID trial. As mentioned previously, first and most importantly, viral enhancer elements are not activated in the SIN Lentiglobin vector, as with the γC vector. Instead, only human β-globin gene–specific promoters and enhancers direct human β-globin gene expression, and these are only active in red blood cells. In addition, DNA sequences called insulators have been added to the Lentiglobin vector to prevent any potential activation of oncogene sequences, and the insertional mutagenesis seen in the X-SCID trial.

In patient PLB, the activation of HMGA2-mediated proliferation of a clone of HSC-like cells was not caused by activation of oncogenes by retroviral elements. The proliferative clone is most likely the effect of the insertion of the Lentiglobin vector directly into the intron of Hmga2 in one of the marrow stem cells during the initial transduction of the patient's HSC. Subsequently, the mutated clone was presumably selected for proliferation; increased HMGA2 protein expression by the clone in PLB's cells has been confirmed in laboratory studies.[24]

Other Lentiglobin Human Gene Therapy Trials

Additional patients with severe thalassemia are currently being recruited to the Paris trial. In addition, Dr Sadelain and his associates have planned a clinical trial with auto-transplantation to begin in the United States in the near future.[18,36] This trial will use a lentiviral human globin gene–containing vector designed by Dr Sadelain that is somewhat different from Lentiglobin.

The only other human gene therapy trial using lentiviral vectors, other than the human globin gene trial, has been reported recently in patients with the neurologic disease, X-linked adrenoleukeukodystrophy (ALD).[37] This is a rare disorder caused by a genetic defect in the ABCD1 receptor gene in which there is deficiency of ALD protein, an ATP-binding cassette transporter protein, required for normal myelination of neurons. The disease is progressive and must be treated early in life to prevent severe neurologic disability.[37]

ALD can be cured by ASCT. Macrophages produced by HSC have been shown to migrate to the central nervous system (CNS), to become functional glial cells capable of producing the normal required protein. In the gene therapy clinical trial of patients with ALD, also performed in Paris, 3 boys with ALD deficiency were treated. CD34+ cells were transduced with an ALD gene–containing lentiviral vector using procedures similar to those used in the Paris human globin gene trial.[37] In all 3 treated ALD patients, there was a lack of progression of CNS demyelination compared with that in untreated patients with ALD.[37] The results are encouraging and comparable with the relative clinical benefit obtained using ASCT. To date, there has been no evidence of specific clonal proliferation in any of the 3 ALD lentiviral vector–treated patients.

A New Homologous Recombination Approach to Thalassemia Gene Therapy

As discussed earlier, ideal human globin gene therapy for Cooley anemia as well as sickle cell anemia would be gene correction: the correction of the single base mutation in the DNA of the mutated human β-globin gene at its normal chromosomal position. This correction can be accomplished by adding a vast excess of DNA containing the normal β-globin DNA sequence to correct the mutant DNA sequence by homologous recombination in the HSC of patients with sickle cell disease and thalassemia. Gene correction has a great advantage compared with gene addition in that there is no possibility of insertional mutagenesis because the corrective piece of DNA used is short, biologically inert, and contains no viral elements; the only change in the patient's chromosomes is that the mutant β-globin gene is corrected.

However, as mentioned earlier, the frequency of gene correction occurring using HSC is currently too low to be clinically useful. This shortcoming is primarily because human HSC are limited in number and cannot be grown to large amounts in culture: they differentiate preferentially into later blood cell elements rather than dividing and reproducing themselves in large enough numbers to be useful for gene therapy.

Homologous recombination with gene correction has been successfully used for many years to correct several gene defects in mice using embryonic stem (ES) cells, the multipotential cells that are capable of producing any tissue of the animal.[38,39] This is because, in contrast with HSC, ES cells can be grown to large numbers without altering their biologic properties. These large numbers of cells are required for gene correction because it is such a rare event, and many individual cells must be isolated and analyzed before sufficient gene-corrected cells can be obtained.

However, in the past 5 years 2 extraordinary advances have occurred that increase the possibility that a gene correction strategy will eventually be used for gene therapy for thalassemia and sickle cell disease. First, Takahashi and Yamanaka[40] and Takahashi and colleagues[41] in Japan showed that human as well as mouse ES cells can be derived by manipulating skin cells from each of these sources. In these experiments, the addition and expression of just 4 genes (Klf4, Oct4, Sox2, and c-Myc) rewire the circuitry of the differentiated skin cells so that they acquire many of the characteristics of true ES cells. These reprogrammed cells are called induced pluripotent stem (iPS) cells. Before this discovery, human ES cells could only be obtained from living human embryos; this has been considered unethical by religious groups because it involves the destruction of embryos. The use of the patients' own skin cells to obtain ES cells greatly diminishes these concerns.

Second, it has been shown that mouse iPS cells derived from skin cells and manipulated in tissue culture can be used to cure mice with the equivalent of human sickle cell anemia.[42] In these experiments, skin cells from these mice were converted to iPS by the addition of the 4 special genes mentioned earlier; short inert pieces of normal human β-globin sequence DNA, containing sequences that correct the sickle cell mutation, were added to the skin-derived iPS of these sickle mice; iPS were grown to large amounts and the rare iPS in which the sickle cell mutation was corrected were isolated; the globin gene–corrected iPS were grown to large amounts and, after being treated in cell culture with growth factors and chemicals, became HSC.[42] These human β-globin gene–corrected HSC, originating from skin cells of mice, were then used to reconstitute the ablated bone marrow of the sickle mice and largely cured their sickle cell anemia, as assessed by correction of anemia and production of normal HbA.[42]

Using an iPS strategy, as with our Lentiglobin gene therapy, there are no immunologic barriers to transplantation because the skin cells originally used are derived from the patient. However, as previously noted, a great advantage of this skin to ES cell approach compared with our Lentiglobin addition gene therapy approach is that it avoids the possibility of insertional mutagenesis because no functional DNA is added to the patient's chromosomes.

One of the genes initially used to convert skin fibroblasts to iPS cells was c-myc, a known oncogene; increased expression of its protein product, c-Myc, is associated with cancer. More recently, several advances, including protocols without increased c-myc, have been made to address the problem.[43–49] Such safer methods of generating iPS cells from skin cells, avoiding c-Myc expression, and using small molecules and/or the required proteins themselves rather than retroviral vectors producing those proteins, may eventually make the use of human iPS cells more feasible for human β-globin gene therapy. It will also be necessary to develop efficient methods for the conversion of human iPS cells to human HSC to accomplish this goal.

Other Approaches to Thalassemia Gene Therapy

Another approach to curing β-thalassemia is to increase human HbF ($\alpha_2\gamma_2$) production. Studies leading to clinical trials using a human γ-globin–containing vector, instead of a human β-globin vector, have been proposed.[50]

Recent success in understanding γ-globin gene regulation and human γ- to β-globin switching in late fetal life has also suggested a different approach to thalassemia and sickle cell gene therapy.[51–53] Earlier, it had been shown that the protein Ikaros was an important regulator of human γ- to β-globin switching from data in mouse models.[51,54] More recently, it has been found that the action of a single human gene, BCL11A, is much more potent than that of Ikaros.[52,53]

Like Ikaros, BCL11A is expressed primarily in adult-type hematopoietic cells and forms chromatin remodeling complexes in these cells that suppress γ-globin production. In mice containing human γ- and β-globin transgenes, it has recently been shown that deletion of BCL11A leads to continued high-level production of HbF.[52] If an antisense strategy can be found to prevent BCL11A action in adult HSC, then continued high-level HbF production might cure β-thalassemia and sickle cell disease. Recent oligonucleotide and antisense RNA strategies may be useful in inhibiting BCL11A expression in human HSC, and provide the basis for such a new globin gene therapy approach.[55–57]

Strategies for the selection and enrichment of HSC containing and expressing a curative human β-globin gene have been of interest for the past 2 decades.[58–61] In this scenario, a retroviral vector plasmid containing both a selectable gene and a human β-globin gene is used. The selectable gene, most commonly the human MDR or methylguanine transferase (MGMT) gene, is one that is normally expressed at low levels in human HSC. Transfer and expression of retroviral vectors that permit high-level expression of MDR or MGMT in HSC then allow the preferential survival of transduced cells, after systemic administration of certain drugs that kill cells expressing only low levels of these proteins. Using this strategy, mouse HSC containing the MGMT and MDR vectors alone have been shown to be preferentially selected by drug administration in intact animals.[59,60]

However, human clinical trials using the human MDR or MGMT genes alone for HSC selection have been unsuccessful in significantly enriching for gene-expressing cells.[7,8] Most recently, a lentiviral vector containing both the human γ-globin gene and the MGMT gene has been shown to select for cells containing and expressing this bicistronic vector in mice.[61]

SUMMARY

ASCT is the only currently available curative option for thalassemia and sickle cell disease. Human β-globin gene therapy with autotransplantation of transduced human HSC is an exciting alternative approach to potential cure. One patient with thalassemia has recently been reported to show clinical benefit after lentiviral human globin gene therapy. He has not required blood transfusions for almost 2 years. Most of the patient's gene correction and new human β-globin gene expression is caused by the expansion of a single clone in which the corrective transgene is inserted into an *Hmga2* gene.

REFERENCES

1. Cavazzana-Calvo M, Hacein-Bey S, de Saint Basile G, et al. Gene therapy of human severe combined immunodeficiency (SCID)-X1 disease. Science 2000; 288(5466):669–72.
2. Cavazzana-Calvo M, Fischer A. Gene therapy for severe combined immunodeficiency: are we there yet? J Clin Invest 2007;117(6):1456–65.
3. Aiuti A, Cattaneo F, Galimberti S, et al. Gene therapy for immunodeficiency due to adenosine deaminase deficiency. N Engl J Med 2009;360(5):447–58.
4. Kacian D, Spiegelman S, Bank A, et al. In vitro synthesis of DNA components of human genes for globins. Nat New Biol 1972;235(58):167–9.
5. Verma IM, Temple GF, Fan H, et al. In vitro synthesis of DNA complementary to rabbit reticulocyte 10S RNA. Nat New Biol 1972;235(58):163–7.
6. Grosveld F, van Assendelft GB, Greaves DR, et al. Position-independent, high-level expression of the human beta-globin gene in transgenic mice. Cell 1987; 51(6):975–85.
7. Hesdorffer C, Ayello J, Ward M, et al. Phase I trial of retroviral-mediated transfer of the human MDR1 gene as marrow chemoprotection in patients undergoing high-dose chemotherapy and autologous stem-cell transplantation. J Clin Oncol 1998;16(1):165–72.
8. Abonour R, Williams DA, Einhorn L, et al. Efficient retrovirus-mediated transfer of the multidrug resistance 1 gene into autologous human long-term repopulating hematopoietic stem cells. Nat Med 2000;6(6):652–8.
9. Markowitz D, Goff S, Bank A. Construction and use of a safe and efficient amphotropic packaging cell line. Virology 1988;167(2):400–6.
10. Markowitz D, Goff S, Bank A. A safe packaging line for gene transfer: separating viral genes on two different plasmids. J Virol 1988;62(4):1120–4.
11. Dzierzak EA, Papayannopoulou T, Mulligan RC. Lineage-specific expression of a human beta-globin gene in murine bone marrow transplant recipients reconstituted with retrovirus-transduced stem cells. Nature 1988;331(6151):35–41.
12. Gelinas RE, Bender MA, Miller AD, et al. Long-term expression of the human beta-globin gene after retroviral transfer into pluripotent hematopoietic stem cells of the mouse. Adv Exp Med Biol 1989;271:135–48.
13. Plavec I, Papayannopoulou T, Maury C, et al. A human beta-globin gene fused to the human beta-globin locus control region is expressed at high levels in erythroid cells of mice engrafted with retrovirus-transduced hematopoietic stem cells. Blood 1993;81(5):1384–92.
14. Raftopoulos H, Ward M, Leboulch P, et al. Long-term transfer and expression of the human beta-globin gene in a mouse transplant model. Blood 1997;90(9): 3414–22.

15. May C, Rivella S, Callegari J, et al. Therapeutic haemoglobin synthesis in beta-thalassaemic mice expressing lentivirus-encoded human beta-globin. Nature 2000;406(6791):82–6.

16. Imren S, Payen E, Westerman KA, et al. Permanent and panerythroid correction of murine beta thalassemia by multiple lentiviral integration in hematopoietic stem cells. Proc Natl Acad Sci U S A 2002;99(22):14380–5.

17. Imren S, Fabry ME, Westerman KA, et al. High-level beta-globin expression and preferred intragenic integration after lentiviral transduction of human cord blood stem cells. J Clin Invest 2004;114(7):953–62.

18. Sadelain M. Recent advances in globin gene transfer for the treatment of beta-thalassemia and sickle cell anemia. Curr Opin Hematol 2006;13(3):142–8.

19. Leboulch P, Huang GM, Humphries RK, et al. Mutagenesis of retroviral vectors transducing human beta-globin gene and beta-globin locus control region derivatives results in stable transmission of an active transcriptional structure. EMBO J 1994;13(13):3065–76.

20. Sadelain M, Wang CH, Antoniou M, et al. Generation of a high-titer retroviral vector capable of expressing high levels of the human beta-globin gene. Proc Natl Acad Sci U S A 1995;92(15):6728–32.

21. Couzin J, Kaiser J. Gene therapy. As Gelsinger case ends, gene therapy suffers another blow. Science 2005;307(5712):1028.

22. Bank A, Dorazio R, Leboulch P. A phase I/II clinical trial of beta-globin gene therapy for beta-thalassemia. Ann N Y Acad Sci 2005;1054:308–16.

23. Anonymous. Beta thalassemia treatment succeeds, with a caveat. Science 2009;326:1468–9.

24. Cavazzana-Calvo M, Payen E, Negre O, et al. Transfusion independence and HMGA2 activation after gene therapy of human thalassemia. Nature 2010;467:318–22

25. Cockrell AS, Ma H, Fu K, et al. A trans-lentiviral packaging cell line for high-titer conditional self-inactivating HIV-1 vectors. Mol Ther 2006;14(2):276–84.

26. Cockrell AS, Kafri T. Gene delivery by lentivirus vectors. Mol Biotechnol 2007;36(3):184–204.

27. Broussau S, Jabbour N, Lachapelle G, et al. Inducible packaging cells for large-scale production of lentiviral vectors in serum-free suspension culture. Mol Ther 2008;16(3):500–7.

28. Throm RE, Ouma AA, Zhou S, et al. Efficient construction of producer cell lines for a SIN lentiviral vector for SCID-X1 gene therapy by concatemeric array transfection. Blood 2009;113(21):5104–10.

29. Stewart HJ, Leroux-Carlucci MA, Sion CJ, et al. Development of inducible EIAV-based lentiviral vector packaging and producer cell lines. Gene Ther 2009;16(6):805–14.

30. Ho C, Willis BF, Shen TJ, et al. Roles of alpha 114 and beta 87 amino acid residues in the polymerization of hemoglobin S: implications for gene therapy. J Mol Biol 1996;263(3):475–85.

31. De Angioletti M, Lacerra G, Pagano L, et al. Beta-thalassaemia-87 C → G: relationship of the Hb F modulation and polymorphisms in compound heterozygous patients. Br J Haematol 2004;126(5):743–9.

32. Michlitsch JG, Walters MC. Recent advances in bone marrow transplantation in hemoglobinopathies. Curr Mol Med 2008;8(7):675–89.

33. Lucarelli G, Gaziev J. Advances in the allogeneic transplantation for thalassemia. Blood Rev 2008;22(2):53–63.

34. Qin S, Ward M, Raftopoulos H, et al. Competitive repopulation of retrovirally transduced haemopoietic stem cells. Br J Haematol 1999;107(1):162–8.
35. Wang GP, Berry CC, Malani N, et al. Dynamics of gene-modified progenitor cells analyzed by tracking retroviral integration sites in a human SCID-X1 gene therapy trial. Blood 2010;115(22):4356–66.
36. Sadelain M, Boulad F, Galanello R, et al. Therapeutic options for patients with severe beta-thalassemia: the need for globin gene therapy. Hum Gene Ther 2007;18(1):1–9.
37. Cartier N, Hacein-Bey-Abina S, Bartholomae CC, et al. Hematopoietic stem cell gene therapy with a lentiviral vector in X-linked adrenoleukodystrophy. Science 2009;326(5954):818–23.
38. Doetschman T, Gregg RG, Maeda N, et al. Targetted correction of a mutant HPRT gene in mouse embryonic stem cells. Nature 1987;330(6148):576–8.
39. Templeton NS, Roberts DD, Safer B. Efficient gene targeting in mouse embryonic stem cells. Gene Ther 1997;4(7):700–9.
40. Takahashi K, Yamanaka S. Induction of pluripotent stem cells from mouse embryonic and adult fibroblast cultures by defined factors. Cell 2006;126(4):663–76.
41. Takahashi K, Tanabe K, Ohnuki M, et al. Induction of pluripotent stem cells from adult human fibroblasts by defined factors. Cell 2007;131(5):861–72.
42. Hanna J, Wernig M, Markoulaki S, et al. Treatment of sickle cell anemia mouse model with iPS cells generated from autologous skin. Science 2007;318(5858):1920–3.
43. Wang Y, Nakayama N. WNT and BMP signaling are both required for hematopoietic cell development from human ES cells. Stem Cell Res 2009;3(2–3):113–25.
44. Maherali N, Hochedlinger K. Tgfbeta signal inhibition cooperates in the induction of iPSCs and replaces Sox2 and cMyc. Curr Biol 2009;19(20):1718–23.
45. Lin T, Ambasudhan R, Yuan X, et al. A chemical platform for improved induction of human iPSCs. Nat Methods 2009;6(11):805–8.
46. Kim PG, Daley GQ. Application of induced pluripotent stem cells to hematologic disease. Cytotherapy 2009;11(8):980–9.
47. Kaufman DS. Toward clinical therapies using hematopoietic cells derived from human pluripotent stem cells. Blood 2009;114(17):3513–23.
48. Ichida JK, Blanchard J, Lam K, et al. A small-molecule inhibitor of tgf-Beta signaling replaces sox2 in reprogramming by inducing nanog. Cell Stem Cell 2009;5(5):491–503.
49. Huang J, Chen T, Liu X, et al. More synergetic cooperation of Yamanaka factors in induced pluripotent stem cells than in embryonic stem cells. Cell Res 2009;19(10):1127–38.
50. Pestina TI, Hargrove PW, Jay D, et al. Correction of murine sickle cell disease using gamma-globin lentiviral vectors to mediate high-level expression of fetal hemoglobin. Mol Ther 2009;17(2):245–52.
51. Bank A. Regulation of human fetal hemoglobin: new players, new complexities. Blood 2006;107(2):435–43.
52. Sankaran VG, Menne TF, Xu J, et al. Human fetal hemoglobin expression is regulated by the developmental stage-specific repressor BCL11A. Science 2008;322(5909):1839–42.
53. Sankaran VG, Xu J, Ragoczy T, et al. Developmental and species-divergent globin switching are driven by BCL11A. Nature 2009;460(7259):1093–7.
54. Lopez RA, Schoetz S, DeAngelis K, et al. Multiple hematopoietic defects and delayed globin switching in Ikaros null mice. Proc Natl Acad Sci U S A 2002;99(2):602–7.

55. Tulpule A, Daley GQ. Efficient gene knockdowns in human embryonic stem cells using lentiviral-based RNAi. Methods Mol Biol 2009;482:35–42.
56. Scherr M, Venturini L, Eder M. Knock-down of gene expression in hematopoietic cells. Methods Mol Biol 2009;506:207–19.
57. Manjunath N, Wu H, Subramanya S, et al. Lentiviral delivery of short hairpin RNAs. Adv Drug Deliv Rev 2009;61(9):732–45.
58. DelaFlor-Weiss E, Richardson C, Ward M, et al. Transfer and expression of the human multidrug resistance gene in mouse erythroleukemia cells. Blood 1992; 80(12):3106–11.
59. Podda S, Ward M, Himelstein A, et al. Transfer and expression of the human multiple drug resistance gene into live mice. Proc Natl Acad Sci U S A 1992; 89(20):9676–80.
60. Allay JA, Davis BM, Gerson SL. Human alkyltransferase-transduced murine myeloid progenitors are enriched in vivo by BCNU treatment of transplanted mice. Exp Hematol 1997;25(10):1069–76.
61. Zhao H, Pestina TI, Nasimuzzaman M, et al. Amelioration of murine beta-thalassemia through drug selection of hematopoietic stem cells transduced with a lentiviral vector encoding both gamma-globin and the MGMT drug-resistance gene. Blood 2009;113(23):5747–56.

BONUS ARTICLES:
Mouse Models of Inherited Cancer Syndromes

Sohail Jahid, BS, Steven Lipkin, MD, PhD

Lower Gastrointestinal Tract Cancer Predisposition Syndromes

Neel B. Shah, MB, ChB, Noralane M. Lindor, MD

Mouse Models of Inherited Cancer Syndromes

Sohail Jahid, BS[a,b], Steven Lipkin, MD, PhD[a,b],*

KEYWORDS

- GEM (Genetically engineered mice)
- Hereditary cancer syndrome • Cancer genetics

MOUSE MODELS AND CANCER

Tumorigenesis is a heterogenous and complex process that involves hundreds if not thousands of genetic and environmental factors. These include both cell autonomous processes (ie, the impact of mutations in the cells that transform into cancer cells) and cell non-autonomous processes involving the tumor niche. Some of the more prominent processes in the tumor niche include adequate oxygenation, nutrition, angiogenesis, and immune surveillance, among others. Historically, this complexity has been challenging to tease apart using in vitro systems. Mouse models are instrumental in studying tumorigenesis in a dynamic physiologic system and have become an integral part of the approach to understanding the mechanistic basis of tumorigenesis. These processes include the action of oncogenes and tumor suppressor genes, the biology and interaction of host and tumor, and potential risk and benefit of chemotherapeutic agents. The laboratory mouse (*Mus musculus*) has become one of the best model system for the study of tumorigenesis, because of their well annotated genome, small size and the ability to breed in captivity, as well as the ease at which they can be manipulate at the genomic level. Due to obvious ethical limitations on the ability to perform studies in human patients—long-term prevention studies or drug screening in uncommon diseases, such as many cancer genetic syndromes—the mouse has become an indispensable tool in mechanistic, therapeutic, and natural history studies

This article was originally planned for publication in the October 2010 issue (24:5) devoted to Genetic Predisposition to Cancer, guest edited by Drs. Kenneth Offit and Mark Robson. To see the rest of the articles in that issue, go to www.hemonc.theclinics.com.

[a] Department of Biological Chemistry, University of California Irvine, Irvine, CA
[b] Department of Genetic Medicine, Weill Cornell College of Medicine, Cornell University, New York, NY 10021, USA
* Corresponding author. Department of Medicine, Weill Cornell College of Medicine, Cornell University, New York, NY 10021.
E-mail address: stl2010@med.cornell.edu

Hematol Oncol Clin N Am 24 (2010) 1205–1228
doi:10.1016/j.hoc.2010.08.011
0889-8588/10/$ – see front matter © 2010 Elsevier Inc. All rights reserved.

of cancer etiology and progression. As the development of more sophisticated models moves forward, different aspects of cancer biology can be examined and better therapeutic agents can be developed.

MOUSE MODELS OF INHERITED CANCER—GENETIC SYNDROMES

There are estimated to be more than 6000 mendelian genetic disorders and more than 50 human familial cancer syndromes.[1,2] Many of these diseases are rare, some vanishingly so, but all are aberrations in a specific gene, including those that involve tumor suppressor genes.[3] This situation applies to many cancer genetic syndromes, some of which have an evolutionary selection against propagation of mutations in the underlying genes from generation to generation. As described in more detail in the article by Powers and colleagues elsewhere in this issue, inherited cancer genetic syndromes can be broadly defined as diseases that involve germline mutations carried throughout the entire body. Using what are current standard techniques, genetically engineered mice (GEM) can be generated to have the precise germline mutations carried by patients. With this approach, loss of function mutations, rare dominant-negative, gain-of-function, and misfunction mutations in the same gene can be studied that reflect the operant mechanisms of these different mutations and to obtain a more complete understanding of allelic heterogeneity in monogenic disorders. Furthermore, many gene interactions, as seen in human tumors, can only be studied under compound mutant animals by crossing different mutant mice. Modifier genes are important in human cancer genetics, and mouse models can tease apart the effect of these genes as well.

GASTROINTESTINAL TUMORS

Several mouse models have been used to study gastrointestinal neoplasias that arise from familial and sporadic syndromes. Mendelian diseases of colorectal cancer (CRC) include familial adenomatous polyposis (FAP), Lynch syndrome, Peutz-Jeghers syndrome (PJS), and Cowden disease (**Tables 1** and **2**).[1,3]

Familial Adenomatous Polyposis

FAP is a rare hereditary syndrome characterized by development of hundreds of colonic polyps during late teens or early twenties of the affected individual. Some of the polyps inevitably transform into colonic carcinomas. Almost all FAP is caused by a mutation in the adenomatous polyposis coli (*APC*) gene. Less frequently, mutations in the base excision repair gene, *MYH*, can cause an attenuated form of FAP.[4] To better mimic common mutations found in FAP patients, several mouse models of *Apc* mutation have been constructed using gene knockout methods other than Apc^{min}. $Apc^{\triangle 716}$ contains a truncating mutation at codon 716, and Apc^{1638N} contains a truncating mutation at codon 1638.[5,6] All three mutations produced different polyp burden in the small intestine on the same background; Apc^{min} producing the most polyps of 100 or more and Apc^{1638} the least number at approximately 3.[7] The polyps were phenotypically indistinguishable from one another in all three mutant models. The advantage of the Apc^{1638N} model for FAP is that with a lower polyp burden, these animals have an increased life span and develop more advanced tumors useful for studying tumor progression and metastasis. They are also useful for looking at positive synergy with mutations in other candidate tumor suppressors, whereas Apc^{Min} are better for testing chemopreventive drugs (eg, assaying for reduced adenoma burden). A confounding finding in the *Apc* deficient mice is that adenomas form in the small intestine instead of colon as seen more commonly in FAP patients. However, *Apc* mouse models have shed much light on the role of Wnt pathway

Table 1
Familial adenomatous polyposis in genetically engineered mice models

Gene	Phenotype	Tumor Incidence	Multiplicity	References
Apc^{min}	Adenoma, small intestine	High	58	5–7,10
Apc^{1638}	Adenoma/carcinoma; small intestine, colon	Low	4	7,9,10
$Apc^{\triangle716}$	Adenoma; small intestine, colon	High	254	5–7,10
Double mutants				
$Apc^{\triangle716}$, Ptgs2 (COX-2)	Adenoma, small intestine	Low	98	9,11
Apc^{min}, Ptgs1 (COX-1)	Adenoma, small intestine	Low	18	8
Apc^{min}, Ptgs2 (COX-2)	Adenoma, small intestine	Low	12	8

in the initiation, development, and progression of CRCs. Furthermore, these mouse models have been useful in studying the effect of modifiers of *Apc* mutations and activated WNT signaling, as well as studying the impact of diet in the process of CRC development. Several modifiers of min-1 have been identified in mice which have provided insight into their epistatic interaction with *APC*. Other mutations that affect the formation of intestinal adenomas in *Apc*[min] mice are genes in archidonic acid pathway.[8] One of these genes is COX-2 Ptgs2, and the double mutant, *Apc*[716]; Ptgs2, has been helpful in interpreting the impact of nonsteroidal anti-inflammatory drugs on mechanisms of colon polyp development. Moreover, the introduction of a cyclooxygenase 1 and 2 (COX-1 an COX-2) mutations in the *Apc*[min] mice had a pronounced effect on the size and number of intestinal polyps.[9–11] This mouse model has been useful for providing a model system for chemoprevention studies, using nonsteroidal anti-inflammatory drugs to treat patients suffering from familial and sporadic polyposis.[12,13]

Lynch Syndrome

Mouse models for DNA mismatch repair (MMR) genes, *MLH1/MSH2/MSH6/PMS2*, have been under investigation for many years; MMR mouse models have been highly valuable in revealing the mechanisms of MMR genes in cancer biology.[14] MMR prevents cancer and suppresses tumors through several mechanisms. These include (1) single base substitution repair, (2) insertion/deletion frameshift repair (also called microsatellite instability), (3) anti-apoptosis, and (4) suppression of promiscuous homeologous recombination. *MLH1* and *MSH2* mutations are responsible for greater than 90% of all cases of Lynch syndrome; other MMR genes mutations are less deleterious.[15] *Msh2* is an essential part of the *MutS* protein complex and several knockout mouse models of *Msh2* have been generated.[16–18] These mice have a reduced life span as a result of aggressive lymphomas, specifically T-cell lymphomas, intestinal tumors, and other tumor types as well as sebaceous gland tumors similar to those in Muir-Torre syndrome patients. Mice with biallelic mutations in *Mlh1/Msh2/Msh6/Pms2* exhibits some of the same malignances seen in humans with biallelic inactivation of the same genes, such as hematologic disorders, that results in shorter life span.[19] One of the hallmarks of MMR deficiency in mice and in humans is the microsatellite instability (MSI) phenotype, reflecting the accumulation of repetitive sequences in the genome. There are, however, differences in the development of the disease in GEM that are deficient in MMR genes as compared to

Table 2
Familial gastrointestinal cancer syndromes in genetically engineered mice models

Gene	Tumor Incidence	Tumor Type/Tumor Site	Repair Defect (MSI)		DNA Damage Response	References
			Mononucleotide	Dinucleotide		
MutS homologs						
Msh2–/–	High	Adenoma, carcinoma; small intestine, colon	High	High	Defective	16,18,19
Msh3–/–	Low	Adenoma	Moderate	High	Normal	21,25
Msh6 –/–	High	Adenoma	None	Low	Defective	22,23
Msh3–/––Msh6–/–	High	Adenoma, carcinoma; small intestine, colon				25
Msh2loxp; Vill-cre	High	Adenoma, colon	N/A	N/A	Normal	17
MutL homologs						
Mlh1–/–	High	Adenoma, carcinoma; stomach, small intestine, colon	High	High	Defective	19,26–29
Pms2–/–	Low	Adenoma; brain	Low	Low	Normal	29–32
Mlh3–/–	Low	Adenoma; small intestine	Moderate	N/A	Defective	32–34
Pms1–/–	None	None	Low	Low	N/A	29
Mlh3–/––Pms2–/–	High	Adenoma, carcinoma; stomach, small intestine, colon	High	N/A	Defective	32,33
Pms2 cre-lox	Low	Adenoma	Low	Low	Normal	35
Knock-in models						
Msh2^G674A/G674A	High	Adenoma; small intestine	High	High	Normal	37,38
Msh6^T1217D/T1217D	High	Adenoma; small intestine	High	High	Normal	38
Mlh1^G67R/G67R	High	Adenoma; small intestine	High	High	Normal	39
Lkb1+/–	N/A	Stomach, small intestine, liver, mammary	N/A	N/A	N/A	53
IBD/somatic inactivation						
IL-2–/–	No tumor/colitis	Colon	N/A	N/A	N/A	43
IL-10–/–	No tumor/enterocolitis	Intestinal	N/A	N/A	N/A	42
Muc2–/–	No tumor/colitis	Colon	N/A	N/A	N/A	44,45
Giv2–/–	Low	Right side colon	High	High	N/A	46,47

human patients; in humans, most of the tumor development occurs in the colon and extracolonic cancers, including endometrium. In order for mice to develop endometrial cancer, MMR-deficient mice must be crossed with *Pten* or other tumor suppressor gene knockout mice.[20] A new mouse model that addresses the difference in tumor development between mice and humans is the conditional mouse line of *Msh2*[loxp]; *Vill*-cre, which directs tumor development to the colon instead of the intestine as was seen in earlier mouse models for Lynch syndrome, and avoids development of lymphomas.[17] *Msh6*-deficient mice show a much later onset of tumor development as compared with *Msh2*[−/−] mice.[21] Since the role of *Msh6* in the MMR system is mostly repair of base substitution and repair of single base IDs, its deficiency does not affect the repair of 2 to 4 base insertion-deletion loops; therefore, mice with *Msh6* mutation mostly accumulate base substitutions mutations as opposed to frameshift mutations seen in *Msh2*[−/−] mice, and the phenotype of MSI is not seen in tumors from these animals. *Msh6*[−/−] mouse models show a similar phenotype of cancer onset and progression seen in Lynch syndrome patients with mutations in *MSH6* gene, where most cancer development and progression occurs at around 60 years or older with variable MSI phenotypes.[22,23] *MSH6* mutation has also been linked to endometrial cancers in Lynch syndrome patients and *Msh6*[−/−] mice are reported to develop endometrial cancers.[21,24] Mouse models for *Msh3* deficiency show a slight predisposition to the development of cancer due to moderate repair defects and display a normal life span. *Msh3*-deficient mouse cells are not able to efficiently repair 1 to 4 base insertion-deletion loops, yet due to the presence of *Msh6* they are efficiently able to repair single base substitution.[25] Similarly, human patients with *MSH3* mutations develop late-onset tumorigenesis. The *MutL* homologs (*MLH* and *PMS* genes) play important roles in DNA excision during repair, acting as molecular scaffold for additional proteins to coalesce. At the heart of the three *Mutl* complexes, *Mlh1/Mlh3*, *Mlh1/Pms2*, and *Mlh1/Pms1*, lies *Mlh1*. MLH1 deficiency in humans is responsible for shortened life span and a strong predisposition to cancer. *Mlh1* knockout mice do not have MMR capacity; therefore, due to the high rate of base substitution, as well as small insertions and deletions in mono- and dinucleotide repeats, these mice have high mutator phenotype similar to *Msh2*[−/−] mice. Mice deficient in *Mlh1* also have a shortened life span and high degree of predisposition for cancer development.[26-29] Combined mutations of *Mlh1* and *Msh2* do not change the tumor suppressor phenotype, consistent with the idea that they both participate in the same complex (M. Liskay, personal communication, 2004). The tumor spectrum of *Mlh1*[−/−] mice includes T-cell lymphomas, intestinal adenomas, and adenocarcinomas as well as skin tumors.[19] PMS2 deficiency in humans is associated with Lynch syndrome as well as Turcot syndrome, a rare genetic condition that also predisposes patients to both multiple adenomatous colon polyps and brain tumors.[30] *Pms2*[−/−] mice exhibit different disease progression; they show a milder mutator phenotype and an increase in mutation frequency at mononucleotide repeat tracts, but they do not develop any intestinal or brain adenomas; rather, they mostly develop lymphomas and sarcomas with a delayed onset.[29,31] Recently characterized *Mlh3* gene deficiency has been shown to have similar effects as *Pms2* deficiency in mice and human patients with the same mutation.[32-34] One major difference between *Pms2*[−/−] and *Mlh3*[−/−] deficiencies is that *Mlh3*[−/−] mice develop small intestinal adenomas and adenocarcinomas as well as extra-gastrointestinal tumors, including lymphomas and basal cell carcinomas of the skin. Similar to *Msh3* and *Msh6* combined inactivation mimicking *Msh2*[−/−], combined inactivation of *Pms2* and *Mlh3* increases the level of mutator phenotype to that of *Mlh1*[−/−]. Thus, *Mlh3*[−/−]*Pms2*[−/−] mice display similar disease development and progression as *Mlh1*[−/−] mice.[25,32] From these mouse models, it has become clear that *Pms2* and *Mlh3* and *Msh3* and *Msh6* have redundant roles in repair and tumor suppression functions and that is the most likely reason penetrance is lower in patients deficient in any one of these genes.[21,25] In a recently reported *Pms2*-cre mouse model, where a cell division–activated cre-lox system for stochastic recombination of Lox-P-flanked loci was used, this system was able to better mimic the spontaneous mutation that occurs in cancer.[35]

MMR deficiency in mice results in DNA repair and DNA damage response defect, where both of these mechanisms are important in suppression of tumorigenesis. To study the role of each mechanism, knock-in mouse models have been generated where the mice carrying a recurrent mutation in a gene renders DNA repair mechanism null. *Msh2*^{G67A} (*Msh2*^{GA}) was one of the first knock-in mutant model with separation-of-function mutation similar to *MSH2* missense mutation seen in patients.[36–38] As predicted, this mutant lost its DNA repair capability but retained its DNA damage response, and *MEFs* from these mice responded to cisplatin, 6-thioguanine (6-TG), and N-methyl-N-nitro-N-nitrosoquanidine (MNNG).[37] Mouse models of *Mlh1*^{G67R} caused a separation of function in the *Mlh1* protein; the DNA damage repair was impaired whereas DNA damage response, including apoptotic response to cisplatin, remained intact. These mice displayed strong cancer predisposition similar to *Mlh1*$^{-/-}$; however, they developed fewer intestinal adenomas.[39] To date, more than 250 different germline mutations have been identified in *MLH1* patients.[40] These new mouse models of different missense mutations, which can elicit different phenotype and, more importantly, different response to therapy, are promising in terms of tailored therapy for variances that exist in patients.

Somatic DNA Mismatch Repair Inactivation

Inflammatory bowel disease (IBD), including ulcerative colitis and Crohn disease, has been linked to the development of cancer.[41] The immune system has been shown to play an important role in colonic inflammation. Several mouse models with deletion of immune-specific genes, such as those for interleukin (IL)-2, IL-10, T-cell receptor chains, and major histocompatibility complex class II molecules, have been generated.[10] These mice have a strong predisposition for developing colorectal adenocarcinomas. IL-2– and IL-10–defective mice display immune system aberrations as well as IBD similar to humans.[42,43] Mucin2 (MUC2) is a secretory protein in the intestinal mucosa, and mice made deficient of Muc2 become prone to inflammation and subsequently develop intestinal adenomas and invasive adenocarcinomas.[44,45] G-protein alpha subunit (Gia2) knockout mouse develops spontaneous colitis and nonpolyposis, right-sided, multifocal CRCs with mucinous histology; and a Crohn-like inflammatory infiltrate. Gia2−/− mice is the first mouse model of somatically acquired MMR deficiency due to inflammation through repression of *Mlh1* promoter.[46,47] These mice also show MSI phenotype as the result of *Mlh1* repression. Treatment of Gia2−/− mice with histone deacetylase inhibitor (HDACi) decreases colitis and relieves epigenetic repression of *Mlh1* expression.[46] IBD mouse models are important because gastrointestinal inflammation is considered a strong risk for developing CRC. Suberoylanilide hydroxamic acid is an HDACi that is currently used in the treatment of cutaneous T-cell lymphoma and is in clinical trial for other cancers; the use of this compound could be extended to treatment of IBD and associated diseases.[48–50]

Peutz-Jeghers Syndrome

PJS is autosomal dominant disease with variable inheritance caused by germline mutation in LKB1/STK11.[51] LKB1/STK11 is a serine/theonine kinase and is considered to be a tumor suppressor. PJS is characterized by hamartomatous polyposis of the gastrointestinal tract, mostly in the small intestine, with a strong predisposition to malignancy, as well as developing mammary tumors and mucocutenous pigmentation.[52] Lkb1/Stk11 null mutation in mice is lethal and Lkb1/Stk11 heterozygous mice exhibit a similar phenotype to PJS patients as they also develop gastrointestinal hamartomatous without wild-type allele inactivation.[53–56] Furthermore, heterozygous mutation of Lkb1 is sufficient for the development of gastrointestinal hamartomas that exhibited histologic features similar to PJS patients.[53] This mouse model has showed that biallelic inactivation is not necessary for hamartoma development and, therefore, it is plausible that LKB1 loss of heterozygosity (LOH) would result in malignant transformation of hamartomas along with other mutations.[56] Furthermore, the life span of a mouse is too short to allow for the inactivation of wild-type allele and any further genetic hits necessary for progression to malignancy as seen in LKB1 inactivation in humans. A proposed mechanism for LKB1's tumor suppression capability is that it is involved in the p53-dependent apoptosis and decreased level of LKB1 protein would suppress growth arrest and apoptosis, which leads to accumulation of somatic mutations.[53] Furthermore, the Wnt pathway is not activated in Lkb1± hamartomas; however, LKB1 LOH adenomatous lesions showed β-catenin mutation, suggesting that mutation in the Wnt pathway is also important for the progression of hamartomas to carcinomas along with LKB1 LOH.[56]

BREAST CANCER AND COWDEN DISEASE

Several genes with germline mutations have been implicated in the development of breast cancer (ie, BRCA1, BRCA2, PTEN [Cowden disease], p53 and STK11/LKB1 [PJS]) (Table 3).[1,57]

Table 3
Familial breast cancer syndromes in genetically engineered mice models

Gene	p53 Comutation	cre-Transgene	Tumor Type	Mean Tumor Latency	References
Brca1 tr/tr	No		Mammary, lymphoma		10,58,75
Brca1 5-6	No		Lymphoma		10,58
Brca1 Δ11 loxp/loxp	No	MMTV-cre	Mammary	>13	59,68
Brca1 Δ11 loxp/loxp	p53Null	MMTV-cre or WAP-cre	Mammary	8	59,67
Brca1 Δ11 loxp/loxp	p53Δ5-6	WAP-cre	Mammary	7	59,84
Brca1 Δ22-24 loxp/loxp	p53Null	BLG-cre	Mammary, lymphoma	7	59,72
Brca1 Δ5-13 loxp/loxp	p53Δ20-10	K14-cre	Mammary	7	59,71
Brca1 Δ1loxp/loxp	No	WAP-cre	Mammary	18	59,61
Brca2 Δ27/27			Lymphoma, sarcoma, carcinoma		10,74
Brca2 Tr2014			Lymphoma		10,58
Brca2 loxp/loxp		WAP-cre	Mammary		10,75
Pten±	No		Mammary tumors		10,20,87,88,91
Pten loxp/loxp	No	Gfap-cre	Non-neoplastic brain lesions		10,89,90
Pten loxp/loxp		MMTV-cre	Mammary tumors		91

Germline mutations in *BRCA1* and *BRCA2* has been confirmed as increasing the rate of breast cancer and ovarian cancer.[58] The risk for other cancers in germline mutations of these two genes is still under investigation. The limitations of homozygous *Brca1/2* mice have been embryonic lethality and the lack of sporadic tumors. Conditional mouse models for *BRCA1* targeted to the breast epithelial cells have been made; these models have been able to shed light on the mechanism of tumor initiation and progression. To date, ten conventional *Brca1* knockout models, each carrying a different mutation, have been generated and none of the heterozygous mice has been able to recapitulate the human heterozygous *BRCA1* germline mutation.[59] Conditional *Brca1* alleles and *Brca2* alleles have also been generated, each displaying a different phenotype. These conditional mice were crossed to either MMTV-cre (mouse mammary tumor virus long terminal repeat), which is active in many tissues, or WAP-cre (whey acidic protein), which is active only in the mammary epithelial cells to generate transgenic lines.[60] In this study, *Brca1* conditional female mice showed abnormal development of the mammary gland, whereas *Brca2* female mice showed reduced ductal side branching in the mammary tissue.[61–63] Mammary tumorigenesis did occur in these mice but with a long latency period; tumors showed genomic instability and altered *p53* expression.[64] Human breast cancer with inactivation of *BRCA1* commonly exhibits *p53* mutation as compared with sporadic tumors.[65,66] Genetic interaction between *BRCA1/2* and the *p53* pathway studies have been possible in mouse models for the *Brac1/2* inactivation and *p53* heterozygosity. For example, the *MMTV-cre; Brca^{co/co}; p53^{±}* mouse closely mimics the *BRCA1*-associated carcinogensis associated with *p53* mutations.[67,68] In humans, *BRCA1*-associated breast tumors fall in the high-grade IDCs that lack the expression of estrogen receptor (ER), progesterone receptor (PR), and ERRB2/HER2, referred to as triple-negative tumors.[69,70] The tumors from these mice were negative for ERα and showed genomic instability at the chromosomal level tested by array comparative genomic hybridization and spectral karyotyping.[64] Association of *p53* and *Brca1* in mammary tumor development has also been shown using *K-14*-cre, which is active in skin, salivary gland, and mammary gland epithelium. Female mice in this model showed aneuploidy, solid carcinomas with ERα-negative, highly proliferative, and poorly differentiated and contact uninhibited tumors.[71,72] *Brca2* is similar to *Brca1* in which homozygous mutant is embryonically lethal, and to better mimic mammary gland–specific tissue affect of the *Brca2* inactivation, a conditional model using Wap-Cre and conventional truncated mutants have given researchers insight into the development of *Brca2* null tumors.[73,74] Female mice in the conditional model developed non-metastatic carcinomas after a long latency period with displaying aneuploidy and genomic instability. The latency period was further reduced in these mice when they were crossed to heterozygous *p53*.[75] Histochemical analysis showed the tumors to be ErbB2/neu negative and usually ERα and cyclin D1 positive.[64,74,76] Together, these results from *BRCA1/2* and *p53* mice indicate cooperative association between *BRCA 1/2* and *p53* in cellular maintenance.

The usefulness of a mouse model for mechanistic studies again becomes clear, because investigation of *Brca1* and 2 mutant mice have showed activation of *Cdkn1a*, *p21* and *p53*, which were analyzed in greater detail in compound mutant animals generated by cross-breeding.[77–80] The *Brca1* and 2 mouse models not only have been instrumental in understanding the disease mechanisms of breast cancer but have also been valuable in testing of novel therapeutics. Current mouse models do have shortcomings in validation studies where the tumors in these mice do not completely mimic the human *BRCA1/2* tumors; however, these models have proven useful in the study of external factors involved in breast cancer, such as hormone dependency of *BRCA1*. A corollary has existed between estrogen and its receptor alpha (ERα) in the *Brca1*-associated mammary tumors. Paradoxically, the majority of human *BRCA1* defective breast cancers are ERα negative as compared to sporadic tumors.[81] Using mouse models, it has been shown that ERα is highly expressed in the precancerous mammary glands; however, its expression lessens as cancer progresses.[82] The *Brca1/p53* conditional model has been valuable in preclinical studies of the poly-(ADP-ribose) polymerase-1 inhibitor (PARP-1).[83] PARP-1 is important in repair of single-strand DNA breaks via the base excision repair pathway and because homologous recombination pathway is defective in *Brca*-deficient cells, these cells would not be able to repair any DNA damage and be marked for cell death due to the accumulation of damaged DNA. The *Brca1/p53* model has also been useful in the study of progesterone antagonist (mifepristone) which prevented mammary tumorigenesis in the mice; this could be used as a chemopreventive therapy.[84]

In summary, the *Brca1/2* mouse models have been useful in studying the mechanisms of *BRCA1/2* tumor suppression. *Brca1* truncation mutants have become important in understanding the role of *Brca1*'s functional domains in the maintenance of the genome and tumor suppression. Improvement on the current *Brca1* mouse model would generate models to study the role of genetic reversion in therapy resistance, and *Brca1* mutations that are similar to known pathogenic *BRCA1* mutations, such as *BRCA1*[C64G]. A knock-in model of *BRCA*[1C64G] (BAC, bacterial artificial chromosome, transgene) into homozygous mutant mice was not able to rescue embryonic lethality where the normal *BRCA1* was able to, this further demonstrate the usefulness of these models for differentiating the pathogenic from non-pathogenic mutations.[85,86]

Cowden disease is a rare genetic disorder characterized by development of hamartomas of the mucous membrane with increased risk of progression to cancer of the breast, thyroid, and endometrium. Genetic mutation of the *PTEN* gene is responsible for this syndrome. *PTEN* is a tumor suppressor and most human tumors display LOH in this gene.[78] *PTEN* encodes a protein with dual-specificity phosphotase that negatively regulates the cell survival signaling of PI3K/Akt. Mutations in *PTEN* are found in many cancers, including breast cancer and CRC. *Pten* homozygous mutant mice are embryonic lethal, and heterozygous mutant animals developed lymphomas, dysplastic intestinal polyps, endometrial complex atypical hyperplasia, prostatic intraepithelial neoplasia, and thyroid neoplasms but the same malignancies are not seen in humans with germline *PTEN* mutations.[87–90] Moreover, consistent with the model that *Pten* is a tumor suppressor, loss of the wild-type allele was frequently observed in mouse lymphomas. Conditional *Pten* mouse models have been used in the study of mammary tumor progression by crossing the mice with MMTV-cre. Female mice from the cross exhibited an increase in ductal branching and increased mammary epithelial cell proliferation.[91] These data suggest that conditional *Pten* knockout mice will be a useful model system for the study of endometrial, prostate, and thyroid cancer in the context of tissue specific cre transgenes.

FAMILIAL ENDOCRINE AND NEURAL TUMOR SYNDROMES

Germline mutations of several genes can result in endocrine or neural cancers. These include neurofibromatosis (*NF1* and *NF2*), multiple endocrine neoplasia type 1 (*MEN1*), retinoblastoma (*RB*), paraganglioma (*SDH*), and Carney complex (PRKAR1A) among others (**Table 4**).[1,57]

Neurofibromatosis (1 and 2)

Neurofibromatosis results from loss of two genes, neurofibromatosis type 1 (*NF1*) and type 2 (*NF2*), and is a common inherited disorder of the nervous system with

Table 4
Familial endocrine and neural cancers in genetically engineered mice models

Gene	Phenotype	Other Conditions	References
$Rb1^{\pm}$	Thyroid, pituitary, adrenal		9,106
$Men1^{\pm}$	Pancreatic islets, thyroid, pituitary, adrenal, accessory sex glands	Hyperparathyroidism	9,102
$Men1^{\triangle N/\triangle N}$, RIP-cre	Pancreatic islets, pituitary		9,102,103
$Nf1^{\pm}$	Phenochromocytoma, leukemia, lymphoma		9,93,99
$Nf1^{flox/-}$; Krox20-cre	Neurofibroma		9,99,100
$Nf1^{-/-}$ Chimera	Plexiform neurofibromas, myelodysplasia, neuromotor defects		95
$Nf1^{\pm}$:$p53^{\pm}$	Malignant peripheral nerve sheath tumors, malignant astrocytomas		95,101
$Nf2^{\pm}$	Osteogenic tumors, fibrosarcoma		9,102,103
$Nf2^{flox/flox}$; P0-cre	Schwann cell hyperplasia, Schwann cell tumors		92,104
$Sdh^{\pm}$	No tumor		112
$Prkar1a^{\triangle\ 2/+}$	Schwannomas, bone tumors, and thyroid neoplasms		89
TEC3; $Prkar1a^{loxP/loxP}$	Facial tumors		89

a strong predisposition to cancer. NF1 mutation results in the development of astrocytomas and peripheral nerve sheath tumors whereas NF2 mutation causes schwannomas and meningiomas.[92,93] The two genes are distinct; NF1 gene product is neurofibromin and NF2 encodes merlin.[93] A mouse model of this disease has been developed to identify the mechanism of tumor suppression of these genes and to develop therapeutics. Mouse models of NF1 have included targeted mutation in the Nf1 gene; in this model the homozygous mutant mice showed embryonic lethality and analysis of heterozygous animals has yielded important insight into the loss of Nf1. $Nf1^{\pm}$ mice are more prone to developing tumors with LOH.[94,95] $Nf1^{-/-}$ chimeric mice, where a subset of cells in the mouse is $Nf1^{-/-}$, developed neurofibromas, similar to plexiform neurofibromas seen in patients with NF1mutation.[96] Several conditional knockout models have been generated; these mice only developed growth abnormalities and failed to develop significant tumors.[97,98] It has been suggested that besides the absence of Nf1 as a tumor suppressor gene, other genetic mutations must occur for the development of brain tumors.[93] Also, cell non-autonomous processes are important in the development of the tumors; when Schwann cells were made null for Nf1 in the setting of Nf1 heterozygosity (ie, Krox-cre; $Nf1^{loxP/-}$), the mice developed schwannomas with 100% penetrance.[99–101] When $NF1^{\pm}$ mice are bred with any tumor suppressor mutant mice (ie, $p53^{\pm}$), they developed malignant tumors.[96,102] Two different models for Nf2-targeted mutation have been reported and the tumor spectrum of the animals was different from NF2 patients.[93,103,104] However, conditional Nf2 knockout models crossed with myelin protein zero promoter (P0-cre) showed similar disease features seen in NF2 patients, including Schwann cell hyperplasia, Schwann cell tumors, cataracts, and cerebral calcifications.[93,105]

Multiple Endocrine Neoplasia Type 1

Multiple endocrine neoplasia type 1 (MEN-1) is an autosomal dominant inherited disorder, characterized by predisposition to pituitary adenomas, parathyroied hyperplasia, and pancreatic endocrine tumors.[106] *MEN1* gene encodes the tumor suppressor, menin. *Men1*$^{-/-}$ mice are embryonic lethal and heterozygous mutant mice exhibit similar phenotype to human *MEN1* phenotype.[107] To further study the role *Men1* in pancreas, conditional knockout *Men1* mice were generated where they developed adenomas.[108] *Men1* mouse model is able to elucidate the role of menin in tumor suppression and possible development of therapeutics.

Retinoblastoma

Loss of the retinoblastoma gene causes familial retinoblastoma in children. *RB1* gene is a tumor suppressor and, based on Knudson's two-hit model of inheritance, one inactive allele results in 90% incidence of retinoblastoma in children and a 10% incidence of osteosarcomas and soft tissue sarcomas.[3,109] Loss of *RB1* gene has also been reported in breast, lung, and bladder carcinomas.[110] *Rb1* gene is required for embryonic development 12 to 15 days post gestation, therefore, different mouse models have been generated with targeted deletion of the gene. One of the first models for *Rb1* inactivation was made by introducing a termination codon in the exon 3 of the gene resulting in a mutant allele. This mouse did not develop any retinoblastoma or retinomas; the mice did develop pituitary tumors.[111] One of the reasons set forth for the lack of similarity between the mouse and human cancer resulting from loss of *Rb1* is that other family members (ie, p107 and p130) of *Rb1* gene have a compensatory effect in mice. To address this problem, the St Jude retinoblastoma (SJ-RBL) mouse, defective both in *Rb1* and p107 was generated. SJ-RBL mouse SJ-RBL mice showed an increase proliferation in the retinal progenitor cells and when they were crossed with *p53*$^{\pm}$ mice, animals lacking *Rb1*, p107, and *p53* developed aggressive metastatic retinoblastoma.[112] These models can be used to further analyze the mechanism of tumorigenesis caused by *Rb1* loss and, more importantly, to test for any potential therapeutics. However, *p53* gene mutations have not been detected in patients with retinoblastoma.

Paraganglioma (Succinate Dehydrogenase)

Paraganglioma is an autosomal dominant disease caused by a germline mutation in the mitochondrial succinate dehydrogenase (SDH). SDH has a role in both tricarboxylic acid cycle and the electron transport chain. It is one of the first proteins in the metabolic process linked to tumorigenesis, both in paraganglioma and pheochromocytomas. Recently, a conventional knockout mouse model was generated by the removal of exon3 of *Sdhd* and crossed with a knockout *H19*, a modifier gene of *Sdhd* tumorigenesis. Only heterozygous animals were studied due to embryonic lethality of the homozygous mutant. The animals did not show hyperplasia nor developed any paragangliomas. The results were surprising because the *SDH* mutation has high penetrance in humans.[113] One reason for this disparity is the chromosomal organization of genetic elements: the locus of the gene in humans is on chromosome 11 and is the main locus for imprinted genes, whereas in the mouse, the two loci are on different chromosomes and it seems that the loss of both elements is required for the development of disease; this also could be the reason that neither paraganglioma nor pheochromocytoma has been detected in mice.[113] The next generation of humanized mouse models would be able to introduce BAC containing the two loci to better model the chromosomal organization seen in humans.

Carney Complex

Carney complex is an autosomal dominant neoplasia syndrome caused by inactivating mutation in *PRKAR1A*, the gene that encodes the type 1A regulatory subunit of protein kinase A. It is characterized by spotty skin pigmentation, myxomatosis, endocrine tumors, and schwannomas.[99,114] Both conventional and conditional mouse models for this disease have been generated to better understand the mechanism of the disease. The spectrum of tumors that developed in these animals overlapped what has been seen in Carney complex patients, specifically schwannomas, bone tumors, and thyroid neoplasms, confirming the validity of this mouse model.[99]

FAMILIAL HEMATOPOIETIC TUMOR SYNDROMES

Hematopoietic cancers arise from germline mutations in *p53* (Li-Fraumeni syndrome, ATM (ataxia telangiectaia), *BLM* (Bloom syndrome), and *FANCA* (Fanconi anemia) **(Table 5)**.[1,3]

Li-Fraumeni Syndrome

Li-Fraumeni syndrome is a rare autosomal dominant cancer syndrome that is caused by mutation in the *p53* gene and confers a predisposition to a variety of tumors with early onset of disease.[57] *p53* plays a critical role in the DNA damage response by delaying the progression of the cell cycle, which proceeds either to DNA repair or apoptosis. Transgenic mice carrying a *p53* mutant allele display an increased incidence of osteosarcomas, soft tissue sarcomas, adenocarcinomas of the lung and adrenal, and lymphoid tumors similar to patients with Li-Fraumeni syndrome.[115,116] Germline *p53* deletion or conditional mutation of *p53* mouse models have resulted in a different spectrum of tumors; moreover, the latter has shown to closely mimic carcinomas seen in human cancers; this is attributed to point mutations that could render a gene hypomorphic or neomorphic and this would more accurately resemble the genetic mutation seen in human tumors.[117] Mouse models are important in the study of pleiotropic genes, such as *p53*, because they associate with many other genes and animal models are the best system to dissect their interactive role in tumorigenesis.

Ataxia Telangiectaia

Ataxia telangiectaia (AT) is a human autosomal recessive disorder with a wide spectrum of clinical manifestations, including progressive cerebellar ataxia, oculocutaneous telangiectasia, lymphoid tumors, and various other abnormalities, including cell-cycle checkpoint defects and chromosomal instability.[3] AT is caused by mutation in

Table 5 Familial hematopoietic tumor syndromes in genetically engineered mice models			
Gene	**Phenotype**	**Other Conditions**	**References**
p53$^{-/-}$ (20% lethality)	Lymphoma, sarcoma, mammary		10,115,116
Atm$^{-/-}$	Lymphoma		10,119,120
Atm$^{\triangle SRI\pm}$	Lymphoma	Neurologic	10,120,121
Atm$^{\triangle SRI-/-}$	Sarcoma		10,120,121
Blm$^{m3/m3}$	Lymphoma, carcinoma		10,122–124
Fanca$^{-/-}$	No tumors	Germ cell defect	10,125

the ATM gene, a Ser/Thr protein kinase and a member for phosphoinositide 3-kinase (PI3K)–related protein kinase (PIKK) family.[118] A mouse model of AT was created using gene targeting techniques; homozygous mutant mice displayed similar neurologic dysfunction, growth retardation, defects in T-lymphocyte maturation, extreme sensitivity to gamma irradiation, and chromosomal abnormalities as seen in AT patients.[119] Heterozygous mutant animals did not display tumor phenotype; however, ATM knock-in ($Atm^{\triangle SR}$) heterozygous mice harboring an in-frame deletion corresponding to the human 7636del9 mutation showed an increased in risk of tumor development.[120,121]

Bloom Syndrome

Bloom syndrome is a rare atuosomal recessive genetic disorder with a predisposition for early onset of hematopoietic, head and neck cancers.[3] BLM is a human homolog of the *Escherichia coli* RecQ helicase and has many potential roles in DNA repair and replication. *Blm* null mice ($Blm^{3m/3m}$) have a fivefold increased risk of developing cancer as compared with *Blm* heterozygous mice ($Blm^{3m/+}$); animals mostly develope hematopoitic cancers similar to those seen in Bloom patients.[122,123] Irradiated *Blm*-deficient mice show accelerated malignancies, especially hematologic malignancies and are a better model for recapitulating many features of the human disease than non-irradiated Blm-deficient mice.[123,124]

Fanconi Anemia

Fanconi anemia is an autosomal recessive disorder caused by mutation in the *FANCA* gene. Disease features include congenital abnormalities, early-onset bone marrow failure, and increased risk of developing myelodysplasia, acute myeloid leukemia, solid tumors, and cellular sensitivity to mitomycin C and ionizing radiation.[3,57] Mouse model for *Fanca* deficiency did not show developmental abnormalities, and hematologic changes in young mice only included a slight decrease in the platelet count and slight increase in the erythrocyte mean cell volume, but did not progress to anemia. Similar to Fanconi anemia patients, both female and male mice showed impaired fertility and, more importantly, the embryonic fibroblasts from these knockout animals displayed spontaneous chromosomal instability and were hyper-responsive to the effect of mitomycin C.[125]

FAMILIAL KIDNEY TUMOR SYNDROMES

Familial kidney tumor syndromes have been linked to several genes: VHL (von Hippel-Lindau disease [VHL]), c-MET (hereditary papillary renal cancer [HPRC]), BHD (Birt-Hogg-Dubé disease), and others (**Table 6**).[126,127]

von Hippel-Lindau Disease

VHL is a rare automosal dominant disease where germline VHL mutation results in hemangioblastomas; precancerous, avernous hemangiomas of the liver; and renal

Table 6
Familial kidney tumor syndromes in genetically engineered mice models

Gene	Phenotype	Other Conditions	References
Vhl±	Hemangioma, hemanioscarcoma	Angiectasis	10,127,128
*Vhl*lf/d/cre	Hepatic vascular tumors		10,128,129
c-Met knock-in	Multiple tumors		10,131,132
Bhd±	Kidney tumor		133,134

cysts and renal cell carcinomas.[127] Conventional heterozygous mutant mice (Vhl[±]) and Vhl conditional knockout mice (actin-cre as a transgene) showed multiple organ and extensive vascularized tumors similar to those seen in humans with VHL mutation.[128,129] However, the mice did not develop the spectrum of disease seen in patients.[130] It has been suggested that the difference is most likely due to lack of modifier gene inactivations. In the future, this model could be better tested in a targeted deletion of Vhl floxed allele in a kidney-specific cre transgenic mouse.

Hereditary Papillary Renal Cancer

HPRC is autosomal dominant with variable penetrance that rises from a mutation in the c-Met oncogene that codes for a membrane bound receptor with an intracellular tyrosine domain.[131] Homozygous mutant mice are embryonic lethal. Mice-targeted mutations in the murine met-locus were generated. The different mutant lines developed unique tumor spectrum, which included carcinomas, sarcomas, and lymphomas. The majority of the tumors from these mice displayed nonrandom duplication of the mutant met allele; this phenomenon has also been seen in HPRC patients. Mouse model for this syndrome shows that different mutations effect downstream signaling.[132]

Birt-Hogg-Dubé Disease

Birt-Hogg-Dubé disease (BHD) is a rare autosomal dominant genetic disorder characterized by mutation in the BHD tumor suppressor gene, and it is associated with a risk of developing kidney cancer. BHD gene encodes folliculin, a protein that may interact with the energy- and nutrient-sensing AMPK-mTOR signaling pathways.[133] Bhd homozygous mutant mice are embryonic lethal and heterozygous mice develop kidney cysts and solid tumors with age. Kidney tumors from Bhd± mice show activation in mTORC1 and mTORC2 similar to human BHD defective kidney tumors.[133,134] Human BHD tumors analyzed showed PI3K-AKT-mTOR activation, regardless of the type of BHD mutation.[134] Furthermore, inhibitors of mTORC1 and mTORC2 are potential therapeutic agents for BHD-associated kidney cancers.

FAMILIAL SKIN CANCER SYNDROMES

Genetic diseases of skin arise from germline mutations in *WRN* (Werner syndrome), *XP* (xeroderma pigmentosum), *PTCH1* (nevoid basal cell carcinoma), and *CDKN2A* (familial melanoma) genes (**Table 7**).[1,57]

Werner Syndrome

Werner syndrome is an autosomal recessive disorder with manifestation of premature aging, genomic instability, and onset of age-related diseases, including

Table 7
Familial skin cancer syndromes in genetically engineered mice models

Gene	Phenotype	Other Conditions	References
Wrn[−/−]	Various tumors	Myocardial fibrosis	10,135,136
Xpa[−/−]	No tumor		10,137–140
Ptch[±]	Medulloblastoma		10,141–144
Ptch[neo67]	Rhabdomyosarcoma		10,142
P16[ink4a−/−]	Lymphoma, sarcoma		10,145–147

myocardial infraction and malignancies.[57] *WRN* gene is a member of Rec-Q–like subfamily of DNA helicases. A *Wrn*-deficient mouse model was generated to further study the cause of the disease.[135] At the cellular level, the fibroblast from the *Wrn*-deficient mice exhibited reduced proliferation and early saturation arrest similar to the fibroblast of Werner syndrome patients. Spontaneous mutation in the *HPRT* locus was found in WRN patients' immortalized cell lines; embryonic stem cells from deficient mice displayed a higher resistant colony count to 6-TG. The deficient mice, at the whole organism level, did not show any signs of premature aging or increased tumor development.[135] However, a mouse model of WRN−/− in a $p53^{-/-}$ background displayed shorter life span and recapitulated many of the phenotypes of WRN.[136] The reasons set forth as to why a better phenotype is seen in the second mouse model is either because *Wrn* and *p53* have been shown to interact physically and, therefore, they might have cooperative role in maintaining genomic integrity, or because $p53^{-/-}$ allows for a more accelerated aging where the phenotype becomes evident.[136]

Xeroderma Pigmentosum

Xeroderma pigmentosum is a rare autosmal recessive disease characterized by lack of UV-induced DNA damage repair due to mutation in the nucleotide excision repair pathway. Xeroderma pigmentosum patients show extreme sensitivity to sunlight and have a 1000-fold increased risk of developing skin cancer. A mouse model with a mutation in the *Xpa* gene which renders the nucleotide excision repair pathway defective and develops skin tumors when exposed to UV light. Mutant animals also show high susceptibility to genotoxic carcinogens, which makes them an attractive model for studying carcinogens.[137–139] A compound mice of *Xpa* and *p53* ($Xpa^{-/-}/p53^{\pm}$) developed tumors earlier than the homozygous mutant ($Xpa^{-/-}$), these mice can be used for short-term carcinogenesis studies.[140]

Nevoid Basal Cell Carcinoma

Nevoid basal cell carcinoma syndrome is an autosomal dominant disorder caused by a mutation in the protein patched homolog 1 (*PTCH1*) gene, which encodes the receptor for sonic hedgehog pathway.[3,57] This syndrome is characterized by developmental abnormalities and a predisposition to cancers, such as basal cell carcinomas, and tumors displaying LOH which suggests that *PTCH1* could be a tumor suppressor gene.[78,141] Heterozygous mutant mice of Ptch1 develop skeletal abnormalities and medulloblastomas, but they do not develop basal cell carcinoma, thus; haploinsufficiency is sufficient for mice to develop medulloblastomas.[142–144]

Familial Melanoma

Germline mutations in *CDKN2A*, which encodes two cell cycle inhibitory proteins, *p16INK4a* and *P14ARF* (*p19Arf* in mice), has been implicated in the development of melanoma as well as other tumors.[145] Mice deficient in *p16Ink4a* are susceptible to developing spontaneous and carcinogen-induced tumors without the loss of *p19Arf*.[146,147] This model shows that loss of one tumor suppressor protein is sufficient for the development of carcinoma.

HUMANIZED MICE

Mouse models of human disease have not been able to recapitulate all aspects of human disease; this is due to the disparate biology of human and mice, especially differences at chromosomal level; however, cancer mouse models have been essential because most of human cancer biology is difficult to study clinically. To improve on current mouse models, the next generation of humanized mouse models can be generated by inserting humans coding and non-coding elements into their genome. Genome-wide association studies have identified many noncoding variants that could affect gene expression and splicing processes that could have dramatic affect on the biology of disease. Since investigators may have to knock in whole introns or large genomic regions to make appropriate models of human disease. Humanized animal models would be able to bridge the gap between preclinical studies and therapeutics. Another mouse model for understanding the role of telomere biology in the context of cancer development and progression is Terc knockout mouse that lacks the RNA subunit of telomerase, and by crossing these mice to the current mouse models of cancer the effect of telomere biology in the context of cancer can be further studied.[148] Finally, differences in drug metabolism and xenobiotic receptor in mice and human can be addressed by crossing mouse models with human cytochrome p450 as well as the model expressing xenobiotic receptor to current mouse models.[149]

SUMMARY AND FUTURE STUDIES

Mouse models have been important in elucidating essential roles of genes, and early embryonic lethal genes are indicative of the important role they play in the development of the organism. It is evident through these different animal models, discussed in this article, that both conventional and conditional models are beneficial in terms of studying the mechanisms of human disease in mice. The new generation of humanized mice will remedy some of the concerns of current models used in research, namely the genomic organizational difference between the two species. Mouse models have been able to elucidate the sufficiency of a single gene's potential in developing cancer as well as the predicted pleiotropic gene role in tumorigenesis.

The naked mole rat (*Heterocephalus glaber*) is a mammal with similar biology as humans which has attracted the cancer research community for many reasons. The naked mole rat is a potential model for tumorigenesis studies because of its longer life span than the current murine models. These long living, colonistic animals are indigenous to the African continent. With a life span of 28 years, they are good candidate for long-term studies, specifically in cancer progression and metastasis. Life span is not the only feature of this animal that would make it a better model for cancer research; they have evolved anticancer defenses similar to humans, which consist of a tight cell cycle regulation, apoptosis, and tumor suppressor genes. Furthermore, their cells show contact inhibition properties similar to human cells.[1] Future studies with genetic manipulation of *Heterocephalus glaber* will be important to study mechanisms related to long-term development of germline cancers.

REFERENCES

1. Offit K. Clinical cancer genetics: risk counseling and management. New York: Wiley-Liss; 1998.
2. McKusick VA. Johns Hopkins University, National Center for Biotechnology Information (U.S.). Omim. Bethesda (MD): The Center; 1987.
3. Vogelstein B, Kinzler KW, Basson CTDIN, et al. The genetic basis of human cancer. 2nd edition. New York: McGraw-Hill; 2002. Medical Pub. Division.
4. Al-Tassan N, Chmiel NH, Maynard J, et al. Inherited variants of MYH associated with somatic G: C–>T: a mutations in colorectal tumors. Nat Genet 2002;30: 227–32.

5. Fodde R, Edelmann W, Yang K, et al. A targeted chain-termination mutation in the mouse Apc gene results in multiple intestinal tumors. Proc Natl Acad Sci U S A 1994;91:8969–73.
6. Oshima M, Oshima H, Kitagawa K, et al. Loss of Apc heterozygosity and abnormal tissue building in nascent intestinal polyps in mice carrying a truncated Apc gene. Proc Natl Acad Sci U S A 1995;92:4482–6.
7. McCart AE, Vickaryous NK, Silver A. Apc mice: models, modifiers and mutants. Pathol Res Pract 2008;204:479–90.
8. Chulada PC, Thompson MB, Mahler JF, et al. Genetic disruption of Ptgs-1, as well as Ptgs-2, reduces intestinal tumorigenesis in Min mice. Cancer Res 2000;60:4705–8.
9. Oshima M, Dinchuk JE, Kargman SL, et al. Suppression of intestinal polyposis in Apc delta716 knockout mice by inhibition of cyclooxygenase 2 (COX-2). Cell 1996;87:803–9.
10. Ward JM, Devor-Henneman DE. Mouse models of human familial cancer syndromes. Toxicol Pathol 2004;32(Suppl 1):90–8.
11. Seno H, Oshima M, Ishikawa TO, et al. Cyclooxygenase 2- and prostaglandin E(2) receptor EP(2)-dependent angiogenesis in Apc(Delta716) mouse intestinal polyps. Cancer Res 2002;62:506–11.
12. Phillips RK, Wallace MH, Lynch PM, et al. A randomised, double blind, placebo controlled study of celecoxib, a selective cyclooxygenase 2 inhibitor, on duodenal polyposis in familial adenomatous polyposis. Gut 2002;50:857–60.
13. Tonelli F, Valanzano R, Messerini L, et al. Long-term treatment with sulindac in familial adenomatous polyposis: is there an actual efficacy in prevention of rectal cancer? J Surg Oncol 2000;74:15–20.
14. Kolodner RD, Marsischky GT. Eukaryotic DNA mismatch repair. Curr Opin Genet Dev 1999;9:89–96.
15. de la Chapelle A. The incidence of Lynch syndrome. Fam Cancer 2005;4:233–7.
16. de Wind N, Dekker M, Berns A, et al. Inactivation of the mouse Msh2 gene results in mismatch repair deficiency, methylation tolerance, hyperrecombination, and predisposition to cancer. Cell 1995;82:321–30.
17. Kucherlapati MH, Lee K, Nguyen AA, et al. An Msh2 conditional knockout mouse for studying intestinal cancer and testing anti-cancer agents. Gastroenterology 2010;138:993.e1–1002.e1.
18. Wei K, Kucherlapati R, Edelmann W. Mouse models for human DNA mismatch-repair gene defects. Trends Mol Med 2002;8:346–53.
19. Edelmann L, Edelmann W. Loss of DNA mismatch repair function and cancer predisposition in the mouse: animal models for human hereditary nonpolyposis colorectal cancer. Am J Med Genet C Semin Med Genet 2004;129C:91–9.
20. Wang H, Douglas W, Lia M, et al. DNA mismatch repair deficiency accelerates endometrial tumorigenesis in Pten heterozygous mice. Am J Pathol 2002;160:1481–6.
21. de Wind N, Dekker M, Claij N, et al. HNPCC-like cancer predisposition in mice through simultaneous loss of Msh3 and Msh6 mismatch-repair protein functions. Nat Genet 1999;23:359–62.
22. Edelmann W, Yang K, Umar A, et al. Mutation in the mismatch repair gene Msh6 causes cancer susceptibility. Cell 1997;91:467–77.
23. Kolodner RD, Tytell JD, Schmeits JL, et al. Germ-line msh6 mutations in colorectal cancer families. Cancer Res 1999;59:5068–74.
24. Wijnen J, de Leeuw W, Vasen H, et al. Familial endometrial cancer in female carriers of MSH6 germline mutations. Nat Genet 1999;23:142–4.

25. Edelmann W, Umar A, Yang K, et al. The DNA mismatch repair genes Msh3 and Msh6 cooperate in intestinal tumor suppression. Cancer Res 2000;60:803–7.

26. Baker SM, Plug AW, Prolla TA, et al. Involvement of mouse Mlh1 in DNA mismatch repair and meiotic crossing over. Nat Genet 1996;13:336–42.

27. Edelmann W, Cohen PE, Kane M, et al. Meiotic pachytene arrest in MLH1-deficient mice. Cell 1996;85:1125–34.

28. Edelmann W, Yang K, Kuraguchi M, et al. Tumorigenesis in Mlh1 and Mlh1/Apc1638N mutant mice. Cancer Res 1999;59:1301–7.

29. Prolla TA, Baker SM, Harris AC, et al. Tumour susceptibility and spontaneous mutation in mice deficient in Mlh1, Pms1 and Pms2 DNA mismatch repair. Nat Genet 1998;18:276–9.

30. Peltomaki P. Lynch syndrome genes. Fam Cancer 2005;4:227–32.

31. Baker SM, Bronner CE, Zhang L, et al. Male mice defective in the DNA mismatch repair gene PMS2 exhibit abnormal chromosome synapsis in meiosis. Cell 1995;82:309–19.

32. Chen PC, Dudley S, Hagen W, et al. Contributions by MutL homologues Mlh3 and Pms2 to DNA mismatch repair and tumor suppression in the mouse. Cancer Res 2005;65:8662–70.

33. Chen PC, Kuraguchi M, Velasquez J, et al. Novel roles for MLH3 deficiency and TLE6-like amplification in DNA mismatch repair-deficient gastrointestinal tumorigenesis and progression. PLoS Genet 2008;4:e1000092.

34. Lipkin SM, Wang V, Jacoby R, et al. MLH3: a DNA mismatch repair gene associated with mammalian microsatellite instability. Nat Genet 2000;24:27–35.

35. Miller AJ, Dudley SD, Tsao JL, et al. Tractable Cre-lox system for stochastic alteration of genes in mice. Nat Methods 2008;5:227–9.

36. Peltomaki P, Vasen H. Mutations associated with HNPCC predisposition—update of ICG-HNPCC/INSiGHT mutation database. Dis Markers 2004;20:269–76.

37. Lin DP, Wang Y, Scherer SJ, et al. An Msh2 point mutation uncouples DNA mismatch repair and apoptosis. Cancer Res 2004;64:517–22.

38. Kelley MR, Tompkinson AE, Williams KJ, et al. Frontiers of mutagenesis and DNA repair: a workshop. Cancer Res 2004;64:3357–60.

39. Avdievich E, Reiss C, Scherer SJ, et al. Distinct effects of the recurrent Mlh1G67R mutation on MMR functions, cancer, and meiosis. Proc Natl Acad Sci U S A 2008;105:4247–52.

40. Silva FC, Valentin MD, Ferreira Fde O, et al. Mismatch repair genes in Lynch syndrome: a review. Sao Paulo Med J 2009;127:46–51.

41. Burstein E, Fearon ER. Colitis and cancer: a tale of inflammatory cells and their cytokines. J Clin Invest 2008;118:464–7.

42. Kuhn R, Lohler J, Rennick D, et al. Interleukin-10-deficient mice develop chronic enterocolitis. Cell 1993;75:263–74.

43. Sadlack B, Merz H, Schorle H, et al. Ulcerative colitis-like disease in mice with a disrupted interleukin-2 gene. Cell 1993;75:253–61.

44. Van der Sluis M, De Koning BA, De Bruijn AC, et al. Muc2-deficient mice spontaneously develop colitis, indicating that MUC2 is critical for colonic protection. Gastroenterology 2006;131:117–29.

45. Velcich A, Yang W, Heyer J, et al. Colorectal cancer in mice genetically deficient in the mucin Muc2. Science 2002;295:1726–9.

46. Edwards RA, Witherspoon M, Wang K, et al. Epigenetic repression of DNA mismatch repair by inflammation and hypoxia in inflammatory bowel disease-associated colorectal cancer. Cancer Res 2009;69:6423–9.

47. Rudolph U, Finegold MJ, Rich SS, et al. Ulcerative colitis and adenocarcinoma of the colon in G alpha i2-deficient mice. Nat Genet 1995;10:143–50.
48. Garcia-Manero G, Yang H, Bueso-Ramos C, et al. Phase 1 study of the histone deacetylase inhibitor vorinostat (suberoylanilide hydroxamic acid [SAHA]) in patients with advanced leukemias and myelodysplastic syndromes. Blood 2008;111:1060–6.
49. Blumenschein GR, Jr, Kies MS, Papadimitrakopoulou VA, et al. Phase II trial of the histone deacetylase inhibitor vorinostat (Zolinza, suberoylanilide hydroxamic acid, SAHA) in patients with recurrent and/or metastatic head and neck cancer. Invest New Drugs 2008;26:81–7.
50. Marks PA. Discovery and development of SAHA as an anticancer agent. Oncogene 2007;26:1351–6.
51. Kelsen D, Fong Y, Gerdes H, et al. Principles and practice of gastrointestinal oncology. 2nd edition. Philadelphia: Wolters Kluwer Health/Lippincott Williams & Wilkins; 2008.
52. Forster LF, Defres S, Goudie DR, et al. An investigation of the Peutz-Jeghers gene (LKB1) in sporadic breast and colon cancers. J Clin Pathol 2000;53: 791–3.
53. Miyoshi H, Nakau M, Ishikawa TO, et al. Gastrointestinal hamartomatous polyposis in Lkb1 heterozygous knockout mice. Cancer Res 2002;62:2261–6.
54. Jishage K, Nezu J, Kawase Y, et al. Role of Lkb1, the causative gene of Peutz-Jegher's syndrome, in embryogenesis and polyposis. Proc Natl Acad Sci U S A 2002;99:8903–8.
55. Miyaki M. [Peutz-Jeghers syndrome]. Nippon Rinsho 2000;58:1400–4 [in Japanese].
56. Miyaki M, Iijima T, Hosono K, et al. Somatic mutations of LKB1 and beta-catenin genes in gastrointestinal polyps from patients with Peutz-Jeghers syndrome. Cancer Res 2000;60:6311–3.
57. Nussbaum RL, McInnes RR, Willard HF, et al. Thompson & Thompson genetics in medicine. 7th edition. Philadelphia: Saunders/Elsevier; 2007.
58. Moynahan ME. The cancer connection: BRCA1 and BRCA2 tumor suppression in mice and humans. Oncogene 2002;21:8994–9007.
59. Drost RM, Jonkers J. Preclinical mouse models for BRCA1-associated breast cancer. Br J Cancer 2009;101:1651–7.
60. Xu X, Wagner KU, Larson D, et al. Conditional mutation of Brca1 in mammary epithelial cells results in blunted ductal morphogenesis and tumour formation. Nat Genet 1999;22:37–43.
61. Shakya R, Szabolcs M, McCarthy E, et al. The basal-like mammary carcinomas induced by Brca1 or Bard1 inactivation implicate the BRCA1/BARD1 heterodimer in tumor suppression. Proc Natl Acad Sci U S A 2008;105: 7040–5.
62. McAllister KA, Haugen-Strano A, Hagevik S, et al. Characterization of the rat and mouse homologues of the BRCA2 breast cancer susceptibility gene. Cancer Res 1997;57:3121–5.
63. McAllister KA, Ramachandran S, Haugen-Strano A, et al. Genetic mapping of the Brca2 breast cancer susceptibility gene on mouse chromosome 5. Mamm Genome 1997;8:540–1.
64. Evers B, Jonkers J. Mouse models of BRCA1 and BRCA2 deficiency: past lessons, current understanding and future prospects. Oncogene 2006;25: 5885–97.
65. Crook T, Crossland S, Crompton MR, et al. p53 mutations in BRCA1-associated familial breast cancer. Lancet 1997;350:638–9.

66. Eisinger F, Jacquemier J, Guinebretiere JM, et al. p53 involvement in BRCA1-associated breast cancer. Lancet 1997;350:1101.

67. Brodie SG, Xu X, Qiao W, et al. Multiple genetic changes are associated with mammary tumorigenesis in Brca1 conditional knockout mice. Oncogene 2001; 20:7514–23.

68. Xu W, Zhu X, Zhang T, et al. [Histological grading in ductal carcinoma in situ of the breast]. Zhonghua Bing Li Xue Za Zhi 1999;28:331–3 [in Chinese].

69. Lee EY. Promotion of BRCA1-associated triple-negative breast cancer by ovarian hormones. Curr Opin Obstet Gynecol 2008;20:68–73.

70. Johannsson OT, Idvall I, Anderson C, et al. Tumour biological features of BRCA1-induced breast and ovarian cancer. Eur J Cancer 1997;33:362–71.

71. Liu X, Holstege H, van der Gulden H, et al. Somatic loss of BRCA1 and p53 in mice induces mammary tumors with features of human BRCA1-mutated basal-like breast cancer. Proc Natl Acad Sci U S A 2007;104:12111–6.

72. McCarthy A, Savage K, Gabriel A, et al. A mouse model of basal-like breast carcinoma with metaplastic elements. J Pathol 2007;211:389–98.

73. Connor F, Bertwistle D, Mee PJ, et al. Tumorigenesis and a DNA repair defect in mice with a truncating Brca2 mutation. Nat Genet 1997;17:423–30.

74. McAllister KA, Bennett LM, Houle CD, et al. Cancer susceptibility of mice with a homozygous deletion in the COOH-terminal domain of the Brca2 gene. Cancer Res 2002;62:990–4.

75. Ludwig T, Fisher P, Murty V, et al. Development of mammary adenocarcinomas by tissue-specific knockout of Brca2 in mice. Oncogene 2001;20: 3937–48.

76. Cheung AM, Elia A, Tsao MS, et al. Brca2 deficiency does not impair mammary epithelium development but promotes mammary adenocarcinoma formation in p53(+/-) mutant mice. Cancer Res 2004;64:1959–65.

77. Lee WY, Jin YT, Chang TW, et al. Immunolocalization of BRCA1 protein in normal breast tissue and sporadic invasive ductal carcinomas: a correlation with other biological parameters. Histopathology 1999;34:106–12.

78. Hakem R, Mak TW. Animal models of tumor-suppressor genes. Annu Rev Genet 2001;35:209–41.

79. Ludwig T, Chapman DL, Papaioannou VE, et al. Targeted mutations of breast cancer susceptibility gene homologs in mice: lethal phenotypes of Brca1, Brca2, Brca1/Brca2, Brca1/p53, and Brca2/p53 nullizygous embryos. Genes Dev 1997;11:1226–41.

80. Hakem R, de la Pompa JL, Sirard C, et al. The tumor suppressor gene Brca1 is required for embryonic cellular proliferation in the mouse. Cell 1996;85: 1009–23.

81. Hosey AM, Gorski JJ, Murray MM, et al. Molecular basis for estrogen receptor alpha deficiency in BRCA1-linked breast cancer. J Natl Cancer Inst 2007;99: 1683–94.

82. Hu Y. BRCA1, hormone, and tissue-specific tumor suppression. Int J Biol Sci 2009;5:20–7.

83. Schultz N, Lopez E, Saleh-Gohari N, et al. Poly(ADP-ribose) polymerase (PARP-1) has a controlling role in homologous recombination. Nucleic Acids Res 2003;31:4959–64.

84. Poole AJ, Li Y, Kim Y, et al. Prevention of Brca1-mediated mammary tumorigenesis in mice by a progesterone antagonist. Science 2006;314:1467–70.

85. Chandler J, Hohenstein P, Swing DA, et al. Human BRCA1 gene rescues the embryonic lethality of Brca1 mutant mice. Genesis 2001;29:72–7.

86. Yang Y, Swaminathan S, Martin BK, et al. Aberrant splicing induced by missense mutations in BRCA1: clues from a humanized mouse model. Hum Mol Genet 2003;12:2121–31.
87. Suzuki A, Itami S, Ohishi M, et al. Keratinocyte-specific Pten deficiency results in epidermal hyperplasia, accelerated hair follicle morphogenesis and tumor formation. Cancer Res 2003;63:674–81.
88. Podsypanina K, Ellenson LH, Nemes A, et al. Mutation of Pten/Mmac1 in mice causes neoplasia in multiple organ systems. Proc Natl Acad Sci U S A 1999;96:1563–8.
89. Marino S, Krimpenfort P, Leung C, et al. PTEN is essential for cell migration but not for fate determination and tumourigenesis in the cerebellum. Development 2002;129:3513–22.
90. Kwon CH, Zhu X, Zhang J, et al. Pten regulates neuronal soma size: a mouse model of Lhermitte-Duclos disease. Nat Genet 2001;29:404–11.
91. Li G, Robinson GW, Lesche R, et al. Conditional loss of PTEN leads to precocious development and neoplasia in the mammary gland. Development 2002;129:4159–70.
92. Friedman JM. Epidemiology of neurofibromatosis type 1. Am J Med Genet 1999;89:1–6.
93. Gutmann DH, Giovannini M. Mouse models of neurofibromatosis 1 and 2. Neoplasia 2002;4:279–90.
94. Jacks T, Shih TS, Schmitt EM, et al. Tumour predisposition in mice heterozygous for a targeted mutation in Nf1. Nat Genet 1994;7:353–61.
95. Brannan CI, Perkins AS, Vogel KS, et al. Targeted disruption of the neurofibromatosis type-1 gene leads to developmental abnormalities in heart and various neural crest-derived tissues. Genes Dev 1994;8:1019–29.
96. Cichowski K, Shih TS, Schmitt E, et al. Mouse models of tumor development in neurofibromatosis type 1. Science 1999;286:2172–6.
97. Gutmann DH, Wu YL, Hedrick NM, et al. Heterozygosity for the neurofibromatosis 1 (NF1) tumor suppressor results in abnormalities in cell attachment, spreading and motility in astrocytes. Hum Mol Genet 2001;10:3009–16.
98. Zhu Y, Romero MI, Ghosh P, et al. Ablation of NF1 function in neurons induces abnormal development of cerebral cortex and reactive gliosis in the brain. Genes Dev 2001;15:859–76.
99. Kirschner LS, Kusewitt DF, Matyakhina L, et al. A mouse model for the Carney complex tumor syndrome develops neoplasia in cyclic AMP-responsive tissues. Cancer Res 2005;65:4506–14.
100. Zhu Y, Parada LF. The molecular and genetic basis of neurological tumours. Nat Rev Cancer 2002;2:616–26.
101. Zhu Y, Ghosh P, Charnay P, et al. Neurofibromas in NF1: Schwann cell origin and role of tumor environment. Science 2002;296:920–2.
102. Vogel KS, Klesse LJ, Velasco-Miguel S, et al. Mouse tumor model for neurofibromatosis type 1. Science 1999;286:2176–9.
103. McClatchey AI, Saotome I, Mercer K, et al. Mice heterozygous for a mutation at the Nf2 tumor suppressor locus develop a range of highly metastatic tumors. Genes Dev 1998;12:1121–33.
104. McClatchey AI, Saotome I, Ramesh V, et al. The Nf2 tumor suppressor gene product is essential for extraembryonic development immediately prior to gastrulation. Genes Dev 1997;11:1253–65.
105. Kalamarides M, Niwa-Kawakita M, Leblois H, et al. Nf2 gene inactivation in arachnoidal cells is rate-limiting for meningioma development in the mouse. Genes Dev 2002;16:1060–5.

106. Harding B, Lemos MC, Reed AA, et al. Multiple endocrine neoplasia type 1 knockout mice develop parathyroid, pancreatic, pituitary and adrenal tumours with hypercalcaemia, hypophosphataemia and hypercorticosteronaemia. Endocr Relat Cancer 2009;16:1313–27.

107. Crabtree JS, Scacheri PC, Ward JM, et al. A mouse model of multiple endocrine neoplasia, type 1, develops multiple endocrine tumors. Proc Natl Acad Sci U S A 2001;98:1118–23.

108. Crabtree JS, Scacheri PC, Ward JM, et al. Of mice and MEN1: insulinomas in a conditional mouse knockout. Mol Cell Biol 2003;23:6075–85.

109. Classon M, Harlow E. The retinoblastoma tumour suppressor in development and cancer. Nat Rev Cancer 2002;2:910–7.

110. Harbour JW. Overview of RB gene mutations in patients with retinoblastoma. Implications for clinical genetic screening. Ophthalmology 1998;105:1442–7.

111. Jacks T, Fazeli A, Schmitt EM, et al. Effects of an Rb mutation in the mouse. Nature 1992;359:295–300.

112. Zhang J, Schweers B, Dyer MA. The first knockout mouse model of retinoblastoma. Cell Cycle 2004;3:952–9.

113. Bayley JP, Devilee P, Taschner PE. The SDH mutation database: an online resource for succinate dehydrogenase sequence variants involved in pheochromocytoma, paraganglioma and mitochondrial complex II deficiency. BMC Med Genet 2005;6:39.

114. Griffin KJ, Kirschner LS, Matyakhina L, et al. A mouse model for Carney complex. Endocr Res 2004;30:903–11.

115. Donehower LA, Harvey M, Vogel H, et al. Effects of genetic background on tumorigenesis in p53-deficient mice. Mol Carcinog 1995;14:16–22.

116. Donehower LA, Harvey M, Slagle BL, et al. Mice deficient for p53 are developmentally normal but susceptible to spontaneous tumours. Nature 1992;356:215–21.

117. Olive KP, Tuveson DA, Ruhe ZC, et al. Mutant p53 gain of function in two mouse models of Li-Fraumeni syndrome. Cell 2004;119:847–60.

118. Lavin MF. Ataxia-telangiectasia: from a rare disorder to a paradigm for cell signalling and cancer. Nat Rev Mol Cell Biol 2008;9:759–69.

119. Barlow C, Hirotsune S, Paylor R, et al. Atm-deficient mice: a paradigm of ataxia telangiectasia. Cell 1996;86:159–71.

120. Spring K, Ahangari F, Scott SP, et al. Mice heterozygous for mutation in Atm, the gene involved in ataxia-telangiectasia, have heightened susceptibility to cancer. Nat Genet 2002;32:185–90.

121. Spring K, Cross S, Li C, et al. Atm knock-in mice harboring an in-frame deletion corresponding to the human ATM 7636del9 common mutation exhibit a variant phenotype. Cancer Res 2001;61:4561–8.

122. Luo G, Santoro IM, McDaniel LD, et al. Cancer predisposition caused by elevated mitotic recombination in Bloom mice. Nat Genet 2000;26:424–9.

123. Chester N, Kuo F, Kozak C, et al. Stage-specific apoptosis, developmental delay, and embryonic lethality in mice homozygous for a targeted disruption in the murine Bloom's syndrome gene. Genes Dev 1998;12:3382–93.

124. Warren ST, Schultz RA, Chang CC, et al. Elevated spontaneous mutation rate in Bloom syndrome fibroblasts. Proc Natl Acad Sci U S A 1981;78:3133–7.

125. Yang Y, Kuang Y, Montes De Oca R, et al. Targeted disruption of the murine Fanconi anemia gene, Fancg/Xrcc9. Blood 2001;98:3435–40.

126. Choyke PL, Glenn GM, Walther MM, et al. Hereditary renal cancers. Radiology 2003;226:33–46.

127. Zbar B, Klausner R, Linehan WM. Studying cancer families to identify kidney cancer genes. Annu Rev Med 2003;54:217–33.
128. Kleymenova E, Everitt JI, Pluta L, et al. Susceptibility to vascular neoplasms but no increased susceptibility to renal carcinogenesis in Vhl knockout mice. Carcinogenesis 2004;25:309–15.
129. Haase VH, Glickman JN, Socolovsky M, et al. Vascular tumors in livers with targeted inactivation of the von Hippel-Lindau tumor suppressor. Proc Natl Acad Sci U S A 2001;98:1583–8.
130. Shen HC, Adem A, Ylaya K, et al. Deciphering von Hippel-Lindau (VHL/Vhl)-associated pancreatic manifestations by inactivating Vhl in specific pancreatic cell populations. PLoS One 2009;4:e4897.
131. Coleman DT, Bigelow R, Cardelli JA. Inhibition of fatty acid synthase by luteolin post-transcriptionally down-regulates c-Met expression independent of proteosomal/lysosomal degradation. Mol Cancer Ther 2009;8:214–24.
132. Graveel CR, London CA, Vande Woude GF. A mouse model of activating Met mutations. Cell Cycle 2005;4:518–20.
133. Menko FH, van Steensel MA, Giraud S, et al. Birt-Hogg-Dube syndrome: diagnosis and management. Lancet Oncol 2009;10:1199–206.
134. Hasumi Y, Baba M, Ajima R, et al. Homozygous loss of BHD causes early embryonic lethality and kidney tumor development with activation of mTORC1 and mTORC2. Proc Natl Acad Sci U S A 2009;106:18722–7.
135. Lebel M, Leder P. A deletion within the murine Werner syndrome helicase induces sensitivity to inhibitors of topoisomerase and loss of cellular proliferative capacity. Proc Natl Acad Sci U S A 1998;95:13097–102.
136. Lombard DB, Beard C, Johnson B, et al. Mutations in the WRN gene in mice accelerate mortality in a p53-null background. Mol Cell Biol 2000;20:3286–91.
137. Berg RJ, de Vries A, van Steeg H, et al. Relative susceptibilities of XPA knockout mice and their heterozygous and wild-type littermates to UVB-induced skin cancer. Cancer Res 1997;57:581–4.
138. de Vries A, van Steeg H. Xpa knockout mice. Semin Cancer Biol 1996;7:229–40.
139. Nakane H, Takeuchi S, Yuba S, et al. High incidence of ultraviolet-B-or chemical-carcinogen-induced skin tumours in mice lacking the xeroderma pigmentosum group A gene. Nature 1995;377:165–8.
140. van Kesteren PC, Beems RB, Luijten M, et al. DNA repair-deficient Xpa/p53 knockout mice are sensitive to the non-genotoxic carcinogen cyclosporine A: escape of initiated cells from immunosurveillance? Carcinogenesis 2009;30:538–43.
141. Gailani MR, Bale AE. Developmental genes and cancer: role of patched in basal cell carcinoma of the skin. J Natl Cancer Inst 1997;89:1103–9.
142. Zurawel RH, Allen C, Chiappa S, et al. Analysis of PTCH/SMO/SHH pathway genes in medulloblastoma. Genes Chromosomes Cancer 2000;27:44–51.
143. Zurawel RH, Allen C, Wechsler-Reya R, et al. Evidence that haploinsufficiency of Ptch leads to medulloblastoma in mice. Genes Chromosomes Cancer 2000;28:77–81.
144. Goodrich LV, Milenkovic L, Higgins KM, et al. Altered neural cell fates and medulloblastoma in mouse patched mutants. Science 1997;277:1109–13.
145. Quelle DE, Zindy F, Ashmun RA, et al. Alternative reading frames of the INK4a tumor suppressor gene encode two unrelated proteins capable of inducing cell cycle arrest. Cell 1995;83:993–1000.
146. Fitzpatrick GV, Soloway PD, Higgins MJ. Regional loss of imprinting and growth deficiency in mice with a targeted deletion of KvDMR1. Nat Genet 2002;32:426–31.

147. Sharpless NE, Bardeesy N, Lee KH, et al. Loss of p16Ink4a with retention of p19Arf predisposes mice to tumorigenesis. Nature 2001;413:86–91.

148. Rudolph KL, Chang S, Lee HW, et al. Longevity, stress response, and cancer in aging telomerase-deficient mice. Cell 1999;96:701–12.

149. Frese KK, Tuveson DA. Maximizing mouse cancer models. Nat Rev Cancer 2007;7:645–58.

Lower Gastrointestinal Tract Cancer Predisposition Syndromes

Neel B. Shah, MB, ChB*, Noralane M. Lindor, MD

KEYWORDS

• Colorectal • Lower GI • Cancer • Genetic syndrome • Risk

Although inherited predisposition to colorectal cancer (CRC) has been suspected for more than 100 years, definitive proof of Mendelian syndromes had to await maturation of molecular genetic technologies. Since the I980s, the genetics of several clinically distinct entities has been revealed. Five disorders that share a hereditary predisposition to CRC are reviewed in this article. They are summarized in **Table 1** .

PEUTZ-JEGHERS SYNDROME
Clinical Overview

Peutz-Jeghers syndrome (PJS) is a rare, highly penetrant, autosomal dominant disorder characterized by hamartomatous polyposis and mucocutaneous pigmentation. Polyps may occur anywhere along the gastrointestinal tract but occur most consistently in the jejunum. Extraintestinal sites of PJS polyps include kidney, ureter, gallbladder, bronchus, and nasal passages. About one-third of patients will develop polyp-related symptoms by age 10 years and close to two-thirds by age 20 years.[1]

The incidence of PJS is estimated to be 1 in 8300 to 1 in 200,000 live births[2]; 25% of cases appear to be nonfamilial. PJS has been reported worldwide[3,4] and occurs in males and females equally. There is variability in both the severity of disease as well as age of onset of symptoms.

The hyperpigmented macules of PJS develop in 95% of affected individuals and arise most commonly in the perioral region, around the eyes and nostrils, on the buccal mucosa, the perianal area, and on the digits of hands and feet. They usually appear by

No conflicts of interest to note.

This article was originally planned for publication in the October 2010 issue (24:5) devoted to Genetic Predisposition to Cancer, guest edited by Drs Kenneth Offit and Mark Robson. To see the rest of the articles in that issue, go to www.hemonc.theclinics.com.

Department of Medical Genetics, Mayo Clinic, 200 First Street SW, Rochester, MN 55905, USA

* Corresponding author.

E-mail address: shah.neel2@mayo.edu

Table 1
Lower gastrointestinal tract cancer predisposition syndromes

Syndrome	Gene	Inheritance	Gastrointestinal Polyp Histology	Extracolonic Cancers	Other Associations	Estimated Cumulative Colorectal Cancer Risk
Peutz-Jeghers syndrome	STK11	AD	Hamartoma +++, Adenoma +	Cervical, uterus, ovarian, breast, sertoli cell tumors, entire GI tract, pancreato-biliary	Hyperestrogenism, Mucosal pigmentation +++, Facial pigmentation +, Polyps in gallbladder, ureter, nasal and bronchial passages	39% by 70 years
Juvenile polyposis	BMPR1A SMAD4 ENG	AD	Hamartoma +++, Adenoma +	Gastric, small intestine, pancreas	HHT	17%–68% by 60 years
Familial adenomatous polyposis	APC	AD	Adenoma +++, Cystic fundic gland polyp	Duodenal, hepatoblastoma medulloblastoma, papillary thyroid	Desmoid tumors, osteomas, CHRPE, dental anomalies, gastric polyps	90% by 45 years (69% by 80 years attenuated FAP)
Lynch syndrome	MLH1 MSH2 PMS2 MSH6	AD	Adenoma +	Endometrial, ovarian, gastric, small intestine, pancreato-biliary, renal pelvis and ureter, sebaceous carcinoma, keratoacanthoma, glioblastoma	Sebaceous adenoma	80% by 75 years
MYH-associated polyposis	MYH	AR	Adenoma +++, Hyperplastic +, Gastric fundic gland polyp	Duodenal	Duodenal adenoma, gastric polyps, CHRPE, osteomas, dental anomalies, desmoid tumors	80% by 70 years

Abbreviations: AD, autosomal dominant; AR, autosomal recessive; CHRPE, congenital hypertrophy of retinal pigment epithelium; GI, gastrointestinal; HHT, hereditary hemorrhagic telangiectasia; +, seen in this condition; +++, very common in this condition.

the end of the first year of life and are almost always present by age 5 years.[5] The macules may be dark blue to dark brown, vary in size from 1 to 5 mm, and may fade in puberty and adulthood, and are not precancerous.

Classical PJS intestinal polyps are hamartomatous and experienced pathologists are capable of distinguishing PJS polyps from juvenile polyps. PJS polyps manifest characteristic hypertrophy or hyperplasia of the smooth-muscle layer branching in tree-like fashion (arborizes) into the superficial epithelial layer. Multiple adenomas may also occur, especially in the colon.[5]

Cancer Risk

PJS carries an increased risk for multiple benign and malignant tumors (see **Table 1**). The cumulative risk of any cancer is 67% to 85% by age 70 and the cumulative risk for CRC is 3% (40 years), 5% (50 years), 15% (60 years), 39% (70 years).[6,7] The risk to age 70 for cancers of the pancreas, uterus/ovary/cervix, breast, and lung were 11%, 18%, 45%, and 17%, in the same series, respectively. An increased risk of primitive biliary cancer was reported in PJS.[8] No correlation has been found between risk of cancer and severity of polyposis or presence of pigmentation.[9]

Molecular Basis of Disease

Germline mutations in STK11 (also known as LKB1) encoding a tyrosine kinase on chromosome 19p13.3 have been identified in nearly all PJS families[10,11] and 94% of patients with PJS overall.[12] Families without an identified mutation do not differ clinically or ethnically from those with a mutation. Only one transcript is known, a 433– amino acid protein that is ubiquitously expressed and present primarily in the cytoplasm and to a lesser extent in the nucleus.[13,14] STK11 is a highly conserved gene with approximately 88% and 84% homology, respectively, with mouse and Xenopus homologs. STK11 is the only tyrosine kinase known to function as a tumor suppressor by physically associating with TP53 to regulate TP53-dependent apoptosis pathways.[15,16] STK11 also interacts with PTEN, which is responsible for other hereditary hamartoma syndromes and also plays a role in the vascular endothelial growth factor (VEGF) pathway and cellular polarity.

Inactivation of STK11 is a critical early event in the development of hamartomas and adenocarcinomas.[17] Adenocarcinomas in Peutz-Jeghers syndrome demonstrate altered TP53 expression and loss of heterozygosity (LOH) in 17p and 18q. Microsatellite instability, LOH near the APC gene, or KRAS mutations have been identified in some tumors,[17] with indications that tumorigenic potential of STK11 mutations is mediated through alternative mechanisms in different tissues, especially those in which hamartoma development is not a feature.

Hamartomatous polyps have generally been considered to have a very low malignant potential and it was uncertain that PJS-associated hamartomas were the premalignant lesions in PJS. However, molecular and histologic studies have confirmed that hamartomatous polyps can undergo malignant transformation in PJS.[18] It is not known whether inactivation of both STK11 alleles is necessary for carcinogenesis or if a 50% decrease in protein expression is sufficient (haploinsufficiency). Data from studies in lkb1 −/+ and lkb1 −/− mice support both possibilities.[19,20]

Clinical Risk Management

The cancer risk with PJS supports efforts at directed surveillance strategies for early detection of tumors. Multiple guidelines based solely on expert opinion exist; none have been validated in controlled trials. **Table 2** shows one set of screening recommendations for PJS.[21] A guiding principle in management is prevention of bowel

Table 2
Cancer screening and surveillance screening guidelines based on expert opinion for Peutz-Jeghers syndrome (no evidence-based data exist to support these guidelines)

Site	Procedure	Starting Age, y	Interval, y
Stomach, small and large bowel	Upper and lower endoscopy Small bowel follow-through / capsule enteroscopy	8 8	2 2[a]
Breast (female only)	Clinical breast examination Mammography	20 20	1 2–3
Testicle	Testicular examination	10	1
Ovary, cervix, uterus	Pelvic examination with cervical cytology Pelvic ultrasound	20 20	21 1
Pancreas	Endoscopic ultrasound or transabdominal ultrasound	30	1–2

[a] Consider laparotomy and intraoperative endoscopy to remove polyps >1.5 cm.
Data from Amos C, Frazier M, McGarrity T. Peutz-Jeghers syndrome. In: Pagon RA, Bird TC, Dolan CR, Stephens K, editors. GeneReviews [Internet]. Seattle (WA): University of Washington, Seattle; 2009.

intussusceptions or obstructions. In one series, laparotomy for bowel obstruction was performed in 30% of individuals by age 10 years and in 68% by age 18 years.[22] Substantial morbidity arises from short-gut syndrome, as a consequence of multiple small-bowel resections for intussusception; therefore, prophylactic removal of small bowel polyps is advised. For small bowel polyps not accessible endoscopically, surgery has been recommended if symptomatic or when larger than 1.5 cm. Intraoperative small bowel endoscopy can allow removal of all identifiable polyps and may decrease the overall frequency of laparotomy.[23,24]

Clinical genetic testing for PJS is available. If a disease-causing mutation has been identified, it is appropriate to offer genetic testing to at-risk relatives and, if positive, surveillance is indicated. If no disease-causing mutation is found in an individual with PJS, then first-degree relatives must be advised that they may still be at risk for PJS and that PJS cancer surveillance is advisable.

JUVENILE POLYPOSIS
Clinical Overview

Juvenile polyposis (JP) is an autosomal dominant disorder characterized by multiple (5–200) hamartomatous polyps of the gastrointestinal tract.[25] It is the most common of the hamartomatous polyp syndromes. Population prevalence is estimated to be between 1 in 16,000 and 1 in 100,000.[26] Twenty percent to 50% of cases are inherited.

Solitary juvenile polyps may be seen in approximately 2% of healthy children but these are seldom dysplastic and are not associated with increased malignancy or extracolonic manifestations.[12,27] In JP, "juvenile" refers to the type of polyp (resembling sporadic inflammatory hamartomatous polyps of childhood) rather than the age of onset, although most affected individuals have some polyps by age 20 years. The hamartomas of JP have a frondlike growth pattern and fewer stroma and dilated glands with more proliferative smaller glands compared with solitary, sporadic juvenile polyps.[28]

Clinical criteria for defining JP have been proposed (**Box 1**). Although only 5 polyps have been proposed as the minimum number for diagnosis, some individuals will have more than 100 polyps. In a review of 272 individuals with JP of undefined genetic subtype, 98% had involvement of the colorectum, 14% of the stomach, 7% of the jejunum and ileum, and 2% of the duodenum.[29] Polyps usually range from 5 to 50 mm in size, can be single or multilobulated, are spherical in shape, and commonly show surface erosion. Clinical symptoms of JP may include bleeding, diarrhea, abdominal pain, intussusceptions, and rectal prolapse and even protein-losing enteropathy. Digital clubbing has been noted, perhaps owing to the overlap with hereditary hemorrhagic telangiectasia and arteriovenous shunting in those patients.[30]

JP may be misdiagnosed, as it shares clinical features with several other colonic hamartomatous polyp syndromes (Cowden, Bannayan-Riley-Ruvalcaba, Peutz-Jeghers, Basal Cell Nevus/Gorlin) so is therefore a diagnosis of exclusion. Physical examination, family history, and molecular testing may help differentiate between these possibilities.[31,32]

Cancer Risk

Most juvenile polyps are benign but malignant transformation may occur resulting in increased lifetime risk for cancers of the colon (10%–40%), stomach (21%), and less commonly involving the small bowel and pancreas. The lifetime risk of cancers has been hard to define and may vary with underlying genetic cause and is likely reduced by screening polypectomies.

Malignant transformation is suspected to follow a juvenile polyp → adenomatous change → dysplasia → carcinoma sequence.[33,34] However, additional work is required to determine if individuals with JP are also predisposed to malignancy separately from the predisposition to polyps.

Molecular Basis of Disease

JP is clinically and genetically heterogeneous. Three genes, *SMAD4*, *BMPR1A*, and *ENG*, have been implicated so far. Each encodes proteins of either transforming growth factor (TGF)-β or bone morphogenetic protein (BMP)-signaling pathways. The low combined mutation detection rate has prompted a search for other candidate genes/proteins within these pathways.

About 20% of individuals with JP have a mutation of *SMAD* (also known as *MADH4* or *DPC*).[32,35,36] *SMAD4* is part of the TGF-β signal transduction pathway. The *SMAD* gene family is on chromosome 18q21.1, adjacent to *DCC* (deleted in colon cancer). *SMAD4* complexes combine with other members of the *SMAD* family of proteins to

---

Box 1
Diagnostic criteria for JP

One or more of the following:

>5 juvenile polyps in the colon/rectum[a]

Juvenile polyps throughout the gastrointestinal tract

Any number of juvenile polyps with a family history of JP

[a] Modified by Giardiello et al, 1991,[12] to 3 or more polyps.
Data from Jass J, Williams C, Bussey H, et al. Juvenile polyposis—a precancerous condition. Histopathology 1988;13(6):619–30.

transmit the TGF-β growth-suppressing signal from the cell surface receptor to nuclear downstream targets, mediating apoptosis and growth inhibition. It has been postulated that the abundant stroma in JP may create an abnormal microenvironment, disrupting TGF-β signaling.[37,38] This theory is supported by the fact that as hamartomatous polyps enlarge and mesenchymal component expands, they take on a serrated or villous-type configuration associated with epithelial dysplasia.

Mutations in *BMPR1A (ALK3)* at 10q22.3, are found in about 20% to 25% of individuals with JP.[32,35,36] *BMPR1A* is a serine-threonine kinase type I receptor of the TGF-β superfamily, which when activated leads to phosphorylation of *SMAD4*. A reduced number of gastric polyps have been observed in *BMPR1A* mutation–positive patients compared with *SMAD4* mutation–positive patients.[35,39,40]

Mutations in *ENG* on chromosome 9q34.1 have been reported in very early onset JP.[41] *ENG* encodes endoglin, an accessory receptor protein that binds to specific TGF-β proteins.[42] Mutations in *ENG* are more often found in individuals with hereditary hemorrhagic telangiectasia (HHT). The combined syndrome of JPS and HHT (termed JPS/HHT) may be present in 15% to 22% of individuals with a *SMAD4* mutation and has also been associated with *ENG* (**Table 3**). The prevalence of *ENG* mutations in patients with JP without HHT has yet to be adequately described.[43]

Clinical Risk Management

No evidence-based guidelines exist to determine optimal screening modalities or intervals in JP. Because of the perceived high risk for malignancies, guidelines based on expert opinion have advised that those affected with or who are at risk for JP receive a complete blood count, upper gastrointestinal endoscopy, and colonoscopy beginning from the onset of symptoms or the age of 15. If no polyps are found, screening should be repeated every 1 to 3 years. Any polyps found should be removed and screening should be annual or based on polyp burden until no polyps are found.[44] For those with extremely numerous polyps, colectomy and/or gastrectomy may be indicated. Colorectal adenocarcinoma should be treated with definitive surgery, and consideration of total colectomy with or without ileorectal anastomosis based on clinical findings.

FAMILIAL ADENOMATOUS POLYPOSIS
Clinical Overview

Familial adenomatour polyposis (FAP) is a highly penetrant, autosomal dominant syndrome caused by germline mutations of the *APC* (adenomatous polyposis coli)

Table 3		
Juvenile polyposis and hereditary hemorrhagic telangiectasia		
Gene (OMIM Number)	**Juvenile Polyposis**	**HHT[a]**
BMPR1A/ALK3 (601299)	Approximately 20%–25%	Not yet reported
SMAD4/MADH4 (600993)	Approximately 20%	<20% some features
ENG (131195)	Reported	30%–40%
ACVR1/ALK1 (601284)	Not reported	30%–40%
Unknown	>50%	>20%

Abbreviation: OMIM, online Mendelian inheritance in man.
[a] HHT = hereditary hemorrhagic telangiectasia (also known as Osler–Weber–Rendu syndrome [OMIM # 187299, 175050, 600376]).
Data from Lindor NM, McMaster ML, Lindor CJ, et al. Concise handbook of familial cancer susceptibility syndromes - second edition. J Natl Cancer Inst Monogr 2008;1–93.

gene[45] at 5q21. FAP has a frequency of 1 in 5000 to 10,000 live births and affects males and females equally.[46] It accounts for 1% of all CRC.[47] Ten percent to 30% of cases arise from de novo mutations.[48] It was the first CRC syndrome to be recognized clinically[49] and the first for which a gene was identified. It offers a model for the adenoma → carcinoma paradigm that is shared by sporadic as well as several familial colorectal cancers and, through this, offers a basis for the concept of all CRC being "genetic."

FAP is the result of an inactivating mutation in *APC* and clinical presentation may be associated with the site of mutation, although it may also be clinically heterogeneous even within the same family. This suggests a role for modifier genes and/or environmental factors in modulating disease expression.[50] Colorectal polyposis, numbering from hundreds to thousands, is nearly pathognomic of FAP. Polyps are generally less than 1 cm and occur throughout the colorectum with a predilection for sigmoid colon and rectum.[51] They may be sessile or pedunculated with histology varying from tubular to villous adenoma.

FAP has multiple extracolonic manifestations involving all 3 embryologic layers. The term Gardner syndrome refers to FAP plus extracolonic features. Endodermal lesions include gastric and small bowel polyps and carcinomas. Mesodermal abnormalities include desmoid tumors, osteomas, and dental abnormalities. Ectodermal lesions can affect the eye, brain, and skin. The combination of CRC and brain tumors was referred to as Turcot syndrome. However, molecular studies have shown that although the combination of colonic polyposis and medulloblastoma is associated with *APC* mutations, the combination of CRC and glioblastoma is associated with defective mismatch repair genes and was also called Turcot syndrome.[52] Hence, there seems to be little clinical value in perpetuating the use of this ambiguous term.

Desmoid tumors are histologically benign clonal neoplasms composed of fibrous tissue. They arise as mostly intra-abdominal soft tissue tumors[53] and occur in approximately 10% to 25% of patients with FAP.[54] Trauma has been suggested to be a factor, as 84% of FAP-associated desmoids developed within 5 years of abdominal surgery in one series.[55] They do not usually metastasize but they can be highly locally invasive and can cause significant mass effect, obstruction, pain, and death. Desmoid tumor may also occur sporadically or in a hereditary manner without colon findings,[56,57] but in cases of families with desmoid tumors or individuals with 2 or more desmoids, attempts should be made to exclude *APC* mutation.

Osteomas may occur in any bone but often localize to the face or skull. Dental abnormalities affect 70% of patients with FAP and include supernumerary teeth, congenitally absent teeth, fused roots, and osteomas of the jaw.[51] Depending on the location, they can lead to symptoms and identification of FAP. Congenital hypertrophy of retinal pigment epithelium (CHRPE) is an asymptomatic hamartoma of the retinal epithelium occurring in 66% to 92% of patients with FAP.[58]

"Attenuated FAP" (AFAP), defined as fewer than 100 synchronous colorectal adenomas, shows a right-sided colonic predilection with rectal sparing and a later presentation.[59] Extracolonic manifestations may occur similar to classic FAP. It has been linked to mutations in exons 1 to 4, 3' regions of *APC* distal to codon 1580, and the alternatively spliced site of exon 9.[45,60–62] However, some patients with this phenotype and no identified *APC* mutation have been shown to have compound heterozygous mutations in the base excision repair gene *MYH*,[63] leaving open the possibility that cases of AFAP may be hitherto unidentified *MYH*-associated polyposis (MAP). If germline *APC* mutation testing is negative in suspected AFAP, testing for *MYH* mutations may be indicated.

Cancer Risk

The age at onset of colorectal adenomas is variable, being present in only 15% of FAP gene carriers at age 10 years, 75% by age 20, and 90% by 30 years[64,65] if untreated. In a review of more than 180 families and 922 affected individuals, the mean age at presentation was 27 and mean age at colectomy was 29.[66]

Extracolonic tumors (**Table 4**) cause significant morbidity in FAP with desmoid tumors and duodenal cancers being the second and third commonest causes of death after CRC.[67] In one series, 88% of patients with FAP developed duodenal polyps, often near the ampulla and papilla,[68] with a lifetime risk of duodenal carcinoma of 4% to 12%.[69] Duodenal polyps may be associated with different germline *APC* mutations than those with severe colonic polyposis.[70] Gastric cystic fundic gland polyps may develop in up to 33% of FAP patients. Gastric carcinoma is rare in FAP but may be higher in Asian populations.[71,72]

Hepatoblastoma occurs in an estimated 0.6% of children before 6 years but is rare thereafter.[73] Thyroid carcinoma may affect 12% of patients with FAP[74] but carries a good prognosis. They are predominantly well-differentiated papillary cancers affecting young women.

Molecular Basis of Disease

APC is a tumor suppressor gene consisting of 15 exons and encodes a protein of 2843 amino acids[75] that is involved in cell adhesion, signal transduction, transcription regulation, cell cycle control, apoptosis, and maintenance of the fidelity of chromosomal segregation. As part of a scaffolding protein complex it negatively regulates Wnt signaling.[75,76]

APC inactivation is the hallmark of the chromosomal instability pathway (CIN) phenotype that occurs in most of CRC. Increasing size, number, and worsening histology of polyps reflect the linear process of carcinogenesis along the CIN pathway.

More than 800 different *APC* germline mutations were reported[62] through 2007 with the vast majority associated with FAP being frameshift or nonsense mutations.[45] *APC* mutations are not distributed evenly, with "hotspots" at codons 1061 and 1309 accounting for approximately 11% and 17%, respectively, of germline mutations. Most lie in the "mutation cluster region" (MCR) between codons 1250 and 1464 in the 5' region of exon 15.[62]

Table 4
Extracolonic tumor risks in familial adenomatous polyposis

Tumor	Relative Risk	Absolute Lifetime Risk, %
Desmoid	852.0	15.0
Duodenum	330.8	3.0–5.0
Thyroid	7.6	2.0 (<12% in women)
Brain	7.0	2.0
Ampullary	123.7	1.7
Pancreas	4.5	1.7
Hepatoblastoma	847.0	1.6
Gastric	—	0.6[a]

[a] The Leeds Castle Polyposis Group.

From National Cancer Institute. Genetics of Colorectal Cancer. Available at: http://www.cancer. gov/cancertopics/pdq/genetics/colorectal/HealthProfessional/Table4. Accessed November 30, 2009. *Data from* Refs.[45,56,170–173]

Clinical Risk Management

Mutation analysis can identify sequence changes in up to 95% of classic FAP cases. However, the early development of adenomas raises special considerations relating to genetic testing of children. Genetic consultation is recommended for newly diagnosed FAP families as this can determine whether genetic testing would be informative for at-risk relatives. A negative test within a family with a known *APC* mutation allows colorectal screening to revert to that recommended to the population with background cancer risk, ie, colonoscopy or equivalent test starting at age 50.

Management can be affected by genotype, as severity of disease and extracolonic tumors may correlate with the location of *APC* mutations. Mutations between codons 1250 and 1464, especially codon 1309, often lead to profuse polyposis with earlier presentations.[77–80]

For those with an FAP phenotype/confirmed mutation or from an affected family but where they have not yet been tested, the following surveillance is advised:

Birth to 6 years:
- Annual hepatoblastoma screening by abdominal ultrasound and alpha-fetoprotein serum concentration.

10 years and up:
- Annual palpation of the thyroid gland.
- Sigmoidoscopy or colonoscopy every 1 to 2 years. Once polyps are detected by either procedure, full colonoscopy should be repeated annually. AFAP family members may begin in the late teens and repeat every 2 to 3 years.
- Esophagogastroduodenoscopy (EGD) with side-viewing endoscope should be performed after the development of colonic polyposis or age 25, whichever is sooner. EGD should be repeated every 1 to 3 years depending on number, size, and degree of dysplasia of duodenal adenomas. Removal of duodenal adenomas is indicated if polyps (1) exhibit villous or severe dysplastic histology, (2) exceed 1 cm in size, or (3) cause symptoms.
  Small bowel contrast studies or computerized tomography (CT) of abdomen and pelvis with oral contrast may also assist in monitoring duodenal and colorectal adenomas. Biopsy of an enlarged but otherwise normal ampullary papilla and endoscopic retrograde cholangiopancreatography (ERCP) to identify duodenal and common bile duct adenomas may also be indicated. Gastric cancer risk may be higher in Asian populations and specific screening may be indicated for these groups.[81]

Prophylactic colectomy before malignant transformation is recommended for classic FAP once polyps have appeared, but timing will depend on adenoma size, number, and degree of dysplasia. Colectomy for AFAP is often deferred until polyps become too difficult to control. For desmoid tumors, as surgery may accelerate growth, a conservative approach may be reasonable.[82,83]

LYNCH SYNDROME OR DEFECTIVE DNA MISMATCH REPAIR TYPE HEREDITARY NONPOLYPOSIS COLON CANCER
Clinical Overview

Lynch syndrome is an autosomal dominant condition caused by a mutation in one of several DNA mismatch repair genes[84,85] that maintain DNA fidelity. These genes encode proteins that form a multimeric DNA mismatch repair (MMR) complex that corrects the small insertions or deletions that frequently occur during somatic replication.[86–88] Defective MMR leads to the so-called "mutator" or "replication error" phenotype where a markedly increased rate of mutation, inevitably involving cell-cycle regulation, increases the potential for malignancy.[89]

Lynch syndrome accounts for approximately 3% to 5% of all CRC[90,91] and 2% of endometrial cancer.[92] It is the commonest inherited colon cancer syndrome. Patients may have synchronous and metachronous CRC with a predilection for right-sided cancer, proximal to the splenic flexure. Other cancers associated with Lynch syndrome include stomach, small intestine, liver, pancreas and biliary tract, brain, ovarian, and transitional cell carcinoma of the ureter and renal pelvis (**Table 5**).[93–96] Small bowel cancer is sufficiently rare in the general population that its diagnosis should instigate a careful history, including pedigree, and physical examination for signs of a cancer syndrome.

Muir-Torre syndrome is a variant of Lynch syndrome that combines colorectal tumors with multiple cutaneous adnexal neoplasms (sebaceous adenomas and carcinomas and keratoacanthomas) and tumors in endometrium, kidney, ovaries, stomach, and small intestine. Mutations in *MSH2* account for most of Muir-Torre syndrome.[97–99] Glioblastoma in Lynch syndrome may be referred to as "Turcot syndrome" but should not be confused with medulloblastoma in familial adenomatous polyposis (FAP), also called Turcot syndrome.

The diagnosis of Lynch syndrome cases has been challenging. The research criteria for identifying Lynch syndrome families were established by the International Collaborative Group (ICG) meeting in Amsterdam in 1990 and are hence known as the "Amsterdam I Criteria," shown in **Box 2**.[100] However, close to half of MMR gene mutation–positive Lynch syndrome families do not meet these criteria,[101] so they were revised in 1999 to Amsterdam II[102–104] to take suspicious extracolonic malignancies into account. An even less stringent third set of criteria have been devised expressly to identify individuals for whom tumor "microsatellite instability" (MSI) (see the section "Molecular Basis of Disease") testing is recommended[105] (Revised Bethesda Guidelines; **Box 3**); broadening the criteria enhances sensitivity but greatly reduces the specificity for Lynch syndrome.

Regarding distinguishing Lynch syndrome from hereditary nonpolyposis colon cancer (HNPCC), many investigators have noted that there are families who fulfill

Table 5
Cancer risks in individuals with Lynch syndrome up to age 70 years

Cancer	General Population Risk	Lynch Syndrome	
		Risks	Mean Age of Onset, y
Colon	5.5%	80%	44
Endometrium	2.7%	20%–60%	46
Stomach	<1%	11%–19%	56
Ovary	1.6%	9%–12%	42.5
Hepatobiliary tract	<1%	2%–7%	Not reported
Urinary tract	<1%	4%–5%	~55
Small bowel	<1%	1%–4%	49
Brain	<1%	1%–3%	~50
Pancreas	1%	4%	~53

Data from Refs.[95,120,174–179]

Box 2
Amsterdam I Criteria (1991)[a]

All criteria must be met:

1. One member diagnosed with CRC before age 50.

2. Two affected generations.

3. Three affected relatives, one of them a first-degree relative of the other two.

4. FAP excluded.

5. Tumors verified by pathologic examination.

Amsterdam II Criteria (1999)[b]

Identical to the Amsterdam I criteria except in broadening the third criterion; it still requires at least 3 affected relatives, but now also requires any of the following recognized Lynch syndrome–related cancers: colorectal, endometrial, small bowel, ureter, or renal pelvis.

[a] *Data from* Vasen H, Watson P, Mecklin J, et al. New clinical criteria for hereditary nonpolyposis colorectal cancer (HNPCC, Lynch syndrome) proposed by the International Collaborative group on HNPCC. Gastroenterology 1999;116(6):1453–56.
[b] *Data from* Llor X, Pons E, Xicola R, et al. Differential features of colorectal cancers fulfilling Amsterdam criteria without involvement of the mutator pathway. Clin Cancer Res 2005;11 (20):7304–10.

---

the classical Amsterdam I criteria but do not have evidence of defects in MMR pathways and who do not appear to have the same risk of syndrome-associated cancers as those with defective MMR. Families meeting Amsterdam I criteria with intact MMR have been classified as "Familial Colorectal Cancer Type X"[106–111] and it is probable that there are, as yet, unidentified genes that are associated with this phenotype. There is a move, therefore, to only refer to Lynch as the syndrome of HNPCC with genomic instability; the term HNPCC remains as an umbrella term including broadly all those who fulfill Amsterdam I or II criteria regardless of MSI status.

Box 3
Revised Bethesda criteria (2004)

Any 1 criterion would support MSI testing:

1. One member diagnosed with CRC before age 50.

2. Presence of synchronous, metachronous CRC or other Lynch syndrome–associated tumor[a] in an individual regardless of age.

3. CRC with MSI-H pathologic features diagnosed in an individual younger than 60 years (presence of tumor-infiltrating lymphocytes, Crohn-like lymphocytic reaction, mucinous/signet-ring differentiation or medullary growth pattern).

4. CRC or Lynch syndrome–associated tumor[a] in at least 1 first-degree relative younger than 50.

5. CRC or Lynch syndrome–associated tumor[a] diagnosed in 2 first-degree or second-degree relatives at any age.

[a] Endometrial, stomach, ovarian, pancreas, small bowel, biliary tract, ureter or renal pelvis, brain, sebaceous gland adenoma or keratoacanthoma.
Data from Valle L, Perea J, Carbonell P, et al. Clinicopathologic and pedigree differences in Amsterdam I-positive hereditary nonpolyposis colorectal cancer families according to tumor microsatellite instability status. J Clin Oncol 2007;25(7):781–6.

Cancer Risk

Lifetime risks for cancers in Lynch Syndrome are shown in **Table 5.**[112] The average age of CRC diagnosis in Lynch syndrome is approximately 44 years, versus 64 years in sporadic cancer, although individuals with mutations in *MSH6* have a mean age at CRC diagnosis of 55 to 57 years.[113] The lifetime risk for developing CRC is 80%, although evidence of differing patterns of penetrance are emerging for each gene,[114–116] with CRC occurring earlier in male *MLH1*-carriers than female.

The commonest extracolonic cancer is endometrial adenocarcinoma, which affects at least one female in about half of all Lynch syndrome families with mean age at diagnosis also in the fifth decade.[112] The lifetime risk for endometrial cancer in women may be 21% to 71% at age 70[113]; risk varies with the underlying gene involved. *MSH2* mutation carriers have higher endometrial cancer risk than do carriers of *MLH1* mutations, for example. Associated endometrial cancer subtypes include endometrioid, clear cell carcinoma, uterine papillary serous carcinoma, and malignant mixed Müllerian tumors.[117]

Molecular Basis of Disease

Lynch Syndrome is caused by germline mutations in 1 of 4 DNA MMR genes that include *MLH1* (human mutL homolog 1) at 3p21.3, *MSH2* (human mutS homolog 2) at 2p21-p22, *MSH6* at 2p16, and *PMS2* (postmeiotic segregation 2) at 7p22. Other DNA MMR genes exist but their roles in Lynch syndrome are unclear. These include *PMS1* at 2q31-q33 and *MSH3* at 5q11-q12.

Microsatellites are short, repeating units of 1 to 3 nucleotides located throughout the genome, primarily in introns.[118] They are particularly susceptible to errors from MMR gene defects. Tumor DNA showing alterations in microsatellite regions is an indicator of defective MMR, which can arise from somatic (restricted to tumor) or germline (Lynch syndrome) mutations.[119] The change in the length of the short repeating units is termed "microsatellite instability" (MSI). For the designation of MSI in an adenocarcinoma, a minimum percentage of unstable loci is required. If a tumor shows more than 30% of markers unstable, it is MSI-high (MSI-H), if less than 30%, it is MSI-low (MSI-L). If no loci are unstable, it is designated microsatellite stable (MSS). Approximately 90% of CRC in Lynch syndrome manifests MSI-H in the tumor.[120,121]

Testing for loss of *MSH2, MLH1, MSH6,* and *PMS2* expression by immunohistochemistry (IHC) in CRC using monoclonal antibodies can help identify the mutated gene.[122–124] Because of the formation of heterodimers in the DNA MMR complex, loss of expression of *MLH1* owing to germline mutation or other mechanisms causes concurrent loss of *PMS2,* whereas loss of expression of *MSH2* causes concurrent loss of *MSH6.* Isolated loss of *MSH6* and *PMS2* suggests mutations in those two genes, respectively. Absent expression has a high predictive value to detect germline mutations although it is not be seen in all MSI-H tumors.[125,126]

MSI-H itself is not specific for a germline MMR defect, as age-related methylation of *MLH1* accounts for the sporadic majority of MSI-H tumors.[102] Clinical testing for tumor promoter methylation of *MLH1* and for somatic *BRAF* mutations can help distinguish sporadic MSI-H cases from those with germline mutations in *MLH1.*

Germline mutation analysis for *MSH2, MLH1, MSH6,* and *PMS2* can be performed for suspected Lynch syndrome, ideally after screening tumors for microsatellite instability and/or absence of protein expression to guide testing.[127,128] Using both screening tests together increases the yield for finding Lynch syndrome mutations.[90,114,116,129] The Revised Bethesda Guidelines[105] describe the clinical indications for MSI and tumor analysis. Up to 90% of Lynch syndrome families have mutations in *MSH2* or *MLH1*.[130,131] Most mutations are detected by sequencing, but deletion and duplication analysis is required to be complete. Using both sequence and deletion testing together may increase sensitivity to 95%.[132–134]

Clinical Risk Management

For those at risk and others with strong family histories but no diagnostic confirmation by genetic or prior tumor testing, colonoscopy every 1 to 2 years, starting at about age 20 or at least 10 years before the earliest CRC in the family, is recommended.[112,135,136] If there is a history of cancer below the age of 25 in the family, this may require genetic testing of children with similar considerations to FAP. Once a mutation is identified in a family, testing can be offered to at-risk relatives and those without the mutation exempted from intensive surveillance. If no mutation can be identified, an inherited cancer predisposition is not excluded but testing of relatives would be uninformative. Members of such families should continue intensive screening.

The progression from normal mucosa to adenoma to cancer may be accelerated in Lynch, and because of the only modest or no increase in number of polyps, it seems a larger proportion undergo malignant transformation.[137,138] This would suggest a requirement for frequent screening and optimal quality examinations to ensure no lesions are missed.

The choice of CRC surveillance techniques has widened in recent years. However, because neoplasms in Lynch syndrome may be subtle, flat lesions, there is evidence that CT colonography (also known as virtual colonoscopy) would have inferior sensitivity compared with standard optical colonoscopy.[139] Chromo-endoscopy using indigo carmine may be used to augment standard screening, as data suggest it aids detection of small but histologically advanced adenomas.[140,141] Unlike for FAP, sigmoidoscopy is not a recommended option because of the preponderance of right-sided cancers. Stool DNA testing for somatic gene mutations cannot replace germline mutation testing and has not been adequately studied in CRC predisposition syndromes.

Polypectomy reduces the incidence of CRC in Lynch syndrome[138]; however, given the shortcomings of screening, some Lynch-syndrome family members will opt for prophylactic colectomy. All Lynch syndrome candidates for prophylactic surgery should be counseled that there have been no controlled studies of such interventions. Moreover, there remains a risk of CRC in the rectal remnant after subtotal colectomy[142] and individuals who have undergone partial resection should continue endoscopic surveillance. Once CRC is found, subtotal or total colectomy with ileorectal anastomosis has been recommended over a partial resection by some experts.

Women at risk for Lynch should be counseled that abnormal or postmenopausal vaginal bleeding warrants further investigation. Endometrial cancer screening may be considered by age 25[135] and options include pelvic examination ± Papanicolaou smear, endometrial biopsy, CA-125 testing, and/or transvaginal ultrasound (TVUS). Studies of the latter so far have been disappointing,[143–146] although TVUS can also help evaluate the ovaries. Endometrial sampling may have better sensitivity[147] and is suggested by a National Institutes of Health task force to begin from age 30 to 35.[136] Oral contraceptives reduce the incidence of sporadic endometrial and ovarian cancer but have not been demonstrated to have a benefit in Lynch syndrome. Women may consider prophylactic hysterectomy and bilateral salpingo-oophorectomy (BSO), but this decision must be taken in light of childbearing plans and potential side effects of long-term hormone replacement therapy. Although a retrospective study suggested hysterectomy and BSO were effective at preventing endometrial and ovarian cancer,[148] all Lynch syndrome candidates for prophylactic surgery should be counseled on the limitations regarding ovarian cancer prevention.

There is no consensus on a role for screening for gastric and small intestinal neoplasms with upper gastrointestinal endoscopy at present. There is also no evidence for annual urinalysis with cytology for urinary tract cancer, but it is noninvasive and inexpensive and hence generally advised. Careful skin examination on an annual basis would appear justified on the same basis, although no screening for cancer of the pancreas, biliary tract, or brain is yet recommended.

Rare patients with biallelic germline MMR mutations have been described with very early onset Lynch tumors, café-au-lait macules, and early-onset hematologic or brain malignancies.[149,150] Management of such individuals is vastly different from that recommended in Lynch syndrome.

MYH-ASSOCIATED POLYPOSIS
Clinical Overview

Mutations in the MYH (or MUTYH) gene on 1p32.1-p34.3 cause an autosomal recessive CRC predisposition syndrome associated with multiple colonic polyps. It may be indistinguishable from classical or attenuated FAP[151] and it has been suggested that MYH-associated polyposis (MAP) is the real attenuated FAP.[63] Duodenal adenomas, gastric fundic gland polyps, CHRPE, osteomas and dental anomalies, and desmoid tumors, previously hallmarks of FAP, have now been reported in MAP. The colorectal polyps range in number from a few to more than 500 and tend to be mainly small tubular or tubulovillous adenomas with mild dysplasia with occasional hyperplastic polyps. Cancer can arise anywhere in the colorectum but the adenomas may show a right colonic predilection.

Cancer Risk

MAP tends to present later than classical FAP. In 2 major series, the mean ages at presentation were 46 and 51 with a range of 13 to 70 and the presenting feature in 50% of cases was CRC.[152,153] Jenkins and colleagues[154] reported cumulative risk to age 70 of 80% representing a 50-fold risk of CRC. There was also a threefold increase in risk in monoallelic carriers (8% cumulative risk to age 70), but other data show no appreciable increase risk in monoallelic MYH carriers.[155–159] Duodenal adenomas with or without duodenal adenocarcinoma have been reported in approximately 5%.[160,161]

Molecular Basis of Disease

MYH is a base-excision repair (BER) gene that repairs mutations caused by reactive oxygen species.[162] It codes for a DNA glycosylase that identifies and removes adenine residues that have been incorrectly paired with 8-oxo-7, 8-dihydro-2′-deoxyguanosine (8-oxodG).[163] Failure to correct this causes an increase in G:C → T:A transversions, particularly at GAA sequences, which leads to a stop codon, TAA. The APC gene is a major downstream target of MYH mutations.[151] MAP tumors are generally microsatellite stable (MSS).

More than 80 germline variants have been reported. Most are missense, but also reported are 6 truncating mutations, splice-site mutations, and several small insertion/deletions.[164] The commonest mutations in whites are Y179C and G396D (formerly called Y165C and G382D, respectively) accounting for 53% and 32% of all mutations respectively. The Y179C mutation is more deleterious than the G396D mutation.[155,160]

Approximately 1% of the general population is heterozygous for an MYH mutation. MYH carriers could acquire a somatic mutation (a "second hit") in the wild-type allele and develop CRC; however, somatic *MYH* mutations are infrequent in CRC.[165] Moreover, the role of somatic mutations in *MYH* in the development of nonfamilial CRC is yet to be understood. It is notable that *MYH* mutations have not yet been implicated in nongastrointestinal cancers in which reactive oxygen species are thought to play a role in carcinogenesis, including lung, breast, kidney, liver, and prostate.[132,166–169]

Clinical Risk Management

Establishing the correct genetic diagnosis will direct cancer surveillance for family members. Classical and attenuated FAP are dominantly inherited with risk for successive generations, whereas only a single generation is at risk for recessively inherited MAP. The National Comprehensive Cancer Network guidelines (http://www.nccn.org/professionals/physician_gls/PDF/colorectal_screening.pdf) from 2009 recommend colonoscopy starting at 25 to 30 years with repeat every 3 to 5 years if negative and upper endoscopy with side-viewing duodenoscope from age 30 to 35. If adenomas are found, then management should proceed as for FAP.

ACKNOWLEDGMENTS

Drs Lindor and Shah thank Cheryl Dowse for her assistance in preparing the manuscript.

REFERENCES

1. Amos C, Keitheri-Cheteri M, Sabripour M, et al. Genotype-phenotype correlations in Peutz-Jegher syndrome. J Med Genet 2004;41(5):327–33.
2. Boardman L. Heritable colorectal cancer syndromes: recognition and preventive management. Gastroenterol Clin North Am 2002;31:1107–31.
3. Anyanwu S. Sporadic Peutz-Jeghers syndrome in a Nigerian. Cent Afr J Med 1999;45(7):182–4.
4. Yoon K, Ku J, Choi H, et al. Germline mutations of the STK11 gene in Korean Peutz-Jeghers syndrome patients. Br J Cancer 2000;82(8):1403–6.
5. Riegert-Johnson D, Boardman L. Peutz-Jeghers syndrome. In: Potter J, Lindor N, editors. Genetics of colorectal cancer. New York: Springer; 2009. p. 193–8.
6. Hearle N, Schumacher V, Menko F, et al. Frequency and spectrum of cancers in the Peutz-Jeghers syndrome. Cancer Res 2006;12(10):3209–15.
7. Mehenni H, Resta N, Park J, et al. Cancer risks in LKB1 germline mutation carriers. Gut 2006;55(7):984–90.
8. Olschwang S, Boisson C, Thomas G. Peutz-Jeghers families unlinked to STK11/LKB1 gene mutations are highly predisposed to primitive biliary adenocarcinoma. J Med Genet 2001;38(6):356–60.
9. Aaltonen L. Peutz-Jeghers syndrome. In: Vogelstein B, Kinzler K, editors. The genetic basis of human cancer. New York: McGraw-Hill; 2002. p. 337–41.
10. Hemminki A, Markie D, Tomlinson I, et al. A serine/threonine kinase gene defective in Peutz-Jeghers syndrome. Nature 1998;391(6663):184–7.
11. Jenne D, Reimann H, Nezu J, et al. Peutz-Jeghers syndrome is caused by mutations in a novel serine threonine kinase. Nat Genet 1998;18:38–43.
12. Giardiello F, Hamilton S, Kern S, et al. Colorectal neoplasia in juvenile polyposis or juvenile polyps. Arch Dis Child 1991;66(8):971–5.
13. Rowan A, Churchman M, Jefferey R, et al. In situ analysis of LKB1/STK11 mRNA expression in human normal tissues and tumours. J Pathol 2000;192(2):203–6.

14. Boudeau J, Baas A, Deak M, et al. MO25alpha/beta interact with STRAD alpha/beta enhancing their ability to bind, activate and localize LKB1 in the cytoplasm. EMBO J 2003;22(19):5102–14.

15. Ylikorkala A, Avizienyte E, Tomlinson I, et al. Mutations and impaired function of LKB1 in familial and non-familial Peutz-Jeghers syndrome and sporadic testicular cancer. Hum Mol Genet 1999;8:45–51.

16. Karuman P, Gozani O, Odze R, et al. The Peutz-Jegher gene product LKB1 is a mediator of p53-dependent cell death. Mol Cell 2001;7:1307–19.

17. Gruber S, Entius M, Petersen G, et al. Pathogenesis of adenocarcinoma in Peutz-Jeghers syndrome. Cancer Res 1998;58:5267–70.

18. Flageole H, Raptis S, Trudel J, et al. Progression toward malignancy of hamartomas in a patient with Peutz-Jeghers syndrome: case report and literature. Can J Surg 1994;37(3):231–6.

19. Nakau M, Miyoshi H, Seldin M, et al. Hepatocellular carcinoma caused by loss of heterozygosity in LKB1 gene knockout mice. Cancer Res 2002;62:4549–53.

20. Jishage K, Nezu J, Kawase Y, et al. Role of Lkb1, the causative gene of Peutz-Jegher's syndrome, in embryogenesis and polyposis. Proc Natl Acad Sci U S A 2002;99(13):8903–8.

21. Amos C, Frazier M, McGarrity T. Peutz-Jeghers syndrome. In: GeneReviews at GeneTests: Medical Genetics Information Resource (database online) Gene reviews 2009, (Updated May 15 2007). Copyright, University of Washington, Seattle 1997–2010. Available at: http://www.genetests.org. Accessed November 30, 2009.

22. Hinds R, Philp C, Hyer W, et al. Complications of childhood Peutz-Jeghers syndrome: implications for pediatric screening. J Pediatr Gastroenterol Nutr 2004;39:219–20.

23. Pennazio M, Rossini F. Small bowel polyps in Peutz-Jeghers syndrome: management by combined push enteroscopy and intra-operative enteroscopy. Gastrointest Endosc 2000;51(3):304–8.

24. Edwards D, Khosraviani K, Stafferton R, et al. Long-term results of polyp clearance by intra-operative enteroscopy in the Peutz-Jeghers syndrome. Dis Colon Rectum 2003;46(1):48–50.

25. Aaltonen L, Jass J, Howe J. Juvenile polyposis. In: Hamilton S, Aaltonen L, editors. Pathology and genetics. Tumours of the digestive system. Lyon (France). IARC Press; 2000. p. 130–2.

26. Burt R, Bishop D, Lynch H, et al. Risk and surveillance of individuals with heritable factors for colorectal cancer. WHO Collaborating Centre for the Prevention of Colorectal Cancer. Bull World Health Organ 1990;68(5):655–65.

27. Nugent K, Talbot I, Hodgson S, et al. Solitary juvenile polyps: not a marker for subsequent malignancy. Gastroenterology 1993;105(3):698–700.

28. Brosens L, van Hattem A, Hylind L, et al. Risk of colorectal cancer in juvenile polyposis. Gut 2007a;56(7):965–7.

29. Hofting I, Pott G, Stolte M. The syndrome of juvenile polyposis. Leber Magen Darm 1993;23:111–2.

30. Chow E, Macrae F. A review of juvenile polyposis syndrome. J Gastroenterol Hepatol 2005;20(11):1634–40.

31. Brosens L, van Hattem W, Jansen M, et al. Gastrointestinal polyposis syndromes. Curr Mol Med 2007b;7(1):29–46.

32. Howe J, Sayed M, Ahmed A, et al. The prevalence of MADH4 and BMPR1A mutations in juvenile polyposis and absence of BMPR2, BMPR1B, and ACVR1 mutations. J Med Genet 2004;41(7):484–91.

33. Merg A, Lynch H, Lynch J, et al. Hereditary colorectal cancer-part II. Curr Probl Surg 2005;42(5):267–333.
34. Roth S, Sistonen P, Salovaara R, et al. SMAD genes in juvenile polyposis. Genes Chromosomes Cancer 1999;26(1):54–61.
35. Sayed M, Ahmed A, Ringold J, et al. Germline SMAD4 or BMPR1A mutations and phenotype of juvenile polyposis. Ann Surg Oncol 2002;9(9):901–6.
36. Pyatt R, Pilarski R, Prior T. Mutation screening in juvenile polyposis syndrome. J Mol Diagn 2006;8(1):84–8.
37. Kim B, Li C, Qiao W, et al. SMAD4 signalling in T cells is required for suppression of gastrointestinal cancer. Nature 2006;441(7096):1015–9.
38. Kinzler K, Vogelstein B. Landscaping the cancer terrain. Science 1998; 280(5366):1036–7.
39. Friedl W, Uhlhaas S, Schulmann K, et al. Juvenile polyposis: massive gastric polyposis is more common in MADH4 mutation carriers than in BMPR1A mutation carriers. Hum Genet 2002;111(1):108–11.
40. Handra-Luca A, Condroyer C, de Moncuit C, et al. Vessels' morphology in SMAD4 and BMPR1A-related juvenile polyposis. Am J Med Genet 2005;138(2):113–7.
41. Sweet K, Willis J, Zhou X, et al. Molecular classification of patients with unexplained hamartomatous and hyperplastic polyposis. JAMA 2005;294(19): 2465–73.
42. Blanco F, Santibanez J, Guerrero-Esteo M, et al. Interaction and functional interplay between endoglin and ALK-1, two components of the endothelial transforming growth factor-beta receptor complex. J Cell Physiol 2005;204(2): 574–84.
43. Howe J, Haidle J, Lal G, et al. ENG mutations in MADH4/BMPR1A mutation negative patients with juvenile polyposis. Clin Genet 2007;71(1):91–2.
44. Howe J, Mitros F, Summers R. The risk of gastrointestinal carcinoma in familial juvenile polyposis. Ann Surg Oncol 1998;5(8):751–6.
45. Galiatsatos P, Foulkes W. Familial adenomatous polyposis. Am J Gastroenterol 2006;101(2):385–98.
46. Rozen P, Macrae F. Familial adenomatous polyposis: the practical applications of clinical and molecular screening. Fam Cancer 2006;5(3):227–35.
47. Lipton L, Tomlinson I. The genetics of FAP and FAP-like syndrome. Fam Cancer 2006;5:221–6.
48. Guillem J, Smith A, Calle J, et al. Gastrointestinal polyposis syndromes. Curr Probl Surg 1999;36(4):217–323.
49. Lockhart-Mummery P. Cancer and heredity. Lancet 1925;205(5296):427–9.
50. Houlston R, Crabtree M, Phillips R, et al. Explaining differences in the severity of familial adenomatous polyposis and the search for modifier genes. Gut 2001; 48(1):1–5.
51. Lal G, Gallinger S. Familial adenomatous polyposis. Semin Surg Oncol 2000; 18(4):314–23.
52. Hamilton S, Liu B, Parsons R, et al. The molecular basis of Turcot's syndrome. N Engl J Med 1995;332(13):839–47.
53. Zippel D, Temple W. When is a neoplasm not a neoplasm? When it is a desmoid. J Surg Oncol 2007;95(3):190–1.
54. Sturt N, Clark S. Current ideas in desmoid tumours. Fam Cancer 2006;5(3): 275–85.
55. Bertario L, Russo A, Sala P, et al. Genotype and phenotype factors as determinants of desmoid tumors in patients with familial adenomatous polyposis. Int J Cancer 2001;95(2):102–7.

56. Lynch H, Fitzgibbons R Jr. Surgery, desmoid tumors, and familial adenomatous polyposis: case report and literature review. Am J Gastroenterol 1996;91(12): 2598–601.
57. Eccles D, van der Luijt R, Breukel C, et al. Hereditary desmoid disease due to a frameshift mutation at codon 1924 of the APC gene. Am J Hum Genet 1996; 59(6):1193–201.
58. Chen C, Phillips K, Grist S, et al. Congenital hypertrophy of the retinal pigment epithelium (CHRPE) in familial colorectal cancer. Fam Cancer 2006;5(4):397–404.
59. Knudsen A, Bisgaard M, Bülow S. Attenuated familial adenomatous polyposis (AFAP). A review of the literature. Fam Cancer 2003;2(1):43–55.
60. Brensinger J, Laken S, Luce M, et al. Variable phenotype of familial adenomatous polyposis in pedigrees with 3' mutation in the APC gene. Gut 1998;43(4): 548–52.
61. Sieber O, Segditsas S, Knudsen A, et al. Disease severity and genetic pathways in attenuated FAP vary greatly but depend on the site of the germline mutation. Gut 2006;55(10):1440–8.
62. Nieuwenhuis M, Vasen H. Correlations between mutation site in APC and phenotype of familial adenomatous polyposis (FAP): a review of the literature. Crit Rev Oncol Hematol 2007;61(2):153–61.
63. Lefevre J, Parc Y, Svrcek M, et al. APC, MYH, and the correlation genotype-phenotype in colorectal polyposis. Ann Surg Oncol 2009;16(4):871–7.
64. Berk T, Cohen Z, Bapat B, et al. Negative genetic test results in familial adenomatous polyposis: clinical screening implications. Dis Colon Rectum 1999;42(3): 307–10.
65. Petersen G, Slack J, Nakamura Y. Screening guidelines and premorbid diagnosis of familial adenomatous polyposis using linkage. Gastroenterology 1991;100(6):1658–64.
66. Rustin R, Jagelman D, McGannon E, et al. Spontaneous mutation in familial adenomatous polyposis. Dis Colon Rectum 1990;33(1):52–5.
67. Arvanitis M, Jagelman D, Fazio V, et al. Mortality in patients with familial adenomatous polyposis. Dis Colon Rectum 1990;33(8):639–42.
68. Church J, McGannon E, Hull-Boiner S, et al. Gastroduodenal polyps in patients with familial adenomatous polyposis. Dis Colon Rectum 1992;35:1170–3.
69. Kadmon M, Tandara A, Herfarth C. Duodenal adenomatosis in familial adenomatous polyposis coli. A review of the literature and results from the Heidelberg Polyposis Register. Int J Colorectal Dis 2001;16(2):63–75.
70. Groves C, Saunders B, Spigelman A, et al. Duodenal cancer in patients with familial adenomatous polyposis (FAP): results of a 10 year prospective study. Gut 2002;50(5):636–41.
71. Park J, Park K, Ahn Y, et al. Risk of gastric cancer among Korean familial adenomatous polyposis patients. Report of three cases. Dis Colon Rectum 1992; 35(10):996–8.
72. Brosens L, Keller J, Offerhaus G, et al. Prevention and management of duodenal polyps in familial adenomatous polyposis. Gut 2005;54(7):1034–43.
73. Cetta F, Mazzarella L, Bon G, et al. Genetic alterations in hepatoblastoma and hepatocellular carcinoma associated with familial adenomatous polyposis. Med Pediatr Oncol 2003;41(5):496–7.
74. Herraiz M, Barbesino G, Faquin W, et al. Prevalence of thyroid cancer in familial adenomatous polyposis syndrome and the role of screening ultrasound examinations. Clin Gastroenterol Hepatol 2007;5(3):367–73.

75. Fearnhead N, Britton M, Bodmer W. The ABC of APC. Hum Mol Genet 2001; 10(7):721–33.
76. Näthke I. The adenomatous polyposis coli protein: the Achilles heel of the gut epithelium. Annu Rev Cell Dev Biol 2004;20:337–66.
77. Bertario L, Russo A, Sala P, et al. Multiple approach to the exploration of genotype-phenotype correlations in familial adenomatous polyposis. J Clin Oncol 2003;21(9):1698–707.
78. Caspari R, Olschwang S, Friedl W, et al. Familial adenomatous polyposis: desmoid tumours and lack of ophthalmic lesions (CHRPE) associated with APC mutations beyond codon 1444. Hum Mol Genet 1995;4(3):337–40.
79. Enomoto M, Konishi M, Iwama T, et al. The relationship between frequencies of extracolonic manifestations and the position of APC germline mutation in patients with familial adenomatous polyposis. Jpn J Clin Oncol 2000;30(2):82–8.
80. Ficari F, Cama A, Valanzano R, et al. APC gene mutations and colorectal adenomatosis in familial adenomatous polyposis. Br J Cancer 2000;82:348–53.
81. Kashiwagi H, Spigelman A. Gastroduodenal lesions in familial adenomatous polyposis. Surg Today 2000;30:675–82.
82. Ferenc T, Sygut J, Kopczyński J, et al. Aggressive fibromatosis (desmoid tumors): definition, occurrence, pathology, diagnostic problems, clinical behavior, genetic background. Pol J Pathol 2006;57(1):5–15.
83. Durno C, Monga N, Bapat B, et al. Does early colectomy increase desmoid risk in familial adenomatous polyposis? Clin Gastroenterol Hepatol 2007;5(10): 1190–4.
84. Nielsen M, Joerink-van de Beld M, Jones N, et al. Analysis of MUTYH genotypes and colorectal phenotypes in patients With MUTYH-associated polyposis. Gastroenterology 2009;136(2):471–6.
85. Jones N, Vogt S, Nielsen M, et al. Increased colorectal cancer incidence in obligate carriers of heterozygous mutations in MUTYH. Gastroenterology 2009; 137(2):489–94.
86. Gruber S, Kohlmann W. The genetics of hereditary non-polyposis colorectal cancer. J Natl Compr Canc Netw 2003;1(1):137–44.
87. Rhyu M. Molecular mechanisms underlying hereditary nonpolyposis colorectal carcinoma. J Natl Cancer Inst 1996;88(5):240–51.
88. Chung D, Rustgi A. DNA mismatch repair and cancer. Gastroenterology 1995; 109(5):1685–99.
89. Lazar V, Grandjouan S, Bognel C, et al. Accumulation of multiple mutations in tumour suppressor genes during colorectal tumorigenesis in HNPCC patients. Hum Mol Genet 1994;3(12):2257–60.
90. Hampel H, Frankel W, Martin E, et al. Screening for the Lynch syndrome (hereditary nonpolyposis colorectal cancer). N Engl J Med 2005;352(18):1851–60.
91. Wijnen J, Vasen H, Khan P, et al. Clinical findings with implications for genetic testing in families with clustering of colorectal cancer. N Engl J Med 1998; 339(8):511–8.
92. Hampel H, Frankel W, Panescu J, et al. Screening for Lynch syndrome (hereditary nonpolyposis colorectal cancer) among endometrial cancer patients. Cancer Res 2006;66(15):7810–7.
93. Watson P, Lynch H. Extracolonic cancer in hereditary nonpolyposis colorectal cancer. Cancer 1993;71(3):677–85.
94. Watson P, Vasen H, Mecklin J, et al. The risk of endometrial cancer in hereditary nonpolyposis colorectal cancer. Am J Med 1994;96(6):516–20.

95. Aarnio M, Mecklin J, Aaltonen L, et al. Life-time risk of different cancers in hereditary non-polyposis colorectal cancer (HNPCC) syndrome. Int J Cancer 1995; 64(6):430–3.

96. Kastrinos F, Mukherjee B, Tayob N, et al. Risk of pancreatic cancer in families with Lynch syndrome. JAMA 2009;302(16):1790–5.

97. Suspiro A, Fidalgo P, Cravo M, et al. The Muir-Torre syndrome: a rare variant of hereditary nonpolyposis colorectal cancer associated with hMSH2 mutation. Am J Gastroenterol 1998;93(9):1572–4.

98. Kruse R, Rütten A, Lamberti C, et al. Muir-Torre phenotype has a frequency of DNA mismatch-repair-gene mutations similar to that in hereditary nonpolyposis colorectal cancer families defined by the Amsterdam criteria. Am J Hum Genet 1998;63(1):63–70.

99. South C, Hampel H, Comeras I, et al. The frequency of Muir-Torre syndrome among Lynch syndrome families. J Natl Cancer Inst 2008;100(4):277–81.

100. Vasen H, Mecklin J, Khan P, et al. The International Collaborative Group on hereditary nonpolyposis colorectal cancer (ICG-HNPCC). Dis Colon Rectum 1991;34(5):424.

101. Syngal S, Fox E, Li C, et al. Interpretation of genetic test results for hereditary nonpolyposis colorectal cancer: implications for clinical predisposition testing. JAMA 1999;282(3):247–53.

102. Liu B, Parsons R, Papadopoulos N, et al. Analysis of mismatch repair genes in hereditary non-polyposis colorectal cancer patients. Nat Med 1996;2(2): 169–74.

103. Beck N, Tomlinson I, Homfray T, et al. Genetic testing is important in families with a history suggestive of hereditary non-polyposis colorectal cancer even if the Amsterdam criteria are not fulfilled. Br J Surg 1997;84(2):233–7.

104. Vasen H, Watson P, Mecklin J, et al. New clinical criteria for hereditary non-polyposis colorectal cancer (HNPCC, Lynch syndrome) proposed by the International Collaborative group on HNPCC. Gastroenterology 1999;116(6): 1453–6.

105. Umar A, Boland C, Terdiman J, et al. Revised Bethesda guidelines for hereditary nonpolyposis colorectal cancer (Lynch syndrome) and microsatellite instability. J Natl Cancer Inst 2004;96(4):261–8.

106. Lindor N, Rabe K, Petersen G, et al. Lower cancer incidence in Amsterdam-I criteria families without mismatch repair deficiency: familial colorectal cancer type X. JAMA 2005;293(16):1979–85.

107. Mueller-Koch Y, Vogelsang H, Kopp R, et al. Hereditary non-polyposis colorectal cancer: clinical and molecular evidence for a new entity of hereditary colorectal cancer. Gut 2005;2005(54):12.

108. Llor X, Pons E, Xicola R, et al. Differential features of colorectal cancers fulfilling Amsterdam criteria without involvement of the mutator pathway. Clin Cancer Res 2005;11(20):7304–10.

109. Valle L, Perea J, Carbonell P, et al. Clinicopathologic and pedigree differences in Amsterdam I-positive hereditary nonpolyposis colorectal cancer families according to tumor microsatellite instability status. J Clin Oncol 2007;25(7):781–6.

110. Jass J. Hereditary non-polyposis colorectal cancer: the rise and fall of a confusing term. World J Gastroenterol 2006;12(31):4943–50.

111. Abdel-Rahman W, Ollikainen M, Kariola R, et al. Comprehensive characterization of HNPCC-related colorectal cancers reveals striking molecular features in families with no germline mismatch repair gene mutations. Oncogene 2005; 24:1542–51.

112. Vasen H, Möslein G, Alonso A, et al. Guidelines for the clinical management of Lynch syndrome (hereditary non-polyposis cancer). J Med Genet 2007;44(6): 353–62.

113. Hendriks Y, Wagner A, Morreau H, et al. Cancer risk in hereditary nonpolyposis colorectal cancer due to MSH6 mutations: impact on counseling and surveillance. Gastroenterology 2004;127(1):17–25.

114. Piñol V, Castells A, Andreu M, et al. Accuracy of revised Bethesda guidelines, microsatellite instability, and immunohistochemistry for the identification of patients with hereditary nonpolyposis colorectal cancer. JAMA 2005;293(16): 1986–94.

115. Choi Y, Cotterchio M, McKeown-Eyssen G, et al. Penetrance of colorectal cancer among MLH1/MSH2 carriers participating in the colorectal cancer familial registry in Ontario. Hered Cancer Clin Pract 2009;7(1):14.

116. Lagerstedt-Robinson K, Liu T, Vandrovcova J, et al. Lynch syndrome (hereditary nonpolyposis colorectal cancer) diagnostics. J Natl Cancer Inst 2007;99(4): 291–9.

117. Broaddus R, Lynch H, Chen L, et al. Pathologic features of endometrial carcinoma associated with HNPCC: a comparison with sporadic endometrial carcinoma. Cancer 2006;106(1):87–94.

118. Weber J, May P. Abundant class of human DNA polymorphisms which can be typed using the polymerase chain reaction. Am J Hum Genet 1989;44(3):388–96.

119. Aaltonen A, Peltomäki P, Leach F, et al. Clues to the pathogenesis of familial colorectal cancer. Science 1993;260(5109):812–6.

120. Boland C, Thibodeau S, Hamilton S, et al. A National Cancer Institute Workshop on Microsatellite Instability for cancer detection and familial predisposition: development of international criteria for the determination of microsatellite instability in colorectal cancer. Cancer Res 1998;58(22):5248–57.

121. Cunningham J, Kim C, Christensen E, et al. The frequency of hereditary defective mismatch repair in a prospective series of unselected colorectal carcinomas. Am J Hum Genet 2001;69:780–90.

122. Thibodeau S, French A, Roche P, et al. Altered expression of hMSH2 and hMLH1 in tumors with microsatellite instability and genetic alterations in mismatch repair genes. Cancer Res 1996;56(21):4836–40.

123. Cawkwell L, Gray S, Murgatroyd H, et al. Choice of management strategy for colorectal cancer based on a diagnostic immunohistochemical test for defective mismatch repair. Gut 1999;45(3):409–15.

124. de La Chapelle A. Microsatellite instability phenotype of tumors: genotyping or immunohistochemistry? The jury is still out. J Clin Oncol 2002;20(4):897–9.

125. Lindor N, Burgart L, Leontovich O, et al. Immunohistochemistry versus microsatellite instability testing in phenotyping colorectal tumors. J Clin Oncol 2002; 20(4):1043–8.

126. Rigau V, Sebbagh N, Olschwang S, et al. Microsatellite instability in colorectal carcinoma. The comparison of immunohistochemistry and molecular biology suggests a role for hMSH6 [correction of hMLH6] immunostaining. Arch Pathol Lab Med 2003;127(6):694–700.

127. Kievit W, de Bruin J, Adang E, et al. Current clinical selection strategies for identification of hereditary non-polyposis colorectal cancer families are inadequate: a meta-analysis. Clin Genet 2004;65(4):308–16.

128. Southey M, Jenkins M, Mead L, et al. Use of molecular tumor characteristics to prioritize mismatch repair gene testing in early-onset colorectal cancer. J Clin Oncol 2005;23(27):6524–32.

129. Baudhuin L, Burgart L, Leontovich O, et al. Use of microsatellite instability and immunohistochemistry testing for the identification of individuals at risk for Lynch syndrome. Fam Cancer 2005;4(3):255–65.

130. Marra G, Boland C. Hereditary nonpolyposis colorectal cancer: the syndrome, the genes, and historical perspectives. J Natl Cancer Inst 1995;87(15): 1114–25.

131. Peltomäki P, Vasen H. Mutations predisposing to hereditary nonpolyposis colorectal cancer: database and results of a collaborative study. The International Collaborative Group on Hereditary Nonpolyposis Colorectal Cancer. Gastroenterology 1997;113(4):1146–58.

132. Charbonnier F, Olschwang S, Wang Q, et al. MSH2 in contrast to MLH1 and MSH6 is frequently inactivated by exonic and promoter rearrangements in hereditary nonpolyposis colorectal cancer. Cancer Res 2002;62(3):848–53.

133. Wagner A, Barrows A, Wijnen J, et al. Molecular analysis of hereditary nonpolyposis colorectal cancer in the United States: high mutation detection rate among clinically selected families and characterization of an American founder genomic deletion of the MSH2 gene. Am J Hum Genet 2003;72(5): 1088–100.

134. Wang Y, Friedl W, Lamberti C, et al. Hereditary nonpolyposis colorectal cancer: frequent occurrence of large genomic deletions in MSH2 and MLH1 genes. Int J Cancer 2003;103(5):636–41.

135. Burke W, Petersen G, Lynch P, et al. Recommendations for follow-up care of individuals with an inherited predisposition to cancer. I. Hereditary nonpolyposis colon cancer. Cancer Genetics Studies Consortium. JAMA 1997; 277(11):915–9.

136. Lindor N, Petersen G, Hadley D, et al. Recommendations for the care of individuals with an inherited predisposition to Lynch syndrome: a systematic review. JAMA 2006;296(12):1507–17.

137. Reitmair A, Cai J, Bjerknes M, et al. MSH2 deficiency contributes to accelerated APC-mediated intestinal tumorigenesis. Cancer Res 1996;56(13):2922–6.

138. Järvinen H, Aarnio M, Mustonen H, et al. Controlled 15-year trial on screening for colorectal cancer in families with hereditary nonpolyposis colorectal cancer. Gastroenterology 2000;118(5):829–34.

139. Renkonen-Sinisalo L, Kivisaari A, Kivisaari L, et al. Utility of computed tomographic colonography in surveillance for hereditary nonpolyposis colorectal cancer syndrome. Fam Cancer 2007;6(1):135–40.

140. Hurlstone D, Karajeh M, Cross S, et al. The role of high-magnification-chromoscopic colonoscopy in hereditary nonpolyposis colorectal cancer screening: a prospective "back-to-back" endoscopic study. Am J Gastroenterol 2005; 100(10):2167–73.

141. Lecomte T, Cellier C, Meatchi T, et al. Chromoendoscopic colonoscopy for detecting preoneoplastic lesions in hereditary nonpolyposis colorectal cancer syndrome. Clin Gastroenterol Hepatol 2005;3(9):897–902.

142. Rodríguez-Bigas M, Vasen H, Pekka-Mecklin J, et al. Rectal cancer risk in hereditary nonpolyposis colorectal cancer after abdominal colectomy. International Collaborative Group on HNPCC. Ann Surg 1997b;225(2):202–7.

143. Ng A, Reagan J, Hawliczek S, et al. Significance of endometrial cells in the detection of endometrial carcinoma and its precursors. Acta Cytol 1974;18(5): 356–61.

144. Yancey M, Magelssen D, Demaurez A, et al. Classification of endometrial cells on cervical cytology. Obstet Gynecol 1990;76(6):1000–5.

145. Dove-Edwin I, Boks D, Goff S, et al. The outcome of endometrial carcinoma surveillance by ultrasound scan in women at risk of hereditary nonpolyposis colorectal carcinoma and familial colorectal carcinoma. Cancer 2002;94(6): 1708–12.

146. Rijcken F, Mourits M, Kleibeuker J, et al. Gynecologic screening in hereditary nonpolyposis colorectal cancer. Gynecol Oncol 2003;91(1):74–80.

147. Renkonen-Sinisalo L, Bützow R, Leminen A, et al. Surveillance for endometrial cancer in hereditary nonpolyposis colorectal cancer syndrome. Int J Cancer 2007a;120(4):821–4.

148. Schmeler K, Lynch H, Chen L, et al. Prophylactic surgery to reduce the risk of gynecologic cancers in the Lynch syndrome. N Engl J Med 2006;354(3): 261–9.

149. Felton K, Gilchrist D, Andrew S. Constitutive deficiency in DNA mismatch repair. Clin Genet 2007;71(6):483–98.

150. Lucci-Cordisco E, Zito I, Gensini F, et al. Hereditary nonpolyposis colorectal cancer and related conditions. Am J Med Genet 2003;122(4):325–34.

151. Al-Tassan N, Chmiel N, Maynard J, et al. Inherited variants of MYH associated with somatic G: C–>T: A mutations in colorectal tumors. Nat Genet 2002; 30(2):227–32.

152. Sampson J, Dolwani S, Jones S, et al. Autosomal recessive colorectal adenomatous polyposis due to inherited mutations of MYH. Lancet 2003;362(9377): 39–41.

153. Sieber O, Lipton L, Crabtree M, et al. Multiple colorectal adenomas, classic adenomatous polyposis, and germ-line mutations in MYH. N Engl J Med 2003;348(9):791–9.

154. Jenkins M, Croitoru M, Monga N, et al. Risk of colorectal cancer in monoallelic and biallelic carriers of MYH Mutations: a population-based case-family study. Cancer Epidemiol Biomarkers Prev 2006;15(2):312–4.

155. Croitoru M, Cleary S, Di Nicola N, et al. Association between biallelic and monoallelic germline MYH gene mutations and colorectal cancer risk. J Natl Cancer Inst 2004;96(21):1631–4.

156. Farrington S, Tenesa A, Barnetson R, et al. Germline susceptibility to colorectal cancer due to base-excision repair gene defects. Am J Med Genet 2005;77(1): 112–9.

157. Webb E, Rudd M, Houlston R. Colorectal cancer risk in monoallelic carriers of MYH variants. Am J Med Genet 2006;79(4):768–71.

158. Lubbe S, Di Bernardo M, Chandler I, et al. Clinical implications of the colorectal cancer risk associated with MUTYH mutation. J Clin Oncol 2009;27(24):3975–80.

159. Avezzù A, Agostini M, Pucciarelli S, et al. The role of MYH gene in genetic predisposition to colorectal cancer: another piece of the puzzle. Cancer Lett 2008;268(2):308–13.

160. Nielsen M, Franken P, Reinards T, et al. Multiplicity in polyp count and extracolonic manifestations in 40 Dutch patients with MYH associated polyposis coli (MAP). J Med Genet 2005;42(9):e54.

161. Nielsen M, Poley J, Verhoef S, et al. Duodenal carcinoma in MUTYH-associated polyposis. J Clin Pathol 2006;59(11):1212–5.

162. Lipton L, Tomlinson I. The multiple colorectal adenoma phenotype and MYH, a base excision repair gene. Clin Gastroenterol Hepatol 2004;2(8):633–8.

163. Holter S, Gallinger S. MUTYH-associated polyposis. In: Potter J, Lindor N, editors. Genetics of colorectal cancer. New York: Springer Science Business Media; 2009. p. 173–81.

164. Cheadle J, Sampson J. MUTYH-associated polyposis—from defect in base excision repair to clinical genetic testing. DNA Repair (Amst) 2007;6:274–9.

165. Halford S, Rowan A, Lipton L, et al. Germline mutations but not somatic changes at the MYH locus contribute to the pathogenesis of unselected colorectal cancers. Am J Pathol 2003;162(5):1545–8.

166. Okamoto K, Toyokuni S, Uchida K, et al. Formation of 8-hydroxy-2'-deosyguanosine and 4-hydroxy-2-nonenal-modified proteins in human renal-cell carcinoma. Int J Cancer 1994;58(6):824–9.

167. Malins D, Haimanot R. Major alterations in the nucleotide structure of DNA in cancer of the female breast. Cancer Res 1991;51(19):5430–2.

168. Jaruga P, Zastawny T, Skokowski J, et al. Oxidative DNA base damage and anti-oxidant enzyme activities in human lung cancer. FEBS Lett 1994;341(1):59–64.

169. DeMarzo A, Nelson W, Isaacs W, et al. Pathological and molecular aspects of prostate cancer. Lancet 2003;361(9361):955–64.

170. Giardiello F, Offerhaus J. Phenotype and cancer risk of various polyposis syndromes. Eur J Cancer 1995;31A(7–8):1085–7.

171. Jagelman D, DeCosse J, Bussey H. Upper gastrointestinal cancer in familial adenomatous polyposis. Lancet 1988;1(8595):1149–51.

172. Sturt N, Gallagher M, Bassett P, et al. Evidence for genetic predisposition to desmoid tumours in familial adenomatous polyposis independent of the germline APC mutation. Gut 2004;53(12):1832–6.

173. Bülow S, Björk J, Christensen I, et al. Duodenal adenomatosis in familial adenomatous polyposis. Gut 2004;53(3):381–6.

174. Davis D, Cohen P. Genitourinary tumors in men with Muir-Torre syndrome. J Am Acad Dermatol 1995;33:909–12.

175. Vasen H, Wijnen J, Menko F, et al. Cancer risk in families with hereditary nonpolyposis colorectal cancer diagnosed by mutation analysis. Gastroenterology 1996;110(4):1020–7.

176. Lin K, Shashidharan M, Thorson A, et al. Cumulative incidence of colorectal and extracolonic cancers in MLH1 and MSH2 mutation carriers of hereditary nonpolyposis colorectal cancer. J Gastrointest Surg 1998;2:67–71.

177. Aarnio M, Sankila R, Pukkala E, et al. Cancer risk in mutation carriers of DNA-mismatch-repair genes. Int J Cancer 1999;81(2):214–8.

178. Watson P, Bützow R, Ht L, et al. The clinical features of ovarian cancer in hereditary nonpolyposis colorectal cancer. Gynecol Oncol 2001;82(2):223–8.

179. Smith R, Cokkinides V, von Eschenbach A, et al. American Cancer Society guidelines for the early detection of cancer. CA Cancer J Clin 2002;52(1):8–22.

Index

Note: Page numbers of article titles are in **boldface** type.

A

Aggresomes, in protein quality control, 1074

Allogeneic cellular gene therapy, for hemoglobinopathies, **1145–1163**
  sickle cell anemia, 1155–1158
  thalassemia, 1147–1155

Alpha (α)-hemoglobin stabilizing protein gene, effect on clinical severity of HbE/β—thalassemia, 1063

Alpha (α)-thalassemia, inheritance of gene for, in patients with HbE/β—thalassemia, 1061
  molecular basis of, competition for the upstream regulatory elements, 1045
    deletions removing both of the duplicated structural genes, 1040–1042
    deletions removing one of the duplicated structural genes, 1040
    deletions removing the upstream regulatory elements of the α-globin gene cluster, 1044–1045
    large deletions extending beyond the α-globin cluster with complex phenotypes (ATR-16 syndrome), 1045–1048
    normal structure and regulation of human α-globin gene cluster, 1034–1035
    normal variation within the human α-globin gene cluster, 1035–1037
    rare mutation via an antisense RNA, 1042–1044
    sequence variations in the structural genes, 1037
    trans-acting mutations, 1048–1049
    translocations and duplications of the α-globin cluster, 1037–1039
  Plasmodium falciparum and, 1022–1024

Antisense RNA, rare mutation causing α-thalassemia via, 1042–1044

Ataxia telangiectasia, mouse models of, 1216–1217

ATR-16 syndrome, causing α-thalassemia, 1045–1048

Autophagy, in protein quality control, 1072
  in erythropoiesis, 1076

B

Beta (β)-thalassemia, hemoglobin E (HbE) type, basis of marked clinical diversity, **1055–1070**
  adaptation to anemia as a modifying factor in, 1064–1065
  clinical severity categories of, 1057–1060
  environmental influences on phenotype of, 1065
  epidemiology, 1055–1056
  factors that influence the clinical severity of, 1060–1064
  pathophysiology, 1056
  recommendations for management of patients, 1065–1066
  understanding the phenotypic heterogeneity of, 1056–1057
  hemoglobin gene therapy for, **1187–1201**
    globin gene therapy, 1188–1190

Hematol Oncol Clin N Am 24 (2010) 1253–1265
doi:10.1016/S0889-8588(10)00149-8
0889-8588/10/$ – see front matter © 2010 Elsevier Inc. All rights reserved.

hemonc.theclinics.com

Moving?

Make sure your subscription moves with you!

To notify us of your new address, find your **Clinics Account Number** (located on your mailing label above your name), and contact customer service at:

Email: journalscustomerservice-usa@elsevier.com

800-654-2452 (subscribers in the U.S. & Canada)
314-447-8871 (subscribers outside of the U.S. & Canada)

Fax number: 314-447-8029

Elsevier Health Sciences Division
Subscription Customer Service
3251 Riverport Lane
Maryland Heights, MO 63043

*To ensure uninterrupted delivery of your subscription, please notify us at least 4 weeks in advance of move.

Printed and bound by CPI Group (UK) Ltd, Croydon, CR0 4YY

03/10/2024

01040445-0006